Documenting Occupational Therapy Practice

THIRD EDITION

Documenting Occupational Therapy Practice

THIRD EDITION

Karen M. Sames, OTD, MBA, OTR/L, FAOTA

*Associate Professor of Occupational Science
and Occupational Therapy
St. Catherine University
St. Paul, Minnesota*

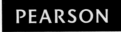

Boston Columbus Indianapolis New York San Francisco Upper Saddle River
Amsterdam Cape Town Dubai London Madrid Milan Munich Paris Montréal Toronto
Delhi Mexico City São Paulo Sydney Hong Kong Seoul Singapore Taipei Tokyo

Publisher: Julie Levin Alexander
Publisher's Assistant: Regina Bruno
Editor in Chief: Marlene McHugh Pratt
Executive Editor: John Goucher
Program Manager: Nicole Ragonese
Editorial Assistant: Ericia Vivani
Director of Marketing: David Gesell
Marketing Manager: Brittany Hammond
Marketing Specialist: Alicia Wozniak
Project Management Lead: Cynthia Zonneveld
Project Manager: Patricia Gutierrez

Operations Specialist: Nancy Maneri-Miller
Cover Art Director: Diane Ernsberger
Cover Designer: Nesbitt Graphics
Art Director Interior: Maria Guglielmo
Cover Art: Agb/Shutterstock; Photo courtesy of Karen M. Sames; Courtesy of www.istockphoto.com
Full-Service Project Management: Revathi Viswanathan
Composition: Lumina Datamatics, Inc.
Printer/Binder: Edwards Brothers, Inc.
Cover Printer: Phoenix Color/Hagerstown
Text Font: 10/12, Meliorand

Credits and acknowledgments for content borrowed from other sources and reproduced, with permission, in this textbook appear on appropriate page within text

Notice: The author and the publisher of this book have taken care to make certain that the information given is correct and compatible with the standards generally accepted at the time of publication. Nevertheless, as new information becomes available, changes in treatment and in the use of equipment and procedures become necessary. The reader is advised to carefully consult the instruction and information material included in each piece of equipment or device before administration. Students are warned that the use of any techniques must be authorized by their medical advisor, where appropriate, in accordance with local laws and regulations. The publisher disclaims any liability, loss, injury, or damage incurred as a consequence, directly or indirectly, of the use and application of any of the contents of this book.

Many of the designations by manufacturers and seller to distinguish their products are claimed as trademarks. Where those designations appear in this book, and the publisher was aware of a trademark claim, the designations have been printed in initial caps or all caps.

Library of Congress Cataloging-in-Publication Data
Sames, Karen M., author.
    Documenting occupational therapy practice / Karen M. Sames. — Third edition.
        p. ; cm.
    Includes bibliographical references and index.
    ISBN-13: 978-0-13-311049-4
    ISBN-10: 0-13-311049-4
I. Title.
    [DNLM: 1. Occupational Therapy—organization & administration. 2. Medical Records—standards.
WB 555
    RM735.4
    615.8'515—dc23
                                                                                            2013037951

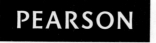

ISBN 10: 0-13-311049-4
ISBN 13: 978-0-13-311049-4

CONTENTS

▼ SECTION II ▼

ETHICAL AND LEGAL CONSIDERATIONS   66

▼ SECTION III ▼

CLINICAL DOCUMENTATION   94

▼ SECTION V ▼

ADMINISTRATIVE DOCUMENTATION   **236**

Please find the below appendices located on Pearson's student resource web site at www.pearsonhighered.com/ healthprofessionsresources.

APPENDIX A: GRAMMAR AND SPELLING REVIEW

APPENDIX B: EXCERPTS FROM MEDICARE STANDARDS

APPENDIX C: MODEL FORMS: IEP, PRIOR WRITTEN NOTICE, EXCERPTS FROM PROCEDURAL SAFEGUARDS, AND IFSP

APPENDIX D: REPRODUCIBLE SAMPLE FORMS

APPENDIX E: SUMMARY OF THE OCCUPATIONAL THERAPY PRACTICE FRAMEWORK

APPENDIX F: ANSWERS TO EXERCISES

PREFACE

For many years, I wished for a book that could be used by students to learn about documentation, while at the same time be used by clinicians to improve the quality of documentation in the field. Eventually, I realized that I could, and should, write that book. As a university professor, I spend a great deal of time reading written work produced by occupational therapy students. As a peer reviewer, I read client charts that insurance companies are unsure about; the charts that are so poorly written that the insurers cannot be certain the services are medically necessary and appropriate.

For these reasons, I decided to begin the long and challenging task of writing this book. Federal rules and professional standards change constantly. Electronic health records have become more common, adding further changes to the way occupational therapy is documented, forcing me to revise and add topics as the book evolved.

My hope for this book is that it gets used; that it is not simply put up on a shelf. I want it to be written in, to have pages flagged, and to have the spine well broken from repeated use. Normally, I would be appalled at the vision of food-stained, rumpled pages in a textbook. But I think this book is different. If it retains its original pristine condition, then it hasn't served its reader well.

The third edition contains updated information and added features including:

- A new chapter focusing on electronic health records has been added to address the skills and information necessary to prepare students for facilities that utilize digital documentation.
- Updates have been made throughout the text to reflect the recent revision to core American Occupational Association documents.
- Chapter 2 has a new section regarding texting as a form of professional communications.
- Guidelines for correcting errors in documentation have been added to Section III.
- Updates have been made throughout the text to reflect changes to Medicare. Additionally, Appendix B outlines several of the new Medicare standards including G-Codes.
- Supplemental materials are available online including answers to exercises, PowerPoints, and a test bank.

REVIEWERS

THIRD EDITION

Kimberly Davis, OTD, MS, OTR/L
Associate Professor
Husson University
Bangor, Maine

Mary Falzarano, PhD
Professor
Kean University
Hillside, New Jersey

Kristin Haas, MOT, OTD, OTR/L
Associate Professor
College of Saint Mary
Omaha, Nebraska

Kerri Hample, OTD, OTR/L
Visiting Assistant Professor
Elizabethtown College
Elizabethtown, Pennsylvania

Shelley Hix, MSOT, OTD, OTR/L, CPAM, CAPS
Fieldwork Coordinator
Belmont University
Nashville, Tennessee

James Lewis, PT, DPT, ATC
Clinical Assistant Professor
Georgia State University
Atlanta, Georgia

Colleen Neumann, BFA, AAS, LMT, COTA
Assistant Professor
Erie Community College
Buffalo, New York

Michelle Sheperd, OTR, M.Ed, Ed.D
Regional Director of Specialty Programs
Brown Mackie College

SECOND EDITION

Diane Anderson, MPH, OTR/L
Chair, Occupational Therapy
College of St. Scholastica
Duluth, Minnesota

Gail Bass, Ph.D., OTR/L
Assistant Professor, Occupational Therapy
University of North Dakota
Grand Forks, North Dakota

Rachelle Dorne, Ed.D., OTR/L
Associate Professor, Occupational Therapy
Nova Southeastern University
Ft. Lauderdale-Davie, Florida

Catherine Emery, MS, OTR/L
Assistant Professor, Occupational Therapy
Alvernia College
Reading, Pennsylvania

Tamera K. Humbert, D.Ed., OTR/L
Associate Professor, Occupational Therapy
Elizabethtown College
Elizabethtown, Pennsylvania

Nancy A Lowenstein, MS, OTR/L, BCPR
Clinical Associate Professor, Occupational
     Therapy
Boston University
Boston, Massachusetts

Lori Reynolds, MOT, OTR/L
Assistant Professor/Fieldwork Coordinator,
     Occupational Therapy
Spalding University
Louisville, Kentucky

Katie L. Serfas, OTD, OTR/L
Clinical Assistant Professor, Occupational
     Therapy and Occupational Science
University of Missouri-Columbia
Columbia, Missouri

Michelle M. Sheperd, MEd, OTR
Program Director, Occupational Therapy
Brown Mackie College
South Bend, Indiana

Janeene Sibla, OTD, MS, OTR/L
Director/Associate Professor Occupational
     Therapy
University of Mary
Bismarck, North Dakota

Barbara J. Williams, OT, OTR
Director/Assistant Professor, Occupational
  Therapy Program
University of Southern Indiana
Evansville, Indiana

FIRST EDITION

Alma R. Abdel-Moty, MS, OTR
Clinical Assistant Professor, Occupational
  Therapy Program
Florida International University
Miami, Florida

Gail S. Bass, OTR/L
Instructor, Occupational Therapy
University of North Dakota
Grand Forks, North Dakota

Estelle B. Breines, Ph.D., OTR, FAOTA
Former Program Chair, Department of
  Occupational Therapy
Seton Hall University
South Orange, New Jersey

Catherine C. Brennan, MA, OTRL/L, FAOTA
Consultant
St. Paul, Minnesota

William R. Croninger, MA, OTR/L
Associate Professor, Occupational Therapy
University of New England
Biddeford, Maine

Anne E. Dickerson, Ph.D., OTR/L, FAOTA
Program Chair and Professor, Occupational
  Therapy
Eastern Carolina University
Greenville, North Carolina

Hahn C. Edwards, MA, MS, OTR
Assistant Professor, Occupational Therapy
  Assistant Program
University of Southern Indiana
Evansville, Indiana

Maria Hinds, JD, MS, OT
Assistant Professor, Occupational Therapy
Florida A&M University
Tallahassee, Florida

Joyce H. McCormick, MS, OTR/L
Fieldwork Coordinator, Occupational Therapy
  Program
Pennsylvania State University—Mont Alto
Mont Alto, Pennsylvania

Deane B. McCraith, MS, OTR/L, LMFT
Clinical Associate Professor, Occupational
  Therapy
Boston University
Sargent College of Health and Rehabilitation
  Science
Boston, Massachusetts

Nichelle L. Miedema, OTR/L
Program Coordinator, Occupational Therapy
  Assistant Program
Kirkwood Community College
Cedar Rapids, Iowa

Candice Jones Mullendore, MS, OTR
Assistant Professor and Academic Fieldwork
  Coordinator, Department of Occupational
  Therapy
Creighton University
Omaha, Nebraska

Kathy Nielson, MPH, OTR/L
Professor and Director, Division of Occupational
  Science
The University of North Carolina at Chapel Hill
Chapel Hill, North Carolina

Karen B. Smith, OTR/L
Program Director, Occupational Therapy
  Assistant Program
Stanly Community College
Albermarle, North Carolina

Kathy Clark Tuminski, MA, OTR/L
Assistant Professor, Occupational Therapy
Eastern Kentucky University
Richmond, Kentucky

Joanne Wright, Ph.D., OTR/L
Program Director, Division of Occupational
  Therapy
University of Utah
Salt Lake City, Utah

INTRODUCTION: THE WHO, WHAT, WHERE, WHEN, AND WHY OF DOCUMENTATION

As occupational therapy practitioners, we work with a variety of clients in a variety of settings. In every setting in which we use our skills as trained professionals, we are asked to document what we do in some way. We may do clinical documentation that becomes part of a medical record. We may contribute to the development of an Individual Education Program (IEP) for a grade school student. We may write a report summarizing our activity as a consultant to a company. It is imperative that our writing demonstrates a high level of professionalism.

▼ WHO ▼

The key to professional writing is to know who we are writing for as well as who we are writing about. As indicated earlier, we write for multiple audiences. Some potential audiences include the intervention team, the client and/or surrogates (caregivers, family, or guardians), facility quality management personnel, third-party payers, peer reviewers, accreditation surveyors, administrators, and lawyers. Because the potential audience for our documentation extends far beyond our peers, it is important that we choose our words very carefully. I know of one occupational therapist who mentally says to herself before putting pen to paper, "Ladies and gentlemen of the jury, . . . " Then she begins her documentation. It forces her to think about how her words may be interpreted by others.

▼ WHAT ▼

On my first occupational therapy job, a director of nursing told me repeatedly, "If it's not documented, it didn't happen." It was like her personal mantra. As much as I got tired of hearing it, I have to admit she was right. It was good advice. If I had to be absent from work, and a substitute had to step in for me, I wanted the substitute to be fully informed about what things have been tried already and in what direction I wanted the intervention to proceed. In order for this to happen, there must be accurate, complete, and clear documentation of what has transpired in occupational therapy thus far. Also, documentation that is written at the time of an event is stronger evidence in a court of law than one's memory. How many of you can remember exactly what you did last Tuesday at 10:00 in the morning? A month ago? Eighteen months ago? Who were you with? What were you doing? Were you successful at whatever you were doing? How much force did you use? You get the picture?

Not only do you want to document what was done, but you also want to document the client's reaction to the intervention. Think of it as painting a verbal picture of the occupational therapy session for the reader. You want to document what instructions were given (e.g., for a home program, splint use and care, adaptive equipment use and care, or instructions to caregivers) and whether the person receiving instructions appeared to understand those instructions. Finally, you want to document what the plan is for future occupational therapy service delivery.

With so much to document, it might become somewhat of a balancing act between working hands-on with a client and documenting that intervention. Most occupational therapists go into the profession because they want to help people. I doubt any become occupational therapy practitioners because they love to write notes all day long. In addition, increasing competition for healthcare dollars have pushed some clinics to develop productivity standards for the amount of billable services each clinician needs to provide each day. This results in less time available for doing documentation. Today, a clinician in a clinical setting will generally spend 6 hours or more (out of an 8-hour day) with clients. The rest of the time is usually for meetings and documentation. In educational or community settings, the time spent with clients may be 7 hours or more in an 8-hour day. However, needing to document so much of what we do does not mean we have to spend a lot of time doing it. Sections III and IV of this book will show you some ways of documenting in an efficient and effective manner.

▼ WHERE ▼

In clinical settings, each client has his or her own health record (chart). The chart may be electronic or paper based. Occupational therapy practitioners may document in a section of the chart dedicated to rehabilitation or therapies. In some settings, integrated notes are done, so that each profession documents progress in a progress note section of the chart that is compiled chronologically regardless of which professional is writing. It is important to follow facility standards for where and when to write in the client's chart, regardless of whether the chart is on a computer or is paper based. Standards for good documentation do not change when the format (electronic or paper) changes.

In educational settings, the Individualized Education Program (IEP) or Individualized Family Service Plan (IFSP) is written annually and reviewed every 6 months. The evaluation report, present levels of performance, and occupational therapy goals are integrated into those documents. The IEP or IFSP then goes into the student's educational record. If the school district is billing third-party payers for occupational therapy services, additional documentation may be required. The school district will have policies for the occupational therapist regarding where any other documentation will be filed and retained.

In addition to the official clinical or educational record, some occupational therapy departments retain copies of everything that is in the official record in a departmental file. These departmental files may also contain test forms, attendance records, and other non-official documents. Chapter 8 will go into more detail about records retention.

▼ WHEN ▼

Documentation is typically done as close to the time of service as possible. Some occupational therapists reserve the last 5 minutes or so of the intervention session to document in the client's chart. This works fine for contact or progress notes, but may not be sufficient for doing larger documents such as evaluation or discontinuation reports. These documents are usually done when there are no clients being treated such as at the beginning or end of the day or over the lunch hour. In some settings, the occupational therapist will dictate evaluation or discontinuation notes to be transcribed by secretarial staff. Others write them out longhand or on a desktop, laptop, or handheld computer.

The longer the time span from when the evaluation or intervention occurred to when the occupational therapist sits down to write about it, the more the chance that something will be forgotten. When possible, writing directly in the client's chart at the time of service delivery is best. However, this is not always possible. Some occupational therapists carry small notebooks or pieces of paper with them in their pockets, and jot quick notes about the clients they see during the day. Others use handheld computers. This does help them remember more clearly what happened with each client. As you can imagine, if an occupational therapist sees 12 clients in a day, by the end of the day it can be difficult to remember who said or did what.

▼ WHY ▼

Occupational therapists document for many reasons. We document to show what has happened to the client in a chronological sequence. We want to show what happened first, then second, then the next thing, and so on. Some regulatory and accrediting bodies want to see that things happened in a clinically sound sequence. For example, if you were working with a client recovering from a severe head injury, you would want to show that the client is aware of safety precautions to take when using a knife before you work on how to use a knife. The client's chart will tell any third-party reviewer the story of that client's recovery following an illness or injury, or a client's development in the case of a developmental delay.

We document to show our high level of clinical reasoning. Someone walking by the occupational therapy clinic could see the occupational therapist watching a client make buttered toast. That person might think, "She went to college for how many years to teach that? I could do that without any training." If that person could read the chart, he or she would see that the occupational therapist was really working on sequencing a task, manipulating utensils, safety awareness, and/or energy conservation. The task of buttering toast represents many different learning opportunities for the client. There is often more to occupational therapy than meets the eye.

We document to inform others on the intervention team about what happened during an intervention session. Everyone is busy, we work different shifts, and there is not always time for each of us to talk to other caregivers about each client. By writing down the essence of what happened in the intervention session, others on the team can be informed in their own time. By the same token, we can read the chart and find out what happened that day in other therapy services, or in the lab, medical imaging, or nursing.

We document to demonstrate the effectiveness of occupational therapy for third-party payers. This is a critically important reason to document well, as payment is often based on the quality of the documentation. Third-party payers such as the government (Medicare, Medicaid, CHAMPUS, and other programs) and private insurers (managed care, worker's compensation, indemnity) want to be sure that they are getting what they paid for—results. A payer virtually never observes the client directly, but relies on the documentation of the services delivered to determine effectiveness. If the payers cannot see progress in the documentation, they will often terminate payment, which in effect terminates services, even if you believe the client could still benefit from further services.

Last, but not least, we document for legal reasons. As stated earlier, the medical record, anything written at the time, is stronger evidence of what happened than anything we can remember from a year or two ago. In many states, a client can bring forward a malpractice case up to 2 years after the incident occurred. In those 2 years, we could have treated more than a hundred other clients. Will we remember exactly what we did with that client on that day, or will all the other clients we have seen since then cloud our memory? Depending on what we write, and how well we write it, the clinical record can be used to protect, or to hurt, us as practitioners. There are ways to ensure that what we write is more likely to help than hurt us, and this book addresses them.

▼ STRUCTURE OF THE BOOK ▼

Section I of this book deals with some of the mechanics of writing. It includes tips on word usage, the use of frames of reference, abbreviations, and jargon. It also takes a broad look at how the language of the profession is ever evolving and describes both internal and external influences on the use of language. This section also includes pointers on professional communication in general.

The second section focuses on the ethical and legal issues around documentation, such as confidentiality, record retention, fraud, and plagiarism. This provides a different yet necessary perspective on documentation: payers, reviewers, and attorneys.

Section III deals with the documentation of the occupational therapy process in a clinical setting. Clinical settings include all occupational therapy practice venues where third-party reimbursement is sought, such as in a hospital, nursing home, clinic, or psychiatric program. Usually, in a clinical setting, there is a physician order or referral, and services are billed for in some way. This is a very broad description of a clinical setting. It excludes services that are paid for with grant money or other funding sources that do not require physician oversight. This section takes you through the occupational therapy process and explains the types of documentation completed at each step of the process. Each chapter describes a type of documentation and includes sections on role delineation and Medicare standards as they apply to that type documentation.

The fourth section is about documentation in school systems. While many school systems are now billing third-party payers to recoup the costs of some therapy services, there are also requirements for certain types of documentation that are unique to school-based services. This section addresses only the documentation requirements of school systems.

The last section deals with administrative documentation. Examples of administrative documentation include policies and procedures, incident reports, meeting minutes, job descriptions, grant writing, and job descriptions. Occupational therapy staff write some of these types of documents, while supervisors and managers generally write others.

If you are reading this book as a required text for a course in an occupational therapy educational program, do not be surprised if your instructor does not require you to read each chapter and do each exercise, in the order in which the chapters appear in this text. In an introductory course in occupational therapy, you may only be assigned the first three or four sections. However, I hope that at some point in your educational program, you will have a chance to work with chapters in the rest of the book. That means that you should hang on to this book even when the course is over. You will undoubtedly have opportunities to practice documentation in several courses in your curriculum, and this book will be a good reference to look back at as you draft your assignments.

If you are a clinician reading this book, I congratulate you on your dedication to the profession and to continuing competence. Depending on how long it has been since you were in school, some of the information in the book will be new to you, some merely a refresher. Each chapter of the book can stand on its own, and you can choose the chapter or chapters on which you want to concentrate. You will also find the material in the appendices especially helpful.

Throughout the book there are exercises to help you develop your skills in documentation. Answers to exercises are included in Appendix F (see Website). While comparing your answers to those in the book can be a good learning experience, it may be even more helpful to get feedback on your answers from an instructor or colleague. An experienced occupational therapist can provide feedback on the subtle nuances that different wording can have on a reader.

As you work through the sections of this book, you will become familiar with principles of good documentation in clinical and educational settings. You will also learn about other types of documentation that occupational therapists may be called on to write during their careers. People form opinions about you as a professional based on how well or how poorly you write. If you want to be thought of as a talented, competent, and skilled professional, you must write like one.

SECTION I

CHAPTER 1

Overview of the Use of Language in Documentation

INTRODUCTION

Documentation requires the use of written words. To document well, one must write well. This involves selecting words that will have meaning to the reader and making the documentation clear, accurate, and relevant to the situation. In the first section of this book, general issues about writing are discussed.

How well you write is one way that others will judge your professionalism. If you write poorly, use outdated terms or excessive jargon, use too many abbreviations, or leave out words, people will think you are either careless or lacking in skill. Appendix A (see website) contains a review of general grammar and spelling considerations that may be a good review for some readers. The American Occupational Therapy Association (2014) has developed a framework for occupational therapy practice that can provide some guidance on the use of terms. Different models or frames of reference used in occupational therapy will shape the way occupational therapists write about clinical or educational progress.

▼ OCCUPATIONAL THERAPY DOCUMENTATION ▼

When documenting occupational therapy practice, it is essential to use language appropriately. Occupational therapy practitioners work in many settings. Some settings, such as hospitals, long-term care, school systems, or home health, have very specific standards for content. Other settings, such as homeless shelters, prisons, or consulting, do not have setting-specific standards, so occupational therapy practitioners may have to create documentation systems to fit the needs of the setting. The American Occupational Therapy Association (AOTA) has guidelines for documentation that can be used in any setting (AOTA, 2013).

In clinical settings such as hospitals, long-term care facilities, home health, outpatient clinics, and psychiatric programs, each step of the occupational therapy process is documented. A referral or physician's order for occupational therapy intervention is typically the first item documented in a clinical record. If an occupational therapy practitioner conducts a screening or makes initial contact with a client, it is documented as a contact note. The occupational therapy evaluation is documented as an evaluation report or evaluation summary. Next, an intervention plan is created. As occupational therapy intervention is provided to the client, the occupational therapy practitioner records progress notes. When occupational therapy intervention is finished, the outcome of that intervention is documented in a discontinuation summary. Section III of this book details these documents.

In educational settings, occupational therapists contribute to team-based documentation of services provided to children with special needs. The services provided to infants and toddlers are documented in an Individualized Family Service Plan (IFSP). The services provided to children between the ages of 3 and 21 are documented in an Individual Education Program (IEP). In addition, every time a team meeting is called, every time a change in the IEP or IFSP is proposed, and every time a child is referred for special education intervention, there are notice and consent forms which document that the child's family has been kept informed of the process. Section IV of this book discusses these documents.

There is also documentation that is necessary, but not related directly to serving clients. We call this documentation administrative documentation. These documents relate to the efficient running of an occupational therapy department. Section V discusses several of these types of documents.

Regardless of setting, occupational therapy practitioners document nearly everything they do. Sometimes, that documentation is very structured; forms tell the occupational therapy practitioner what to document and where. In other situations, the documentation may be less structured; the occupational therapy practitioner uses a blank page to record his or her actions in a narrative format. Sometimes, the documentation is handwritten or done using a word processor, although that is becoming much less common. In more and more settings, the occupational therapy practitioner enters evaluation, intervention, and outcome data on a computer or mobile device.

Electronic documentation is now more common than handwritten or word-processed documentation. Electronic documentation makes the data that is entered instantly available to other members of the healthcare or educational team. Read more about electronic health records in Chapter 12.

▼ STRUCTURE OF THIS SECTION OF THE BOOK ▼

Chapter 2 presents an overview of the types of communication one might use on the job, including memos, letters, e-mails, and phone calls. This chapter discusses the importance of using the proper tone, voice, and language when communicating with other professionals in the workplace. While memos, letters, and e-mails are not generally considered documentation for the purpose of documenting occupational therapy practice, they are an essential part of the work of occupational therapy practitioners. Effectively communicating in writing with referral sources, coworkers, supervisors and supervisees, and colleagues is a skill everyone needs to master.

Chapter 3 will deal with use of language, including buzzwords, jargon, and abbreviations. Lists of common abbreviations are included. This chapter is very specific to occupational therapy practice. Just as certain phrases used in everyday conversations can be trendier than others, so can certain phrases used in occupational therapy.

Chapter 4 relates the language used in documentation to the language used in the primary documents that guide the profession of occupational therapy. These documents are written by the American Occupational Therapy Association and the World Health Organization.

Chapter 5 suggests that the words chosen for documenting occupational therapy services will reflect the model or frame of reference used with a particular client. It includes a brief summary of several different models and frames of reference.

Finally, Chapter 6 includes a checklist for ensuring careful documentation. It deals specifically with documenting clearly and accurately, making the documentation relevant and documenting any exceptions to the way the therapist expected things to go.

The lessons learned in these chapters will help improve documentation regardless of the setting in which the occupational therapy clinician or student works. What is important to remember is that you must always choose your words carefully.

REFERENCES

American Occupational Therapy Association. (2014). Occupational therapy practice framework: Domain and process (3rd ed.). *American Journal of Occupational Therapy, 68*(Suppl. 1), S1–S48. http://dx.doi.org/10.5014/ajot.2014.682006

American Occupational Therapy Association. (2013). Guidelines for documentation of occupational therapy. Retrieved from http://www.aota.org/Practitioners/Official/Guidelines/41257.aspx?FT=.pdf

Visit **www.pearsonhighered.com/healthprofessionsresources** to access the student resources that accompany this book. Simply select Occupational Therapy from the choice of disciplines. Find this book and you will find the complimentary study tools created for this specific title.

CHAPTER 2

Professional Communication

Occupational therapy practitioners communicate with others in the workplace using several methods, including face-to-face discussions, letters, memos, e-mails, and phone calls. The word choices and tone of the writing or speech used in professional, or formal, communication are very different from those used with friends.

Professional communication requires a level of respect and formality that is not required while e-mailing or talking to friends. In formal writing, the reader may be unknown to the writer; for example, while you might know the nursing staff who read your progress notes on a client, you might not know the client's attorney or family members who might also read the document (Lincoln University, n.d.). Professional communication avoids slang, contractions, cliché's, sexist or racist terms, and profanity (Lincoln University, n.d.; Word-mart.com, 2010). Informal communication may be written in the first, second, or third person, while formal communication is usually written in the third person. Formal communication often uses longer and more complex sentences and paragraphs. Be careful, however, to not go overboard by using big words and complex sentences just to try to sound impressive because then the writer might start to sound pompous (Lincoln University, n.d.; Word-mart.com, 2010). This textbook is written in a more informal voice, however, clinical, school, or administrative documentation are written in a more formal voice (Table 2.1). When writing a letter to appeal a denial of coverage, an evaluation report, a notice and consent form, or a discontinuation summary, the writer may or may not know the person reading it, so formal writing is called for.

TABLE 2.1 Formal and Informal Writing Examples

	Informal Writing	Formal Writing
Slang or jargon	The guy freaked out when he found out he had to wear the splint every night.	The client yelled and threw his splint when he heard that he had to wear it every night.
Person	I told him he had to wear the splint every night.	The client was told to wear the splint every night.
Sentence structure	He was told to wear the splint every night.	To prevent contractures, the client was instructed to wear the splint every night, watching for any signs of skin breakdown.
Emotion	I knew he'd be upset, and I felt bad about it, but I told him to wear the splint every night anyway.	The client was told to wear his splint every night.
A known reader (or not)	Kerry, my patient, refuses to wear his splint every night.	Mr. Mortez stated he refused to wear his splint nightly.

Specific standards may govern the contents of formal documentation. For example, the Individuals with Disabilities Education Act (IDEA) requires that specific items be included on the Individual Education Program (IEP), and Medicare requires specific documentation elements for occupational therapy reimbursement in long-term care. The Joint Commission (2012) recommends avoiding the use of certain abbreviations because of the likelihood of medical errors caused by misreading abbreviations that are remarkably close in appearance to each other. In addition, one's employer may further direct the method (electronic or paper and pen), timing, placement, and word choices of documentation.

▼ TONE ▼

Tone is the most important consideration in professional communication, whether it is spoken or written. In writing, the message has to stand alone, without the benefit of facial expression or gestures that convey meaning in oral communication. Readers will interpret what is written through their own lens, depending on their own practice setting, educational level, and cultural background. The writer has to consider how the reader is likely to interpret the message. Try to be confident, honest, and respectful (OWL at Purdue University, 2010a). At the same time, try not to be condescending (OWL at Purdue University, 2010a). For example, which of the following statements sounds more professional?

- I am appealing this coverage determination because, based on my clinical judgment, it is critical that Mrs. Rameriz receive additional occupational therapy services. I know when a client has reached her full potential, and this client has NOT yet reached her full potential.
- I am appealing this coverage determination because this client has not achieved her goal of independence in meal preparation, which is essential if she is to return to her previous living situation.

Clearly, the second statement is less condescending, yet honest and respectful. The first statement screams that the writer knows more than the reader, and has some under lying angry feelings toward the person who made the initial coverage decision.

The example also shows emphasis in the form of a word in all capital letters. Using all capitals in writing is like shouting in oral communication (Yale University, n.d.). If you want to emphasize a word or a point, some people suggest putting an *asterisk* around the word or words (Yale University, n.d.). Another way to show emphasis is to put the most important idea first in the letter, paragraph, or sentence (OWL at Purdue University, 2010a). The amount of space you devote to a particular idea also conveys importance (OWL at Purdue University, 2010a).

▼ ACTIVE VOICE ▼

In professional writing, an active voice is preferred to a passive voice. Using active voice in a sentence means that the person doing the action comes first, then the action (OWL at Purdue University, 2011). Active voice is usually more direct and clear than passive voice. Typically, a sentence written in passive voice will have a verb phrase using a "be" word (e.g., have been) (OWL at Purdue University, 2011). Following are two sentences that say essentially the same thing; the first is written in a passive voice, whereas the second uses an active voice.

- Self-care skills have been a concern of this client.
- This client has been concerned with his self-care skills.

▼ NONDISCRIMINATORY LANGUAGE ▼

It is important to use nondiscriminatory language in professional writing (American Psychological Association, [APA] 2010; Lunsford, 2009; OWL at Purdue University, 2010b). This may seem like an obvious statement, but sometimes word a creep into our speech or writing that reflect personal biases in subtle ways. All professional writing, whether it is a progress note, thank-you letter to a referral source, or policy and procedure, needs to be free of language that might be interpreted as sexist, racist, ageist, or otherwise biased on such factors as ethnicity, religion, disability, or sexual orientation (OWL at Purdue University, 2010b). Avoid broad categorizations such as *hemiplegics, stroke victims*, or *the blind* when discussing a population (APA, 2010). "Person first" language (e.g., people with hemiplegia, a person with visual deficits) is preferred when discussing a population or a person with a disability (APA, 2010; The ARC, 2012). Use the adjective form of population descriptors rather than the noun form (e.g., elderly people rather than the elderly) (APA, 2010).

It is no longer acceptable to use masculine pronouns (e.g., he, his) to refer to both genders or to refer to all occupational therapists as she (APA, 2010). Other words that can be substituted include *person, one*, and *individual*. Another way to get around this difficulty is to restructure the sentence to use plural forms of pronouns such as *they, their*, and *them* (APA, 2010; Lunsford, 2009). The last option is to simply eliminate the pronoun, or replace it with an article (APA, 2010; Lunsford, 2009)—for example, a departmental policy might say, "Remove shoes before jumping in the ball pit" rather than "Everyone must remove their shoes before jumping in the ball pit." Of course, if you are writing in a specific person's clinical or educational record, and you know the person's gender, it is fine to use the appropriate gender-specific pronoun.

What is the best way to refer to occupational therapists and occupational therapy assistants? When referring to them in combination, the term *occupational therapy practitioner* may be used (AOTA, 2010). Some people prefer to spell out both levels of practice, and that is fine; it just takes a second or two longer to write out both terms. Be cautious about dropping the adjective *occupational* when talking about occupational therapy practitioners or occupational therapy program. The term *therapist* can refer to a psychologist, a social worker, a marriage and family counselor, and a variety of other professionals. The term *therapy* can refer to physical therapy, psychotherapy, nutrition therapy, or any number of other therapy programs. If, as a profession, we want other disciplines to know and respect us, we need to use our complete title at all times.

▼ MEMOS ▼

Sometimes, an occupational therapy practitioner needs to communicate with people who work on another shift or another building, coworkers who are not available at the time the critical information needs to be conveyed, or the occupational therapist wants to confirm in writing a conversation that took place. The best way to do this is through a memo. The overall purpose of a memo is to convey information in an effective way (OWL at Purdue University, 2010c). A memo may also be used in place of a cover letter when sending a packet of documents to people you know to tell them what is in the packet and why you sent it (Sabath, 2002). A formal letter is preferred if the packet is going to people you do not know.

The first part of a memo is the heading. This is what makes the memo different from a letter. According to OWL at Purdue University (2010c), the heading usually contains four elements:

To: (reader's full name; sometimes includes job titles with proper capitalization)
From: (your name; sometimes includes job title)
Date: (month, day, year the memo was written)
Subject or Re: (brief explanation of the point of the memo; re is the abbreviation for regarding)

Some word processing programs have templates for writing memos that automatically enter the date. Check the spelling of names, and be sure that you are writing to the right person. Make sure the subject is stated concisely and cannot be construed to mean something other than what you intended. You do not want to unnecessarily alarm the reader, but you also do not want to put the entire content of the memo in the subject line (OWL at Purdue University, 2010c).

Bravemen (2006) suggests a basic five-paragraph structure for memos:

- **Introduction:** explain the reason for the memo.
- **Background:** establish the context.
- **Recommendation or request:** what you want the reader to do or what you want to have happen.
- **Rationale:** explain your reasoning behind your recommendation or request.
- **Conclusion:** restate your position.

Make the memo both look good and sound good (Sabath, 2002). Pay attention to the rules of good grammar, such as capitalization, punctuation, and sentence construction. (See Appendix A [see website]). Use one reasonably sized font style that looks professional. Be consistent in your format, such as the indentation of the first line of each paragraph, throughout the document. Although it is generally a good rule to limit a memo to one page, do not squish everything together, decrease font size, or use smaller margins, just to make it fit on one page (OWL at Purdue University, 2006). If it does not look good on one page, then make it two, well-spaced pages (Sabath, 2002). It is most common for a memo to be written with 1-inch margins on all sides, and to use 10- to 12-size font (OWL at Purdue University, 2006). Font style is a matter of personal preference. If your memo is intended to be read on a screen, then a sans serif font such as Arial or Calibri is easier to read. If your memo is on paper, then a serif font such as Times New Roman is a good choice. Whatever font you use, be sure that you use just one font throughout the memo (OWL at Purdue University, 2006). To add emphasis to certain words, use italics rather than all capital letters. Underlining is fine for a print memo, but if the memo will be read on a screen, then underlining looks like a link that could be clicked to take the reader somewhere else.

▼ LETTERS ▼

Much of the advice for writing memos also applies to writing formal letters. Because the recipient of the letter may not be an acquaintance of the writer, letters often take on an even more formal tone. In a formal letter, the heading is replaced by more detailed information. Often a letter is written on company or organization letterhead. When word processing a letter, make sure that you start the letter down far enough on the page that what you write will not print over the letterhead. A good rule of thumb is that you should start the letter at least 2 inches down the page when using letterhead.

The first part of the formal letter is the sender's address. This is optional, because if the letter is printed on letterhead, the address may already be there. If you do choose to type in your address, leave one empty line after your address before adding the date (OWL at Purdue University, 2010c). The date is usually in the format of month, date, year (May 19, 2012) in the United States, and is left justified (OWL at Purdue University, 2010d).

After the date, include the name, title, and address of the person to whom the letter is addressed (OWL at Purdue University, 2010d). This is called the inside address (OWL at Purdue University, 2010d). According to OWL at Purdue University (2010d), the inside address is typed one line below the sender's address or 1 inch below the date, and it is always left justified. Make sure you use the proper title of the person to whom you are sending the letter.

Between the inside address and the body of your letter, you need to greet your reader. This is called the salutation (OWL at Purdue University, 2010d). If you know the person to whom you are sending the letter, it is fine to greet the person by starting the letter with Dear Maria (or whatever the person's first name is). If the letter is going to someone you do not know, or to someone who holds a higher position than yours, then use the person's full name, including

Mr., Dr., Ms, Professor, or other personal title. In a business letter, use a colon after the name rather than a comma (OWL at Purdue University, 2010d). Things get a little dicey when you do not know the gender of the person to whom you are writing, and therefore do not know whether to say Mr. or Ms. When this happens, you have two choices. You can just leave off the personal title and use the person's whole name, or you can use a generic term like "To Whom It May Concern" or "Dear Appeals Review Coordinator" (OWL at Purdue University, 2010d).

There are several formats for business letters; the important thing is to be consistent in the format (Sabath, 2002). A block format uses a blank line between paragraphs but does not indent the first line of each paragraph (OWL at Purdue University, 2010d). A semi-block format also used a blank line between paragraphs, but the first line of each paragraph is indented (OWL at Purdue University, 2010d). A less formal format indents first lines of each paragraph but does not include a blank line between paragraphs.

Because a letter does not include a subject line in the heading, it is good to get right to the point and state the purpose of the letter in the first paragraph (OWL at Purdue University, 2010d). The following paragraphs can include justification for the main point, and background information the reader needs. The last paragraph restates the purpose of the letter, and may include the action you are requesting the reader take (OWL at Purdue University, 2010d).

The closing begins one line below the last paragraph (OWL at Purdue University, 2010d). A typical closing would simply be the word "Sincerely," but "Thank you," or "Respectfully," could also be used. Notice that there is a comma after the closing word(s), and that only the first word is capitalized. Leave 3–4 lines of blank space, then type in your name and title. This allows room for your signature (OWL at Purdue University, 2010d). If you are including other documents with the letter, it is helpful to list those at the bottom of the letter; underneath the signature, type Enc., which is a short for enclosure, or use the whole word Enclosure and then list each enclosed document.

▼ E-MAIL ▼

Most of us have been using e-mail for years, but its use in healthcare is evolving. There are still questions about the security of electronic transmissions, particularly between healthcare providers and their clients. Programs that encrypt e-mails are considered more secure than those that do not. The American Medical Association ([AMA], 2003) has advised its physicians that while e-mail has many advantages, the disadvantages must be addressed. The AMA recommends that prior to using e-mail to communicate with patients, physicians need to make sure that they let patients know about the risks to privacy of any e-mail communication (AMA, 2003). Healthcare providers, including occupational therapy practitioners, need to be conscious of adhering to codes of ethics, particularly to those standards relating to privacy and confidentiality, and to principles of good communication when communicating via e-mail.

E-mail, instant messaging, and text messaging have evolved to create new words, phrases, acronyms (e.g., LOL or CU), and emoticons (e.g., :-) [smile] or <g> [grin]), which are fine to use among friends but should be used sparingly in the workplace (Braveman, 2006; OWL at Purdue University, 2010e). Professional communication, as stated earlier, is more formal. E-mails to colleagues for work purposes need to follow certain conventions. On the other hand, acronyms and emoticons can help convey your intent or help the reader understand the spirit in which the communication was intended (OWL at Purdue University, 2010e).

When replying to an e-mail, think about who should see your reply. You have two options: reply and reply all. Some e-mail systems are automatically set to send the reply to everyone on the original e-mail. Evaluate your response and determine if the response is best sent to one person or everyone in the group, and then choose reply or reply all, as appropriate. Be aware that anything you write in an e-mail can be forwarded, without your knowledge, to others (Scott, 2013). If you are responding to an e-mail that is part of a listserv, but the sender asks for e-mails to come to his or her personal e-mail account, you need to copy and paste that person's e-mail address into the "To" box rather than simply clicking "reply" (OWL at Purdue University, 2010e).

Sabath (2002, p. 55) suggests five e-mail commandments:

E-mail only those people to whom your messages actually pertain (rather than entire address groups).

Make a point of responding to messages promptly.

Always use spell-check and grammar-check before sending messages.

Include your telephone number in your messages.

Learn that e-mail should be used for business rather than personal use.

E-mail is often used in place of memos, letters, phone, and face-to-face conversations; however, it can create as many problems as it can solve in the workplace. E-mails allow the reader to interpret the message in ways the sender never intended; they are open to misinterpretation by the reader. If they are long with few, if any, breaks in the text, they are hard to read. They are easily distributed either by forwarding or by printing and circulating, so they can end up in the hands of people the sender did not want to receive the message. A final consideration is that every e-mail system is different, and what looks properly formatted on one system may look different on another system (Sherwood, n.d.). Box 2.1 lists some tips that can help minimize the potential for misunderstandings.

BOX 2.1   E-Mail Tips

- Never put something in an e-mail at work that would embarrass you if your boss read it.
- Include a clear subject heading, so your message gets attention. "Update" is pretty vague unless it is followed by a description of what is being updated.
- Address the recipient in the body of the message by starting the message with a salutation that includes the person's name.
- Create a signature that includes your name, title, and contact information. You may also include the organization's vision or slogan, or an appropriate quote.
- Be concise but clear.
- When replying to someone's message, include part or all of the sender's message to help the originator remember what he or she said. Do not include entire back-and-forth conversations; delete long strings of past messages.
- Respect the confidentiality of the sender. Remove unnecessary names and e-mail addresses before forwarding it on to someone else.
- Use proper spelling and grammar. Many e-mail systems have a spell-checker option.
- Respond in a timely manner. A good habit to get into is to check your work e-mail at least twice a day.
- Don't SHOUT by using all capital letters. Don't underutilize capital letters, either. If a word or name would be capitalized in printed material, it should be capitalized in e-mail.
- Use Cc and Bcc appropriately. Cc is for including people in the message who have a stake in the topic of discussion; everyone who gets the message knows who else got a copy of the message. Bcc is for e-mailing several people who do not know each other. It is a way to protect each person's confidentiality by not sharing their e-mail addresses with strangers.
- Don't use "Reply to All" unless everyone really does need to see your response. If you are part of a listserv and want to reply just to the sender of a message, do not hit reply at all. Copy the sender's e-mail address and paste it into the To: line of a new message.
- Be careful about sending attachments, especially large ones that take up a lot of space on the system. When you are replying to an e-mail that contains an attachment, use the "Reply without attachment" option if you have it. If that is not an option on your system, delete the attachment before you hit "send." The person who sent you the attachment already has a copy of the document, so he or she does not need another copy of it.

- Do not overuse the "highest priority" option. It ceases to be a priority if it is used daily.
- Keep business e-mails short, a paragraph or two, with sentences that are less than 20 words each. Use bullet points or numbered lists to make the messages easy to read.
- If you are angry when writing an e-mail, save it as a draft and go back and edit it when you have calmed down. Once it's sent, you can't take it back. Expression of extreme emotion in an e-mail is called flaming. Flaming is never a good practice.
- Keep a copy of the e-mails you send. You can set your e-mail system to automatically save all sent mail.

Sources: Oliu, Brusaw, & Alred (2010); OWL at Purdue University (2010e); Scott (2013); Sherwood (n.d.).

▼ PHONE CALLS ▼

When an occupational therapy practitioner needs to communicate with a physician or other team member about a client, a phone call is one of the fastest ways to communicate. It allows the caller and receiver to interact immediately, to ask questions of each other and clarify the actions needed. When using the phone to communicate information about a client, be sure that you are in a place where your side of the conversation cannot be overheard by people who do not have a need to know about the client.

Many healthcare facilities are using a system called "SBAR" (pronounced es-bar) to facilitate communication between departments and between staff and physicians (Guise & Lowe, 2006; "SBAR Initiative," 2005; "SBAR for Students," 2007; Velji et al., 2008). This method of communication can be used in person as well as on the phone. It organizes what a healthcare professional needs to communicate so that it is done quickly and efficiently.

SBAR stands for

- **S**ituation
- **B**ackground
- **A**ssessment
- **R**ecommendations

If this sounds like something the military would use, that's because it was developed by the military years ago to try to standardize communication between soldiers and commanders ("SBAR Initiative," 2005). It was adapted by Bonacum, Graham, and Leonard at Kaiser Permanente as a means to improve patient safety during transfers of responsibility such as during patient hand-offs at shift change or when a patient moves from one unit to another ("SBAR Checklist," 2006). It is now being used for telephone communication in hospitals, nursing homes, clinics, rehabilitation centers, and home care settings.

Let's say that you have to call a client's physician because you noticed that the client has made significant gains in self-feeding. Using SBAR, you would say

Situation: "Hello Dr. Gonzales, my name is Karen Person and I am the occupational therapist working with Phoebe Finch at the Pediatric Rehabilitation and Feeding Center."

Background: "Phoebe is a 4-year-old, born 3 months prematurely, who is being weaned off tube feedings. She has been making great progress and is now chewing and swallowing soft foods consistently."

Assessment: "She has not had any incidents of choking, pocketing, or spitting out food in our last three sessions. She appears to want to eat."

Recommendation: "I would like to try introducing more solid and crunchy foods such as chips, boxed cereals, apple slices, and the like. Would you be willing to sign off on changing the order to include solid foods?"

SBAR can also be used to communicate quickly with nursing staff when a client has a sudden change in condition. If you notice that your client is not behaving normally, it is important to share this information with the client's primary caregiver. Writing a note in the clinical record is important, but the note might not be read for hours, which could endanger client safety. Here's an example of an occupational therapy assistant talking (either in person or on the phone) with the floor nurse in a long-term care center.

"Hi Beth. I was just in Hilda McBride's room, working with her on her morning cares. I have been working with her for five days in a row, and she has always remembered me and what I am there to do. Today she acted as if she had never seen me. She did not know where she was or why she was here. She did not remember having a stroke. She was very lethargic and stopped doing self-cares right in the middle of them, saying she was too tired. When I asked her to squeeze my hands, she was very weak with both hands. Has she had a medication change?"… "No? I wonder if something new is going on with her. I'll document this in her chart, but you may want to check her vitals and alert her doctor if you agree with me that something is not right."

Exercise 2.1

For the example of Hilda McBride, identify each part of SBAR

Situation:

Background:

Assessment:

Recommendation:

This system of communication might also be helpful when occupational therapy assistants are working with a client and notice something that needs to be brought to the occupational therapist's attention. It enables clear, efficient, and structured communication (Guise & Lowe, 2006; SBAR Checklist, 2006).

The SBAR system has been adapted by some to include a second R—Repeat, Read back, or Response (Guide & Lowe, 2006; Velji et al., 2008). The benefit of the SBARR system is that once the receiver and sender agree on the action to be taken, the sender repeats what they both agreed to; a double check that the action is correct. In their study of the SBARR system, Velji et al. (2008) demonstrated significant improvements in incident reporting, overall perceptions of safety, teamwork within units, and patients reported better continuity and transitions.

Exercise 2.2

Create an SBAR script for the following situations:

1. To nurse: You were working on toilet transfers with a client who had a hip transplant. During the transfer, the client lost her balance and you lowered her to the floor.

   S:

   B:

   A:

   R:

2. To physician: A client who missed his last two appointments comes to the clinic at a time other than his scheduled appointment, slurring his speech, and he does not remember how he got there.

   S:

   B:

   A:

   R:

3. To teacher: A child you are working with has improved by leaps and bounds. She is now tying her shoes independently, writing her name legibly, and engaging in age-appropriate play.

   S:

   B:

   A:

   R:

4. To OT supervisor: A client has had a tendon transfer and needs a specific splint. When you go to the supply closet, the material that you need is not there.

   S:

   B:

   A:

   R:

▼ TEXTING ▼

Texting (text messaging) is a very popular way to communicate with friends and family, but is just beginning to be used in healthcare settings. The Centers for Disease Control and Prevention (CDC) recognizes that more adults use a mobile device than use the Internet (CDC, 2009). Terry (2008) reports that on "January 1, 2008, 43 billion text messages were sent globally" (p. 520). He argues that text messaging is not the elephant in the room, but it is trying to get into the room, even though the healthcare industry is not sure how big it is or what we'll do with it once it's in. The sheer number of people texting every day means that it will find its way into professional communication.

Texting could be used for health promotion by allowing users to text questions to health information providers. One example of this is the Internet Sexuality Information Services, Inc. (ISIS), of Oakland California (Terry, 2008). The text number is posted on billboards around town. Text users can submit text questions to that phone number and receive a response within minutes, right on their phones (Terry, 2008). A search of the Medline database shows that texting is being used as a method to increase compliance with a number of health-related programs such as smoking cessation, sexually transmitted diseases, medication and vaccination compliance, blood-glucose monitoring, eating disorders, brain injury, weight loss, and sunscreen use, as well as a tool for data collection in behavior health studies. Texting is seen as a cost-effective way to manage chronic diseases (Fischer et al., 2012).

Another way that texting could be used is to send reminders to clients of upcoming appointments, medication reminders, or other reminders (Terry, 2008). Intelecare Compliance Solutions, Inc., is developing communications systems that can be tailored to several kinds of communication tools, including texting. Clients and caregivers can determine the kinds of messages they want to send or receive. Smile Reminder is another service that physicians and dentists can use to send appointment reminders, birthday greetings, and special offers (Terry, 2008).

One of the concerns about texting is that text messaging uses abbreviations and often ignores normal grammatical rules for written communication, leading to bad habits in writing. Another concern is related to client privacy. How easy is it for someone to pick up and read text messages on another person's phone?

As more healthcare and education related uses for text messaging are developed, we can look forward to more uses in occupational therapy. For example, text messaging could be used as a way of providing off-site supervision of occupational therapy assistants (between face-to-face visits), or to remind clients with short-term memory loss about daily activities and goals. They could be used to send appointment reminders to outpatients.

SUMMARY

In this chapter we examined several means of professional communication: memos, letters, e-mails, phone calls, and text messages. Memos are short, structured, written notices meant to convey limited information. Letters are a more formal form of written professional communication. General letter formats were presented in this chapter; a more detailed presentation of appeal letters will be presented in Chapter 25. E-mails are a form of electronic communication that is an efficient way to send the same message to multiple recipients, or when a response is needed more rapidly than the typical response time for a memo or letter. Phone calls are used when the message is more urgent. The SBAR method of communicating in a clinical setting was presented as a good way to organize a phone call to a physician or for a face-to-face conversation about a client. Finally, texting was suggested as an up and coming way to communicate messages quickly in a health-related setting. Each of these methods of communication has uses that are more appropriate under certain conditions than others. As always in professional communication, regardless of the delivery system, the communication needs to be made in a professional manner using appropriate tone, active voice, and nondiscriminatory language.

REFERENCES

American Medical Association. (2003). *Opinion 5.026: The use of electronic mail.* Retrieved from http://www.ama-assn.org/ama/pub/physician-resources/medical-ethics/code-medical-ethics/opinion5026.page

American Occupational Therapy Association (AOTA). (2010). *Standards of practice for occupational therapy.* Retrieved from http://www.aota.org/Practitioners/Official/Standards/36194.aspx?FT=.pdf

American Psychological Association. (2010). *Publication manual of the American Psychological Association (6*th *ed.).* Washington, DC: Author.

Braveman, B. (2006). *Leading and managing occupational therapy services: An evidence-based approach.* Philadelphia: F. A. Davis.

Centers for Disease Control and Prevention. (2009). *Mobile e-health data brief.* Retrieved Nov. 19 from http://www.cdc.gov/healthmarketing/ehm/databriefs/

Fischer, H. H., Moore, S. L., Ginosar, D., Davidson, A. J., Rice-Peterson, C. M., Durfee, M. J., & ... Steele, A. W. (2012). Care by cell phone: Text messaging for chronic disease management. *American Journal of Managed Care, 18*(2), e42–e47.

Guise, J., & Lowe, N. (2006, May). Do You Speak SBAR?. *JOGNN: Journal of Obstetric, Gynecologic & Neonatal Nursing,* 313–314. doi:10.1111/j.1552-6909.2006.00043.x.

Joint Commission (2012). *Official "do not use" list.* Retrieved from http://www.jointcommission.org/assets/1/18/Do_Not_Use_List.pdf

Lincoln University. (n.d.). *Editing for formality: Find your academic voice.* Retrieved from http://www.lincoln.edu/mhs/owl/formality.html

Lunsford, A. (2009). *The everyday writer* (4th ed.). New York: Bedford/St. Martin's.

Oliu, W. E., Brusaw, C. T. & Alred, G. J., (2010). *Writing that works with 2009 MLA and 2010 APA updates: How to write effectively on the job* (10th ed.). New York, NY: St. Martin's Press.

OWL at Purdue University. (2006). *HATS: A design procedure for routine business documents*. Retrieved from http://owl.english.purdue.edu/owl/resource/632/1/

OWL at Purdue University. (2010a). *Tone in business writing*. Retrieved from http://owl.english.purdue.edu/owl/resource/652/1/

OWL at Purdue University. (2010b). *Stereotypes and biased language*. Retrieved from https://owl.english.purdue.edu/owl/resource/608/05/

OWL at Purdue University. (2010c). *Memos*. Retrieved from http://owl.english.purdue.edu/owl/resource/590/1/

OWL at Purdue University. (2010d). *Basic business letters*. Retrieved from http://owl.english.purdue.edu/owl/resource/653/1/

OWL at Purdue University. (2010e). *Email etiquette*. Retrieved from http://owl.english.purdue.edu/owl/resource/636/01/

OWL at Purdue University. (2011). *Active versus passive voice*. Retrieved from http://owl.english.purdue.edu/owl/resource/539/02/

Sabath, A. M. (2002). *Business etiquette.* New York, NY: Barnes and Noble.

"SBAR checklist can cut risk at patient handoff." (2006) *Healthcare Risk Management.* Retrieved April 5, 2009 from accessmylibrary: http://www.accessmylibrary.com/coms2/summary_0286-17346447_ITM

"SBAR initiative to improve staff communication." (2005). *Healthcare Benchmarks and Quality Improvement*, *12*(4), 40–41. Retrieved from MEDLINE database.

"SBAR for students." (2007). *Nursing Education Perspectives*, *28*(6), 306. Retrieved from Health Source: Nursing/Academic Edition database.

Scott, R.W. (2013). *Legal, ethical, and practical aspects of patient care documentation: A guide for rehabilitation professionals* (4th ed.). Boston, MA: Jones and Bartlett.

Sherwood, K. D. (n.d.). *Context.* Retrieved March 22, 2006, from http://www.webfoot.com/advice/email.top.html

Terry, M. (2008). Text messaging in healthcare: The elephant knocking at the door. *Telemedicine Journal and E-Health: The Official Journal of the American Telemedicine Association*, *14*, 520–524. http://dx.doi.org/10.1089/tmj.2008.8495

The ARC. (2012) *What is people first language?* Retrieved from http://www.thearc.org/page.aspx?pid=2523

Velji, K., Baker, G., Fancott, C., Andreoli, A., Boaro, N., & ... Sinclair, L. (2008). Effectiveness of an adapted SBAR communication tool for a rehabilitation setting. *Healthcare Quarterly (Toronto, Ont.)*, *11*(3 Spec No.), 72–79.

Word-mart.com. (2010). *Formal and informal writing*. Retrieved from http.//www.word-mart.com/html/formal_and_informal_writing.html

Yale University (n.d.). *Netiquette*. Retrieved March 22, 2006, from http://www.library.yale.edu/training/netidquette

---

Visit **www.pearsonhighered.com/healthprofessionsresources** to access the student resources that accompany this book. Simply select Occupational Therapy from the choice of disciplines. Find this book and you will find the complimentary study tools created for this specific title.

CHAPTER 3

Buzzwords, Jargon, and Abbreviations

INTRODUCTION

The longer you write progress notes and intervention plans, the more you fall into certain patterns. You learn what words get the attention of reviewers in positive and negative ways. There are lists floating around, developed by experienced occupational therapists, containing words one should never use, and other lists with words that one should be sure to use. If your supervisor hands you such a list, he or she will expect you to use it. Go ahead and use these lists. Do not, however, depend on them as your sole source for good words. If you do, all your documentation will sound the same.

▼ BUZZWORDS ▼

Buzzwords are words that are currently popular or trendy. They let the reader or listener know that you are up-to-date. Some current buzzwords include *collaborative*, *embedded*, *function*, *sustainable*, and *community*. There may be others that are specific to different regions of the country.

"Function" is a special buzzword. It is a necessary word to occupational therapy practice. Occupational therapy practitioners must show that their services result in functional changes in their clients. This is true of other providers such as physical therapists and speech language pathologists as well. In most settings, demonstrating improvement in function is essential to receiving payment for services. This means that as occupational therapists document their services, it is not enough to say that someone's range of motion increased. So what? Just because Mrs. Smith can bend more at the elbow, it does not automatically mean that she can do more because of it. Can she now feed herself or fasten the top button on her blouse? If a person can now follow three-step directions, what does it mean? Can this person now prepare a meal? Function is the difference between a client tolerating being in water for 3 minutes and taking a bath. Documentation must be explicit in its descriptions of functional activities.

Evidence and *evidenced-based* are buzzwords that appeal to third-party payers. When an occupational therapy practitioner says that the evidence says such and such, it gives credibility to the rationale for choosing a particular intervention. This is good. Payers are calling for evidence-based practice. An occupational therapy practitioner should be ready to support the claim of evidence, if asked. Although the most current definitions of evidence-based practice include not only the best research evidence but also clinician expertise and client preferences, a payer is most likely to expect evidence to be found in the literature. Upon request, a payer will expect to see well-designed clinical studies that demonstrate the effectiveness of the intervention rather than anecdotal evidence.

Sustainable is another buzzword. Sustainable means that the outcomes of the interventions will persist after occupational therapy services end. Payers want to pay for services that will make a lasting difference in the client's life. For example, an occupational therapy practitioner in a clinic setting worked for months with a 4-year-old with autism, teaching him to dress himself. After several months, this child was successfully dressing himself every time she worked with him, so she discontinued working on that goal. The child's family received reports and instructions throughout those months to assist in carry-over to the home setting.

Then, after 2 months of working on other self-care and play skills, the occupational therapy practitioner decided to see if the boy could still dress himself. He could not. The occupational therapy intervention was not sustainable given the child's home situation. If you were responsible for paying this child's therapy bill, would you think it was money well spent?

Interprofessional is another buzzword. The literal definition of interprofessional is between professions. Related terms are *intraprofessional* (within one profession, such as when occupational therapists and occupational therapy assistants collaborate) and *uniprofessional* (one profession). Countries all over the globe are calling for more interprofessional collaboration in practice. The World Health Organization (WHO, 2010) says practitioners trained in interprofessional team collaboration will reduce error rates, shorten lengths of stays, be a more satisfied and stable workforce, and improve the quality of healthcare. WHO (2010) goes on to define interprofessional collaborative practice as "When multiple health workers from different professional backgrounds work together with patient, families, carers, and communities to deliver the highest quality of care" (p. 7). In order to show interprofessional collaboration, practitioners need to document that they have communicated with other members of the care delivery team.

Red-Flag Words

Just as there are buzzwords, there are what I call *red-flag words*. These words will cause the reader to stop and perhaps not read any further. They serve as big signs of trouble. An example of a red-flag word is *continued* or *maintained* when read by a payer who pays only for occupational therapy services as long as there is demonstrable progress.

Some payers will also view documentation with an eye toward discontinuing service if they read that a client was *seen* in occupational therapy rather than *participated in* the occupational therapy session. If the writer says that a client was seen in occupational therapy today, the payer may interpret it to mean that the client was seen in the room but did not necessarily do anything while in the room. *Participated* implies some action on the part of the client.

For years, clinicians have refrained from writing goals that deal with the client's need to participate in cultural, religious, or spiritual activities. It seemed that culture, religion, and spirituality were red-flag words. Clinicians were hesitant to address issues of participation in cultural, religious, or spiritual activities, primarily because they were sure payers would not pay for such services (they may be viewed as diversionary activities, which are usually not reimbursable). One occupational therapist told me that even though she was working with an elderly priest who had had a stroke, the payer would not pay for her to work toward the goal that he be able to conduct the mass, so she never again tried to get any services involving religion or spirituality covered. While completing the tasks of the mass does relate to religion, perhaps if she had stated the goal in terms of regaining the skills required to return to work, she might have gotten paid for her services.

That was several years ago, and maybe things have changed since then. If what is important to your client is participation in religious or spiritual life, then that is what you should work on with him or her. Instead of anticipating the reaction of payers to red-flag words, use them and then appeal the case if it is denied. We may find that we are no longer being denied coverage. The *Occupational Therapy Practice Framework* (AOTA, 2014) can provide an occupational therapy practitioner with wording that is consistent with best practice. However, just because AOTA says an occupation or intervention activity is within the scope of occupational therapy practice, it does not mean a third-party payer will pay for it.

▼ JARGON ▼

Jargon is terminology widely understood by one profession or group of people but not understood by others outside the group or profession (Lunsford, 2009). Occupational therapy practitioners are notorious for their use of jargon, so are many other healthcare professionals. Sadly, each profession uses jargon unique to itself, and it can create a lot of unnecessary confusion.

If we all document using common terminology, we can all help each other carry out interventions that support each other for the good of the client. As mentioned in the introduction to this book, occupational therapy practitioners (and other professionals) need to consider the audience they are addressing. Often, the people making decisions about whether or not to pay for occupational therapy services are not occupational therapy practitioners themselves. Physicians and nurses may be called on to translate our documentation for clients, and if they cannot understand our jargon, then we have put them in a bad spot. Although occupational therapy practitioners know what bilateral integration is, most people do not.

Here is an example of a narrative note written with lots of buzzwords, jargon, and abbreviations:

> Pt. seen for 3 units for ADLs. Patient sat at EOB with min assist. Pt. told to perform upper body hyg/grmg. Needed min assist and s/u. Pt. showed a poor bilateral integration due to L hemiplegia and L hemianopsia. Pt's SO instructed by this therapist in comp techniques and cuing patterns. SO return demonstration not adequate. Will need additional instruction.

Here is the same paragraph written in relatively plain English:

> Patient participated in a 45-minute bedside session this morning for self-care activities. The pt. sat at the edge of the bed with minimal assistance. With minimal assistance following setup, the patient washed his face and trunk, brushed his teeth, and combed his hair. He did not wash his L arm or the L side of his face. The pt's wife was instructed in ways to set up tasks and verbally cue the patient to compensate for left visual field cut. She tended to try to do the task for her husband; she will need more instruction.

Both paragraphs describe the same client doing the same activities. The second one is easier for most people to read and understand. Note that it does not eliminate every abbreviation or word of jargon. To do so would make it sound too simplistic and unprofessional. It is a question of balance and of which terms are likely to be understood by every professional in the program and by payers.

Exercise 3.1

Translate these narrative notes into plain English.

1. Jennifer attended 3 sessions this wk. She needed enc. to engage in the group discussion. She rarely made eye contact with the OT or other group members. She mumbled incoherently and occasionally picked at something unseen in the air around her, possibly hallucinating. When given a cognitive task to do, she completely disengaged. Her attention span was < 2 min. She appeared to respond +ly to classical music, the mumbling and picking at the air ceased and she smiled. Pt. oriented x1.

2. Ling was seen for a three-unit session today. She selected the 30-inch ball as the first thing she wanted to try. She positioned herself prone on the ball and proceeded to rock in a linear pattern. Then she went to the bolster swing and engaged in circular vestibular stimulation. Ling alternated between these two activities for 15 minutes. Next she asked to draw in the shaving cream on a mirror. She attended to this task for 5 minutes, then ran to the sink to wash and dry her hands. Next she wrapped herself up tightly in a parachute. Following that, she quietly played with puzzles. She is demonstrating improved tactile and vestibular processing. Plan is to continue working on SI activities to improve sensory processing as outlined in POC.

▼ ABBREVIATIONS ▼

One way to shorten the time it takes to write notes is to use abbreviations. It takes less time to write "bid" than it does to write "two times per day." However, the problem with abbreviations is that not everyone knows what the abbreviations mean. Sometimes the same abbreviation can mean different things. In one setting "hoh" might mean hard of hearing, but in another it could mean hand over hand (as a form of assisting a client to complete a task). Most facilities have a list of acceptable abbreviations for use at that facility. It is important to use such a list if it exists, and not assume that other people understand your abbreviations. The Joint Commission (2012) has published a list of abbreviations that should not be used. It did this because errors related to misreading abbreviations were leading to adverse events involving patients (Joint Commission, 2012).

Here is a narrative note written by a practitioner, using abbreviations when possible and then rewritten using as few abbreviations as possible. Using abbreviations saved three lines of type, but made it harder to read.

Client partic. in OT bid 5x/wk. He partic. in a w.u. Ax consisting of ROM ex. for BUE including ✓/–, ab/ad, & IR/ER. Client shows ↑ in ROM and # reps all directions. He is dressing himself with fewer vc's. He prog from max to min assist in making sandwiches. The sandwiches required him to use bilat integ. skills & cog abilities. Client is showing ↑ in these skills & abilities. Plan to ↑ # and complexity of BUE Ax.

Client participated in OT twice daily for 5 days this week. He participated in a warm-up activity consisting of ROM exercises for both arms including flexion/extension, ab-/adduction, and internal/external rotation. Client shows increase in ROM and number of repetitions of movements in all directions. He is dressing himself with fewer verbal cues. He progressed from max to min assistance in making sandwiches. The sandwiches required him to use both hands together & plan, sequence, and problem solve. Client is showing an increase in these skills & abilities. The plan is to increase the number and complexity of upper extremity activities per session.

In some instances, people expect abbreviations to be used. When signing your name on any formal documentation, it is common practice to identify yourself by putting your professional credentials after your name in the form of an abbreviation. Common abbreviations for professional credentials are listed in Box 3.1. There are many others, but these are the most common. Abbreviations are also used to document the frequency with which something occurs. Box 3.2 shows a list of such abbreviations. Abbreviations can refer to parts of the body, injuries, or illnesses. Box 3.3 is a partial list; however, inclusion in this list does not guarantee that anyone who reads these abbreviations knows what they mean. There are other abbreviations referred to in the jargon of the profession as the "x" abbreviations (Box 3.4). These have varied use and acceptability in different parts of the country. Occupational therapists and other medical professionals use a variety of abbreviations to identify types of range of motion, as shown in Box 3.5. Clinical procedures and common clinical terminology are abbreviated in letters and with symbols (Box 3.6). The first part of Box 3.6 contains those terms with letter abbreviations and the symbols follow. Box 3.7 shows abbreviations most commonly used when payment is being discussed. Finally, Box 3.8 contains a list of abbreviations related to education. Please note that not all possible abbreviations are included in these lists and, conversely, inclusion in this book does not mean that an abbreviation is acceptable in all settings. In most settings, there will be a list of approved abbreviations.

BOX 3.1   Professional Credentials and Job Titles

AP	Advanced Practitioner, for OTAs or COTAs only
APE	Adaptive Physical Education
ATC	Athletic Trainer Certified
ATP	Assistive Technology Professional
BCG	Board Certified in Gerontology (AOTA)
BCMH	Board Certified in Mental Health (AOTA)
BCP	Board Certified in Pediatrics (AOTA)
BCPR	Board Certified in Physical Rehabilitation (AOTA)
CAPS	Certified Aging in Place Specialist
CCC	Certificate of Clinical Competence [for speech-language pathologists]
CCM	Certified Case Manager
CEO	Chief Executive Officer
CFO	Chief Financial Officer
CHT	Certified Hand Therapist
CI	Clinical Instructor
COO	Chief Operating Officer
COTA	Certified Occupational Therapy Assistant
COTA/L	Certified Occupational Therapy Assistant, Licensed
CPE	Certified Professional Ergonomist
CST	Craniosacral Therapist
D/APE	Developmental and Adaptive Physical Education
DC	Doctor of Chiropractic
DDS	Doctor of Dental Surgery
DMD	Doctor of Medical Dentistry
DO	Doctor of Osteopathy
DPT	Doctor of Physical Therapy
EBD	Emotional or Behavioral Disorder (teacher)
EdD	Education, Doctor of
ENT	Ear, Nose, and Throat Doctor (otolaryngologist)
FACP	Fellow of the American College of Physicians
FACS	Fellow of the American College of Surgeons
FAOTA	Fellow of the American Occupational Therapy Association
FWE	Fieldwork Educator
HHA	Home Health Aide
LD	Learning Disability
LMFT	Licensed Marriage and Family Therapist
LP	Licensed Psychologist
LPN	Licensed Practical Nurse
LSW	Licensed Social Worker
MAOT	Master of Arts in Occupational Therapy
MD	Medical Doctor
MOT	Master of Occupational Therapy
MPH	Master of Public Health
MSOT	Master of Science in Occupational Therapy
MSW	Master of Social Work
NDT	Neurodevelopmental Therapist
OT/L	Occupational Therapist, Licensed
OTA	Occupational Therapy Assistant
OTA/L	Occupational Therapy Assistant, Licensed
OTAS	Occupational Therapy Assistant Student
OTD	Occupational Therapist, Doctor of [clinical doctorate]
OTD/L	Doctor of Occupational Therapy, Licensed

OTIP	Occupational Therapist in Independent Practice—Medicare
OTR	Occupational Therapist, Registered
OTR/L	Occupational Therapist, Registered and Licensed
OTS	Occupational Therapy Student
PA	Physician Assistant
PCA	Personal Care Attendant
PharmD	Doctor of Pharmacy
PhD	Doctor of Philosophy
PT	Physical Therapist
PTA	Physical Therapist Assistant
QMHP	Qualified Mental Health Professional
QMRP	Qualified Mental Retardation Professional
QRC	Qualified Rehabilitation Consultant
RD	Registered Dietician
RN	Registered Nurse
ROH	Roster of Honor
RRT	Registered Recreation Therapist or Registered Respiratory Therapist
RT	Recreation Therapist or Respiratory Therapist
ScD	Doctor of Science
SCDCM	Specialty Certification in Driving and Community Mobility (AOTA)
SCEM	Specialty Certification in Environmental Modification (AOTA)
SCFES	Specialty Certification in Feeding, Eating, and Swallowing (AOTA)
SCLV	Specialty Certification in Low Vision (AOTA)
SLP	Speech-Language Pathologist

Source: AOTA (2012).

BOX 3.2 Abbreviations Related to Time and Frequency

ad lib	at liberty; as desired
ASAP	as soon as possible
bid	twice a day
BIN	twice at night
eod	every other day
noc	at night
prn	as needed
PTA	prior to admission
qd	once a day
qid	four times a day
qod	every other day
STAT	immediately
tid	three times a day
i	once a day
ii	twice a day
iii	three times a day
1x/wk	once a week
2x/wk	twice a week
3x/wk	three times a week (*continues up to 7x/wk*)
1x/mo	once a month
2x/mo	twice a month
3x/mo	three times a month (*continues up to 12x/mo or more*)

BOX 3.3   Abbreviations Related to Body Parts, Diagnoses, and Tests

AA	atlantoaxial; adjusted age; or active assist
AAA	abdominal aortic aneurysm
AAOX3	alert, awake, and oriented to person, place, and time [times three]
ABG	arterial blood gasses
ABN	abnormal
AC	joint acromioclavicular joint
ACA	anterior communicating artery; anterior cerebral artery
ACL	anterior cruciate ligament
ACVD	acute cardiovascular disease
ADD	attention deficit disorder
ADHD	attention deficit hyperactivity disorder
Adm	admitted on; admission
AE	above elbow
AEA	above elbow amputation
AF	atrial fibrillation
AGA	appropriate for gestational age
AI	aortic incompetence; aortic insufficiency
AIDS	acquired immunedeficiency disorder
AK	above knee
AKA	above knee amputation; also known as
ALL	acute lymphocytic leukemia; anterior longitudinal ligament
ALS	amyotrophic lateral sclerosis
ant.	anterior
AP; A/P	anterior-posterior
APGAR	appearance, pulse, grimace, activity, respiration
ARDS	acute respiratory distress syndrome; adult respiratory distress syndrome
ARF	acute renal failure; acute respiratory failure
AS	aortic stenosis; ankylosing spondylitis
As & Bs	apnea and bradycardia
ASCVD	arteriosclerotic cardiovascular disease
ASD	atrial septal defect
ASHD	atherosclerotic heart disease
ASIS	anterior superior iliac spine
ATNR	asymmetrical tonic neck reflex
AV	arteriovenous; atrioventricular; aortic valve
BBB	bundle-branch block; blood brain–barrier
BE	below elbow
BEA	below elbow amputation
Bi-PAP	bi-level positive airway pressure
BK	below knee
BKA	below knee amputation
bl	blood; bleeding
BLE	both lower extremities
BMI or bmi	body mass index
BMP	basic metabolic panel
BMR	basal metabolic rate
BP	blood pressure
BPD	bronchopulmonary disease
bpm	beats per minute
BS	breath sounds; blood sugar; bowel sounds
BUE	both upper extremities
BUN	blood urea nitrogen

bw	birth weight
c̄	with
CA; Ca	cancer; carcinoma
CABG	coronary artery bypass graft
CAD	coronary artery disease
Cal	calories
CAT	computerized axial tomography
cath	catheter
CBC	complete blood count
CBI	closed brain injury
CC, C/C or cc	chief complaint; carbon copy
CCU	cardiac care unit; critical care unit
C-diff	C. difficile (bacteria)
CF	cystic fibrosis
CFS	chronic fatigue syndrome
chemo	chemotherapy
CHF	congestive heart failure
CHI	closed head injury
CICU	cardiac intensive care unit
CLD	chronic liver disease
CMC	carpometacarpal (joint)
CMV	cytomegalovirus
CN	cranial nerve, usually followed by the number of the nerve using Roman numerals
CNS	central nervous system
CO	cardiac output; carbon monoxide
c/o	complains of
COD	co-occurring disorder [psychiatric diagnosis with a chemical misuse diagnosis]
COLD	chronic obstructive lung disease
Cont.; cont.	continued
COPD	chronic obstructive pulmonary disorder
CP	cerebral palsy; chest pain
CPAP	continuous positive airway pressure
CPR	cardiopulmonary resuscitation
CRF	chronic renal failure
C&S	culture and sensitivity
CSF	cerebrospinal fluid
CT	chest tube; computerized axial tomography
CTR	carpal tunnel release
CTS	carpal tunnel syndrome
CVA	cerebral vascular accident—stroke
CVP	cerebral vascular pressure
DD	developmental disabilities; dual diagnosis
DDD	degenerative disc disease
DDH	developmental dysplasia of the hip
DF	dorsiflexion
DIP	distal interphalangeal (joint)
DJD	degenerative joint disease
DM	diabetes mellitus
DMD	Duchenne muscular dystrophy
DNR	do not resuscitate
DOB	date of birth
DOE	dyspnea on exertion
DT	delirium tremens

(Continued)

BOX 3.3   Continued

DTR	deep tendon reflex
DVT	deep vein thrombosis
EBV	Epstein Barr virus
ECG; EKG	electrocardiogram
ECHO; echo	echocardiogram
ED	erectile dysfunction
EEG	electroencephalogram
EENT	ears, eyes, nose, and throat
EID	easily identified depression
ELBW	extremely low birth weight
EMG	electromyelogram
EOM	extraocular movement
ER	emergency room; external rotation
ESRD	end-stage renal disease
ETOH; EtOH	alcohol [use or abuse]
FAE	fetal alcohol effects
FAS	fetal alcohol syndrome
FBS	fasting blood sugar
FTT	failure to thrive
F/U; f/u	follow up
FUO	fever of unknown origin
G	good
G-tube	gastrostomy tube
GA	gestational age
GB	gall bladder
GBS	Guillain-Barré syndrome
GCS	Glasgow coma scale
GERD	gastroesophageal reflux disease
GI	gastrointestinal
G#P#A#	number of births, pregnancies, and abortions
Grava	gravida [number of births]
GSW	gunshot wound
GU	genitourinary
GYN	gynecologic; gynecology
H/A or HA	headache
HAC	hospital acquired condition
Hams	hamstrings
HB, Hb or Hgb	hemoglobin
HBP	high blood pressure
HBV	hepatitis B virus
HC	heel cords
HCVD	hypertensive cardiovascular disease
HEENT	head, ear, eyes, nose, throat
HIB	haemophilus influenza B [vaccine]
HIV	human immunodeficiency virus
HLT	heart lung transplant
HNP	herniated nucleus pulposus
HOH	hard of hearing; hand over hand
H & P	history and physical
HPI	history of present illness
HR	heart rate
HSV	herpes simplex virus
Ht	height
HT	heart transplant

HTN	hypertension
IBS	irritable bowel syndrome
ICA	internal carotid artery
ICH	intracranial hemorrhage; intracerebral hemorrhage
ICP	intracranial pressure
ICU	intensive care unit
ID	infections disease
I&D	incision and drainage
IDDM	insulin-dependent diabetes mellitus
Ig	immunoglobulin
IM	intramuscular
imp.	impression
Indep or I	independently
inf	inferior
IP	interphalangeal
IQ	intelligence quotient
IR	internal rotation
IV	intravenous
IVC	inferior vena cava
JRA	juvenile rheumatoid arthritis
jt	joint
KUB	kidneys, ureter, bladder
lap	laparoscopy; laparotomy
lat	lateral
LBBB	left bundle branch block
LBP	low back pain
LBW	low birth weight
LCA	left carotid artery
LD	learning disability
LE	lower extremity—leg
LG	limb-girdle dystrophy
LLE	left lower extremity
LLQ	left lower quadrant [abdomen]
LMN	lower motor neuron
LMP	last menstrual period
LOC	loss of consciousness
LP	lumbar puncture
LT	lung transplant
LUE	left upper extremity
LUQ	left upper quadrant [abdomen]
MAP	main arterial pressure
MCA	middle cerebral artery
MCL	medial collateral ligament
MCP or MP	metacarpal phalangeal
MD	muscular dystrophy
med	medial
meds	medications
mets	metastasis
MH	mental health
MI	myocardial infarction; mental illness
MP	metacarpal phalangeal (joint)
MRI	magnetic resonance imaging
MRSA	methicillin-resistant staphylococcus aureus
MS	multiple sclerosis or mitral stenosis
MV	mitral valve

(Continued)

BOX 3.3   Continued

MVA	motor vehicle accident
MVP	mitral valve prolapse
N	normal; nausea
N/A	not applicable; not available
NAD	no appreciable disease; nothing abnormal detected; no acute distress
nc	nasal cannula
Neg	negative
NG	nasogastric
NGT	nasogastric tube
NICU	neonatal intensive care unit
NIDDM	non-insulin-dependent diabetes mellitus
NKA	no known allergies
NKDA	no known drug allergies
nl	normal
nn	nerve
NOS	not otherwise specified
NPO	nothing per mouth
NSAID	nonsteroidal anti-inflammatory drugs
NSR	normal sinus rhythm
N & V; N/V	nausea and vomiting
O2	oxygen
OA	osteoarthritis
OB	obstetrics
OBS	organic brain syndrome
OD	overdose
OI	osteogenesis imperfecta
OM	otitis media [ear infection]
ORIF	open reduction, internal fixation
p	post; after
PA	pulmonary artery
PARA; para	paraplegia
PCA	patient controlled analgesia; personal care attendant
PCL	posterior cruciate ligament
PD	Parkinson's disease
PDD	pervasive developmental disorder
PE	pulmonary embolus; pulmonary edema
PEDI	Pediatric Evaluation of Disability Index
PEEP	positive end expiratory pressure
PEG	percutaneous endoscopic gastrostomy
peri	perineal
PERRLA	pupils equal, round, reactive to light, and accommodation
PET	positron emission tomography
PFT	pulmonary function test
PH	past history
Phys Dys	physical disabilities
PI	present illness
PICA	posterior inferior cerebellar artery; posterior inferior communicating artery
PICU	pediatric intensive care unit
PID	pelvic inflammatory disease
PIP	proximal interphalangeal (joint)
PKU	phenylketonuria
PLF	prior level of function
PMH	past medical history

PNI	peripheral nerve injury
PNS	peripheral nervous system
POA	present on admission
Pos	positive
post	posterior
postop	postoperatively; after surgery
preop	preoperatively; before surgery
PSIS	posterior superior iliac spine
Psych	psychology; psychiatry; psychiatric
PTCA	percutaneous transluminal coronary angioplasty
PTSD	posttraumatic stress disorder
PVC	premature ventricular contraction
PVD	peripheral vascular disease
PWA	person with AIDS
PWB	partial weight bearing
QUAD; quad	quadriplegia; quadriplegic
RA	rheumatoid arthritis; right atrium
RAS	reticular activating system
RBBB	right bundle branch block
RBC	red blood count
RCA	right carotid artery
RD	retinal detachment
Resp	respiration
RF	renal failure
RHD	rheumatoid heart disease
RLE	right lower extremity
RLQ	right lower quadrant [abdomen]
r/o	rule out
ROS	review of symptoms
rr	respiratory rate
RSD	reflex sympathetic dystrophy
RSV	respiratory syncytial virus
RUE	right upper extremity
RUQ	right upper quadrant [abdomen]
RV	right ventricle
SAD	season affective disorder
SC	subcutaneous
SC joint	sternoclavicular joint
SCD	sickle cell disease
SCI	spinal cord injury
SCM	sternocleidomastoid [joint]
SD	seizure disorder
SDH	subdural hematoma
SED	seriously emotionally disturbed; suberythemal
SF-36	short-form 36
SICU	surgical intensive care unit
SIDS	sudden infant death syndrome
SIJ	sacroiliac joint
SLE	systemic lupus erythematosus
SOB	shortness of breath
S & S; S/S	signs and symptoms
S/P	status post; after
STD	sexually transmitted disease
STNR	symmetrical tonic neck reflex

(Continued)

BOX 3.3   Continued

str	strength
sup	superior; supine
SVC	superior vena cava
Sz	schizophrenia
T & A	tonsils & adenoids; tonsillectomy and adenoidectomy
TB	tuberculosis
TBI	traumatic brain injury
TD	tardive dyskinesia
TEE	transesophageal echocardiogram
THA	total hip arthroplasty
THR	total hip replacement
TIA	transient ischemic attack
TKA	total knee arthroplasty
TKR	total knee replacement
TMJ	temporal mandibular joint
TNR	tonic neck reflexes [ATNR, STNR]
TPN	total parenteral nutrition
TPR	temperature, pulse, & respiration
TSA	total shoulder arthroplasty
TUR	transurethral resection
TV	tidal volume
UA	urine analysis; urinalysis
UE	upper extremity—arm
UMN	upper motor neuron
URI	upper respiratory infection
UTI	urinary tract infection
VC	vital capacity
VD	venereal disease
vent.	ventilator
VLBW	very low birth weight
VSD	ventricular septal defect
VT	ventricular tachycardia
v.s.	vital signs
WBC	white blood count

Sources: Gartee (2011); Gately & Borcherding (2012); Jacobs & Jacobs (2009); Kettenback (2004); Shamus & Stern (2011).

BOX 3.4   "X" Abbreviations

Ax	activity
Dx	diagnosis
Fx	fracture
Hx	history of
PMHx	past medical history
Px	physical examination
Rx	therapy
Sx	symptom
Tx	treatment; traction; tests (performed)

BOX 3.5   Range of Motion Abbreviations

AAROM	active assisted ROM
AROM	active ROM
CPM	continuous passive motion
FROM	functional ROM
PROM	passive ROM
ROM	range of motion
RROM	resisted ROM

BOX 3.6   Abbreviations for Clinical Procedures

A	assessment; assist; assistance
ABD or abd	abduction
ABR	absolute bed rest
ac	before meals
ADD or add	adduction
ADL	activities of daily living
ad lib	at liberty, as desired
AFO	ankle-foot orthosis
ALF	assisted living facility
ALOS	average length of stay
a.m. or AM	morning
ama or AMA	against medical advice
amb	ambulation; ambulates
a p	Before dinner
amt or am't	amount
ASA	aspirin
ASAP	as soon as possible
AT	assistive technology
B or bilat.	bilateral or both
BADL	basic activities of daily living
b/c	because
b/4	before
bm	body mechanics
BP	bed pan
bpm	beats per minute
BRP	bathroom privileges
B/S	bed side
C	centigrade
cal	calories
CAT	computer-assisted tomography
CBR	complete bed rest
CBT	cognitive behavioral therapy
cc	chief complaint
CGA	contact guard assist
CIMT	constraint-induced movement therapy
cm	centimeter

(Continued)

BOX 3.6 Continued

c/o	complains of
cont.	continue
CP	cold pack
CPAP	continuous positive airway pressure
CPM; CPMM	continuous passive motion machine
CPR	cardiopulmonary resuscitation
CT	computerized tomography
CVP	continuous venous pressure
D, dep	dependent
DAFO	dynamic ankle foot orthosis
D/C	discontinuation; discharge
Dept.	department—may also be written with a small d
DME	durable medical equipment
DNR	do not resuscitate
DOB	date of birth
DOE	dyspnea on exertion
DRS	disability rating scale
EBP	evidence-based practice
e.g.	for example; such as
eob	edge of bed
ES or e-stim	electrical stimulation
etc.	et cetera, and so forth
eval	evaluation
ex	exercise
ext.	extension
F or f	fair
f	female
FCE	functional capacity evaluation
FES	functional electrical stimulation
FEV1	forced expiratory volume in 1 second
FIM	Functional Independence Measure
flex	flexion
FRG	functional related groups
ft	feet; foot as in a measurement, not a body part
f/u	follow-up
FW I	fieldwork one
FW II	fieldwork two, also called affiliation experience
FWB	full weight bearing
G	good as in muscle strength
g	gram
GM&S	general medicine and surgery
GSR	galvanic skin response
GT	gait training
h or hr.	hour
H&P	history and physical
Hemi	hemiplegia
HEP	home exercise program
HH	home health; handheld
HHA	hand hold assist
HKAFO	hip knee ankle foot orthosis
HME	home medical equipment
HOB	head of bed
HOH/hoh	hand over hand; hard of hearing

HP	hot pack
HR	heart rate
hr.	hour
hs	at night, hours of sleep
ht	height
I	independently
ICU	intensive care unit
I & O	intake and output
IADL	instrumental activities of daily living
ICD-9	International Classification of Diseases, Ninth Edition
ICD-10	International Classification of Diseases, Tenth Edition
ICF	intermediate care facility; International Classification of Function
ICU	intensive care unit
i.e.	that is; in other words
ILC	independent living center
IM	intramuscular
imp	impression
in.	inches
inhal	inhalation
Inj	injection
IP	inpatient
ITB	intrathecal baclofen
IV	intravenous
KAFO	knee-ankle-foot orthosis
kg.	kilogram
KJ	knee jerk
L	left
L or l	liter
l/m	liters per minute
LAD	language acquisition device
lb.	pound
LBQC	large-based quad cane
LLB	long leg brace
llq	left lower quadrant
LOS	length of stay
LP	lumbar puncture
LTC	long-term care
LTG	long-term goal
LUQ	left upper quadrant
L&W	living and well
m	male
MAO	monoamine oxidase
max	maximum or maximal
MED	minimal effective dose; minimal erythemal dose
meds	medications, medicines
MET	metabolic level; maximal
MFR	myofascial release
MFT or mft	muscle function test
mg	milligram
MH	moist heat
MHP	moist hot pack
min	minutes; minimum
ml	milliliter
mm	millimeter

(Continued)

BOX 3.6 Continued

mm-Hg	millimeters of mercury
MMSE	Mini-Mental Status Exam
MMT	manual muscle test
mo.	month
mob	mobility; mobilization
mod	moderate
MRI	magnetic resonance imaging
MSQ	Mental Status Questionnaire
MVC	maximum voluntary contraction
N	normal, as in muscle grade
na or N/A	not applicable; not available
NaC	normal saline
NBQC	narrow-based quad cane
NDT	neurodevelopmental treatment
neb	nebulizer
neg.	negative
NICU	neonatal intensive care unit
NKA	no known allergy
NKDA	no known drug allergy
NMES	neuromuscular electrical stimulation
noc	nocturnal, at night
NPO	nothing per mouth
nt	not tested
NWB	non-weight bearing
O	objective
O2	oxygen
OBS	observation
od	once daily; right eye
OH	occupational history
OOB	out of bed
OP	outpatient
OR	operating room
os	left eye
OTC	over the counter
ou	both eyes
Ox3	oriented times three [person, place, time]
Ox4	oriented times four [person, place, time, and situation]
oz.	ounce
P	plan; poor; pulse
$\bar{p}$	after
PADL	personal activities of daily living
PAMS	physical agent modalities
para	paraplegic
pc	after meals
PEDI	Pediatric Evaluation of Disability Index
per	by or through
PLOF	past level of function
PLOP	present level of performance
p.m. or PM	between noon and midnight
PMR: PM&R	physical medicine and rehabilitation
PNF	proprioceptive neuromuscular facilitation
po	per mouth, orally
P/O; post-op	after surgery

POC	plan of care
POD	post-op day number
POMR	problem-oriented medical record
pos	positive
poss	possible
post	posterior
post-op	after surgery
PPE	personal protective equipment
PRE	progressive resistive exercise
pre-op	before surgery
pro; pron	pronation
PRN; prn	per as needed
Pt; pt.	patient; pint; point
PTA	prior to admission
PTB	patellar tendon bearing [prosthesis]
PVE	prevocational evaluation
PWB	partial weight bearing
q	every
qt.	quart
quad	quadriceps
R	right
RA	reasonable accommodation
Re: or re:	regarding
rehab	rehabilitation
REM	rapid eye movement
reps	repetitions
resp	respiratory, respiration
RET	rational emotion therapy
rlq	right lower quadrant
RM	repetition maximum
RPE	rating of perceived exertion
RTC	return to clinic
RTI	Routine Task Inventory
RTO	return to office
ruq	right upper quadrant
RW	rolling walker
S	subjective
SBA	stand by assist
SE	side effects
sec	seconds
SH	social history
SI	sensory integration
sig	directions for use, give as follows
SLB	short leg brace
SLR	straight leg raise
SNF	skilled nursing facility
SOAP	subjective, objective, assessment, plan; progress note format
SOB	shortness of breath
SOC	start of care
SOP	standard operating procedure
SPEM	smooth pursuit eye movement
stat	immediately
STG	short-term goal
STM	short-term memory

(Continued)

BOX 3.6   Continued

STNR	symmetrical tonic neck reflex
sup	supination
SWD	short wave diathermy
T	trace as in muscle strength; temperature
Tbsp.; tbsp.	tablespoon
TCU	transitional care unit
TDD	telecommunications device for the deaf
TDWB	touch down weight bearing
TEDS	thromboembolic disease stockings
TENS, TNS	transcutaneous electrical nerve stimulation
ther ex	therapeutic exercise
TLSO	thoracic lumbar spine orthosis
TO; t.o.	telephone order
TOS	thoracic outlet syndrome
TPN	total parenteral nutrition
trng.	training
tsp.	teaspoon
TTWB	toe touch weight bearing
TWB	total weight bearing
un	unable
US	ultrasound
UV	ultraviolet
VC	vital capacity
v.o.	verbal order
vol.	volume
VS; v.s.	vital signs; vestibular stimulation
W	walker
WB	weight bearing
WBAT	weight bearing as tolerated
WBQC	wide base quad cane
W/C; w/c	wheelchair
WFL	within functional limits
Wk	week
WN	well nourished
WNL	within normal limits
w/o	without
WP or wpl	whirlpool
wt.	weight
X; x	times
$\bar{x}$	except [for]
y/o; y.o.	year old, as in a 5 y/o girl
yd	yard
yr	year
°	degree
'	feet
"	inches
↑	increased; up
↓	decreased, down
→	toward
↔	to and from
+	positive, plus, and
−	negative, minus
=	equal

~ or ≈	approximately
%	percent
Δ	change
♀	female
♂	male
#	number, pound
&	and
@	at or each
/	per
<	less than
>	greater than
✓	flexion
/	extension; per
c̄	with
p̄	post, after
s̄	without
1°	primarily, primary
2°	secondary, secondary to
ψ	psychology; psychological
‖	Parellel bars

Sources: Gately & Borcherding (2012); Jacobs & Jacobs (2009); Kettenback (2004); Shamus & Stern (2011).

BOX 3.7 Abbreviations Related to Administration and Reimbursement

ABN	Advance Beneficiary Notice
ACA	Affordable Care Act
ACO	Accountable Care Organization
ADA	Americans with Disabilities Act
appt	appointment
ARRA	American Recovery and Reinvestment Act
BBA	Balanced Budget Act
BCBS	Blue Cross Blue Shield
CARF	Commission on Accreditation of Rehabilitation Facilities
CDC	Centers for Disease Control and Prevention
CHAMPUS	Civilian Health and Medical Program of the Uniformed Services
CMS	Center for Medicare and Medicaid Services, formerly HCFA
COB	coordination of benefits
COLA	Cost of living adjustment
CORF	certified outpatient rehabilitation facility
CEU	Continuing Education Unit [10 contact hours]
CQI	Continuous Quality Improvement
CPT	Current Procedural Terminology, a coding system used to bill for medical procedures
DHHS	Department of Health and Human Services
DOE	Department of Education
DOL	Department of Labor

(Continued)

BOX 3.7 Continued

DOT	Dictionary of Occupational Titles
DRG	diagnostic-related group
DSM-V	Diagnostic and Statistical Manual, Fifth Edition
EHR	electronic health record
EMR	electronic medical record
FDA	Food and Drug Administration
FI	fiscal intermediary
GAO	Governmental Accounting Agency
HCFA	Health Care Financing Administration [part of the U.S. Department of Health and Human Services, now the Centers for Medicare and Medicaid Services]
HCPCS	Healthcare Common Procedures Coding System
HIM	Health information management
HIPAA	Health Insurance Portability and Accountability Act
HITECH	Health Information Technology for Economic and Clinical Health
HMO	Health maintenance organization
HHA	Home health agency
HIPAA	Health Insurance Portability and Accountability Act
ICD-9	International Classification of Diseases, Ninth Edition
ICD-10	International Classification of Diseases, Tenth Edition
IDEA	Individuals with Disabilities Education Act
IEP	Individualized education program
IFSP	Individualized family service plan
IOM	Institute of Medicine
IPA	Independent Practice Association
IPO	Independent Practice Organization
IRB	Institutional Review Board
IT	Information technology
JCAHO	Joint Commission on Accreditation of Health Organizations (now called simply the Joint Commission)
MCH	Maternal and Child Health [DHHS]
MDS	Minimum Data Set
MOU	Memorandum of understanding
NBCOT	National Board for Certification in Occupational Therapy
NCLB	No Child Left Behind
NIH	National Institutes of Health
NIOSH	National Institute for Occupational Safety and Health
NLM	National Library of Medicine
OASIS	Outcome and Assessment Information Set
OBRA '87	Omnibus Budget Reconciliation Act of 1987
OCR	Office of Civil Rights [Department of Health and Human Services]
OIG	Office of the Inspector General [Department of Health and Human Services]
OMB	Office of Management and Budget
OOT	Outpatient occupational therapy
OSEP	Office of Special Education Programs [DOE]
OSERS	Office of Special Education and Rehabilitation Services [DOE]
OSHA	Occupational Safety and Health Administration
OTPP	Occupational Therapist in Private Practice
PCMH	Patient-Centered Medical Home
PDR	Physicians' Desk Reference [medication information]
PHI	Protected Health Information
PHR	Personal health record
PIN	Personal identification number
PPO	Preferred Provider Organization
PPS	Prospective Payment System

PSRO	Professional Standards Review Organization
QA	Quality Assurance
QI	Quality Improvement
QM	Quality Management
RBRVS	Resource-Based Relative Value Scale [Medicare]
RSA	Rehabilitation Services Administration [DOE]
RUGS	Resource Utilization Groups
SAMHSA	Substance Abuse and Mental Health Services Administration [DHHS]
SSA	Social Security Administration [DHHS]
SSN	Social Security number
TEFRA	Tax Equity and Fiscal Responsibility Act
TQM	Total quality management
UR	Utilization Review
URQA	Utilization Review Quality Assurance
VA	Veterans Administration
VAMC	Veterans Affairs Medical Center
WHO	World Health Organization

Sources: Administrative and Management Special Interest Section (2000); Gartee (2011); Jacobs & Jacobs (2009); Meyer & Schiff (2004).

BOX 3.8 Educationally Related Abbreviations

APE	adapted physical education
AT	assistive technology
CFR	Code of Federal Regulations
D/APE	developmental and adaptive physical education
DOE	Department of Education
ECFE	early childhood family education
ECSE	early childhood special education
EI	early intervention
FAPE	free and appropriate public education
IDEA	Individuals with Disabilities Education Act
IEP	Individualized Education Program
IFSP	Individualized Family Service Plan
LD	Learning disability
LEA	local education agency
LRE	least restrictive environment
NCLB	No Child Left Behind
OHI	other health impaired
OSEP	Office of Special Education Program, U.S. Department of Education
OSERS	Office of Special Education and Rehabilitation Services [DOE]
PI	physically impaired
PLEP	present level of educational performance
RSA	Rehabilitation Services Administration [DOE]
SEA	state education agency
SI	sensory integration
USC	United States Code

Source: Jackson (2007)

SUMMARY

Buzzwords, jargon, and abbreviations can give the appearance that you know what you are doing. However, they can also become barriers to effective communication. As with most things in life, using buzzwords, jargon, and abbreviations in moderation is fine, but do not overdo it.

In documenting occupational therapy practice, regardless of the setting, choosing your words carefully is a critical step in the writing process. There are words that are trendy or send positive messages to the reader, and there are other words that send up red flags to the reader. Sometimes occupational therapists use abbreviations to the extent that they make the note hard to read. Always remember who the readers of the documentation could be so that you write for all audiences.

REFERENCES

Administration and Management Special Interest Section. (2000). *Occupational therapy administrative reimbursement algorithm*. Retrieved January 5, 2000, from www.aota.org/members/area2/docs/industrial.pdf

American Occupational Therapy Association. (2014). Occupational therapy practice framework: Domain and process (3rd ed.). *American Journal of Occupational Therapy*, *68*(Suppl. 1), S1–S48. http://dx.doi.org/10.5014/ajot.2014.682006

American Occupational Therapy Association (2012). Board and Specialty Certification. Retrieved from http://www.aota.org/Practitioners/ProfDev/Certification/certified.aspx

Gartee, R. (2011). *Electronic health records: Understanding and using computerized medical records*. Upper Saddle River, NJ: Pearson Education.

Gateley, C. A., & Borcherding, S. (2012). *Documentation manual for occupational therapy: Writing SOAP notes* (3rd ed.). Thorofare, NJ: Slack.

Jackson, L. L. (Ed) (2007). *Occupational therapy services for children and youth under IDEA* (3rd ed.). Bethesda, MD: American Occupational Therapy Association.

Jacobs, K., & Jacobs, L. (2009). *Quick reference dictionary for occupational therapy* (5th ed.). Thorofare, NJ: Slack.

Joint Commission (2012). Official "do not use" list. Retrieved from http://www
.jointcommission.org/assets/1/18/Do_Not_Use_List.pdf

Kettenback, G. (2004). *Writing SOAP notes* (3rd ed.). Philadelphia, PA: F. A. Davis.

Lunsford, A. A. (2009). *The everyday writer.* (4th ed.). Boston, MA: Bedford/St. Martin's.

Sabath, A. M. (2002). *Business etiquette.* New York: Barnes and Noble.

Shamus, E. & Stern, D. (2011). *Effective documentation for physical therapy professionals*
(2nd ed.). New York, NY: McGraw Hill.

World Health Organization [WHO]. (2010). *Framework for action on interprofessional education and collaborative practice.* Retrieved from http://whqlibdoc.who.int/hq/2010/
WHO_HRH_HPN_10.3_eng.pdf

CHAPTER 4

The Occupational Therapy Practice Framework and Important Other Documents

INTRODUCTION

The language of the profession of occupational therapy is ever evolving. As the leaders of the profession review and revise the documents that guide the profession, the terminology used to describe occupational therapy changes. In addition, organizations external to occupational therapy, such as the World Health Organization, have changed the way words are used to describe the human condition. In this chapter, we explore the changes that have occurred in the last 10 years or so.

▼ INTERNATIONAL CLASSIFICATION OF FUNCTIONING, DISABILITY, AND HEALTH ▼

The World Health Organization (WHO) has changed the way in which it looks at disability and functioning. With this new look comes a set of words to describe disability and functioning. Instead of looking at the source of the dysfunction, WHO is looking at the outcomes of the dysfunction, the body structures and functions, activities and level of participation in life, and the environmental factors affecting performance (WHO, 2013). WHO suggests that instead of diagnosing a person with a particular disease, condition, or injury, the clinician should describe the client's level of functioning, demonstrating the impact of the disease, condition, or injury. This will enable health professionals and payers to determine if progress is being made. The document *International Classification of Functioning, Disability and Health* (ICF) issued by WHO (2013) is intended to standardize the terminology used across health professions the world over. This document provides a numerical coding system for every possible body part, body function, activity one can participate in, and environments and personal factors that can affect a person's ability to actively participate in life situations. This system is seen as more universal (not specific to any particular culture), more integrative (not just medical or social), more context inclusive (not just the person), and more interactive (not linear) than previous models (WHO, 2013).

There are two parts within the structure of the ICF. The first part highlights functioning and disability, and the second focuses on contextual factors. Table 4.1 shows the basic structure of the ICF. Each item in the ICF has a corresponding code number, and the qualifiers also have numeric value. For example, if a person needed moderate assistance putting on his clothes, the code for that would be d5400.22. In the United States, few, if any, occupational therapy practitioners use the ICF to assign code numbers. For billing purposes, different coding systems are used.

The ICF identifies more than 1,400 terms that can help clinicians think globally while labeling the tasks and activities that their clients engage in on a daily basis. At the

TABLE 4.1 Structure of the International Classification of Functioning, Disability and Health (ICF)

Components	Body Functions and Structures	Activities and Participation	Environmental Factors	Personal Factors
Constructs	Functions Structures	Capacity Performance	Barriers Facilitators	
Examples	*Functions* • Vision • Hearing • Breathing *Structures* • Nerves • Muscles • Lungs	• Learning • Self-care • Interpersonal interactions • Community, social, and civic life	• Products and technology • Natural environment • Attitudes • Systems and policies	• Gender • Age • Coping style • Education
Qualifiers	*Function: Extent of impairment* • No impairment • Mild • Moderate • Severe • Complete *Structure: Nature of change* • No change • Total absence • Partial absence • Additional part • Aberrant dimensions • Discontinuity • Deviating position • Qualitative changes • Not specified	*Capacity:* • No problem • Mild • Moderate • Severe • Complete *Function:* • No problem • Mild • Moderate • Severe • Complete	*Barriers* • No barriers • Mild • Moderate • Severe • Complete *Facilitators* • No facilitator • Mild • Moderate • Severe • Complete	

Source: WHO (2013).

WHO Web site there is a sample checklist to aid in gathering data about a client's function (http://www.who.int/classifications/icf/training/icfchecklist.pdf). The American Occupational Therapy Association (AOTA) used the ICF during the development of the *Occupational Therapy Practice Framework-III*, which helps illustrate the importance of this document (AOTA, 2014).

▼ OCCUPATIONAL THERAPY PRACTICE FRAMEWORK ▼

In 2002, AOTA created a document called the *Occupational Therapy Practice Framework: Domain and Process* (AOTA, 2002). Often referred to simply as *The Framework*, it was revised in 2008 and again in 2013. *The Framework* describes the domain (scope of practice) of occupational therapy and the processes involved in interactions between occupational therapists and clients (AOTA, 2014). It describes the process of occupational therapy with an emphasis on the use of occupations as therapeutic agents. *The Framework-III* begins with an understanding of the occupational needs of any client (a client can be an individual, a group, or a population) and ends with achieving occupational therapy outcomes that are focused on "achieving health, well-being, and participation in life through engagement in occupation" (AOTA, 2014, p. S2).

While *The Framework-III*, is summarized here, it is not a sufficient substitute for the original document (AOTA, 2014). *The Framework-III* is available from AOTA through its online store (www.aota.org), in the March–April 2014 supplement issue of the *American Journal of Occupational Therapy* (free for members to download), and at some campus bookstores and libraries.

One point that *The Framework-III* makes is that the concept of independence may be viewed differently by occupational therapy practitioners and others outside the profession (AOTA, 2014). To an occupational therapy practitioner, a client may be considered independent when performance of a given occupation is controlled by the client, regardless of whether any assistance is needed. Some occupations are done alone and some are done with others. *The Framework-III* also recognizes the concept of co-occupation, in which two or more people share an occupation, which requires interaction between the people engaged in it (AOTA, 2014).

In *The Framework-III* the term *client* means a person, group, or population (AOTA, 2014). Occupational therapy practitioners use the power of engagement in occupations when working with individuals, families, groups of people, or communities (AOTA, 2014). A client can be a person who has been injured on the job, the family of a child with a disability, a group of residents of a group home learning to plant a garden, a company seeking to reduce the incidence of workplace injuries, or a city developing ways to safely shelter people in the wake of a natural disaster.

Domain of Occupational Therapy

The Framework-III uses the phrase "achieving health, well-being, and participation in life through engagement in occupation" (AOTA, 2014, p. 3S4) to represent the overall domain of occupational therapy practice. There are five aspects within the domain of occupational therapy, and no one aspect is of greater importance than any other. The relationship among these aspects is illustrated in Figure 4.1.

OCCUPATIONS Occupations are the "daily life activities in which people engage" (AOTA, 2014, p. 9). Within these areas are eight categories:

- *Activities of daily living:* Those things we do to take care of ourselves, including, bathing/showering, bowel and bladder management, dressing, eating, feeding, functional mobility, personal device care, personal hygiene and grooming, sexual activity, and toilet hygiene.
- *Instrumental activities of daily living:* Those things we do in our daily life at home and in the community such as care of others, care of pets, childrearing, communication management, community mobility, financial management, health management and maintenance, home establishment and management, meal preparation and cleanup, safety and emergency maintenance, and shopping.
- *Rest and sleep:* Those things we do to restore ourselves such as resting, sleep preparation, and sleep participation.
- *Education:* Those things we do as students or to participate in a learning environment, including exploring and participating in both formal and informal learning situations.

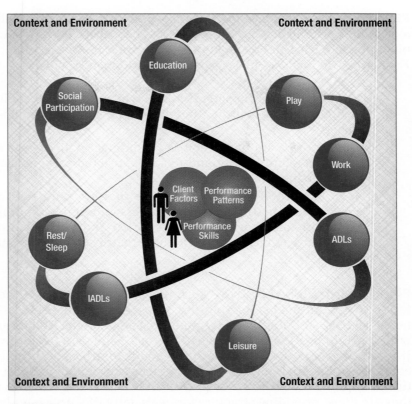

FIGURE 4.1 Domain of Occupational Therapy.
Source: AOTA (2014).

- *Work:* Those things we do to engage in paid employment or volunteer experiences such as exploring, identifying, seeking, and obtaining paid work; performing at work; preparing for and adjusting to retirement, and exploring and participating in volunteer experiences.

- *Play:* Those things we do simply for "enjoyment, entertainment, amusement, or diversion" (Parham & Fazio, 1997, as cited in AOTA, 2014, p. 45), including both exploration and participation in play.

- *Leisure:* Those things we do when we are not obligated to do anything else, including both exploration and participation in leisure.

- *Social participation:* Those things we do when we are interacting with others, whether that interaction takes place between friends/peers, family, or community. They may occur in person or via technology (AOTA, 2014).

CLIENT FACTORS In *The Framework*, there are three main client factors (AOTA, 2014). One client factor is the set of **body structures**—anatomical parts and systems that make up the person. **Body functions** are the mental, sensory, neuromuscular, cardiovascular, vocal, digestive, genitourinary, and skin-related processes that occur inside a person. Specific examples of body functions include, but are not limited to, orientation, temperament, memory, proprioception, and muscle tone and reflexes. **Values**, **beliefs**, and **spirituality** are the third client factor. These factors help us understand what clients find meaningful, what they think is important, and what they hold as true (AOTA, 2014).

PERFORMANCE SKILLS In *The Framework-III*, performance skills are actions that enable a person's performance in occupation (AOTA, 2014). Performance skills are the building blocks of activities and occupations. They are small, observable, and purposeful. In *The Framework-III*, there are five categories of performance skills:

- *Motor skills* are those skills involved in moving, such as bending, reaching, turning, pacing, coordination, balancing, maintaining posture, and manipulating objects.
- *Process skills* are those required to interact with objects and tasks. They include the skills required to attend to a task, use tools, sequence the steps of a task, and terminate the task.
- *Social interaction skills* are those that are required for getting one's wants, needs, and intentions across to others and understanding the wants, needs, and intentions of others, including verbal and nonverbal communication, giving and receiving messages, and participating in appropriate relationships (AOTA, 2014).

PERFORMANCE PATTERNS Performance patterns reflect the ways in which behavior occurs including habits, routines, roles, and rituals (AOTA, 2014). Performance patterns can be seen in individuals, groups, or populations. **Habits** are things individuals do without thinking; they are automatic. Some habits are useful in that they contribute to life satisfaction; others are dominating and interfere with daily life, as in obsessive–compulsive disorder. Impoverished habits either do not support daily life or need practice to improve. **Routines** are sequences of behavior that occur in the same way each time they are done, providing structure for one's daily life. An example of this might be always taking a particular route to work, regardless of traffic delays. An organization might demonstrate routine in the way that its employees follow corporate policies and procedures. **Roles** are "sets of behavior expected by society, shaped by culture, and may be further conceptualized by the client" (AOTA, 2014, p. S8). Examples of roles include those of parent, teacher, coach, or patient, and are tied very closely to a person's sense of identity. A group or organization may have a role in society such as the role of the American Red Cross in providing assistance to people in the aftermath of natural disasters. **Rituals** are symbolic actions associated with spiritual, cultural, or social meaning. Habits, routines, roles, and rituals can, depending on the circumstance, be helpful or hinder health and well-being (AOTA, 2014).

CONTEXT AND ENVIRONMENT Contexts are conditions that exist within or around a person and have an influence on the individual's performance (AOTA, 2014). Environments surround a client in the physical and social realms; they are the people, spaces, and objects with whom people interact. While some people use the terms *context* and *environment* interchangeably, *The Framework-III* uses both so as to capture the widest possible interpretations of the terms. *The Framework-III* names seven kinds of contexts and environments:

- *Cultural contexts* represent the customs, beliefs, activity patterns, and behavioral expectations and standards of the community in which the client is a member. They can include health, political, legal, economic, educational, and employment opportunities.
- *Physical environments* are natural and human-made spaces, terrains, buildings, objects, plants, and animals.
- *Social environments* concern groups of people and the influences that they have on the performance of each other. People can include relatives, friends, caregivers, and members of an organization in this context.
- *Personal contexts* are unique to the individual and include age, gender, economic status, employment status, educational status, and living situation.

- *Temporal contexts* include aspects of performance that relate to time, such as developmental age, life stages, seasonal considerations, and time of day.
- *Virtual contexts* are those where communication takes place without physical contact between people, such as via computers, radio, or telephone (AOTA, 2014).

A more detailed breakdown of *The Framework* can be found in Appendix E (see website).

Process

The process of occupational therapy, at its most simple, involves evaluation, intervention, and outcomes (AOTA, 2014). It describes the client-centered delivery of occupational therapy services. While there is a fixed starting point (the occupational profile), the other parts of the process interact with and influence other parts throughout occupational therapy service delivery. The focus of the occupational therapy process is to "achieving health, well-being, and participation in life through engagement in occupation" (AOTA, 2014, p. S2). Figure 4.2 shows the occupational therapy process as outlined by *The Framework-III*.

Woven throughout the entire occupational therapy process are key concepts that separate occupational therapy from other professions. First is the focus on using occupations as a therapeutic tool to "promote health, well-being, and participation in life" (AOTA, 2014, p. S11). Next is the clinical reasoning used by occupational therapy practitioners. The therapeutic use of self enhances the client-centeredness of occupational therapy practice. Activity analysis is used to identify the demands that occupations place on the client and match an activity to the skills and abilities of the client. All of these combine to give occupational therapy a different perspective on the client than others who may be working with the same client (AOTA, 2014).

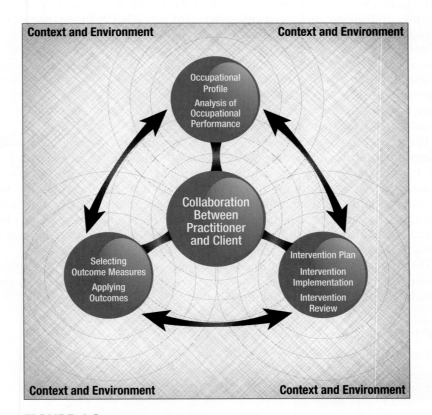

FIGURE 4.2 Process of Occupational Therapy.
Source: AOTA (2014).

The evaluation process begins with the first interactions with the client and evolves as new information is obtained during each interaction with the client (AOTA, 2014). The evaluation has two substeps: the **occupational profile** and the **analysis of occupational performance**. The occupational profile helps the occupational therapist understand "the client's perspective and background" (AOTA, 2014, p. S13). The analysis of occupational performance uses information gathered from the client's health or educational record, assessment tools, and observations to more fully understand the nature of the occupational performance problem (AOTA, 2014). The occupational profile starts when the occupational therapist engages in a shared process of data gathering with the client or client's surrogate (e.g., a parent when the client is a child or the adult child of an older adult with Alzheimer's disease). Clients bring information about their history, interests, values, wants, and needs, and the occupational therapist brings information about the power of engagement in occupation, disease or conditions, theoretical perspectives, and clinical reasoning, to the discussion (AOTA, 2014). The type of questions the occupational therapist might ask is influenced by the frame of reference and/or theories employed by the occupational therapist. Knowledge of disease processes, medical and psychiatric conditions, and human anatomy and physiology are also used to help guide the occupational therapist in gathering information and forming a hypothesis about the client. While the occupational profile is the first step in the evaluation process, it is adjusted as the client moves through the process and new data comes to light (AOTA, 2014). You can see that this is a very client-centered process.

The second step of the evaluation is the analysis of occupational performance (AOTA, 2014). In this step, more data is gathered about the client, the relevant contexts and environments, the occupations and activities the client engages in, and the client's occupational performance. The process of analyzing occupational performance includes identifying both barriers and facilitators to successful engagement in occupations. The frame of reference and models of practice used by the occupational therapist will influence the type of and method by which this data is gathered. (See Chapter 5 for more information on frames of reference and models.) A more thorough description of the evaluation process is described in Chapter 14 of this text.

Intervention is a process of planning, delivering, and evaluating the effectiveness of skilled occupational therapy services (AOTA, 2014). Occupational therapy intervention is provided to clients (individuals, groups, or populations) "to promote health, well-being, and participation" (AOTA, 2014, p. S2). As with the evaluation phase of the occupational therapy process, the intervention phase is informed by the theory, model, or frame of reference used by the occupational therapist (AOTA, 2014).

There are three substeps in the intervention process: the **intervention plan, intervention implementation,** and **intervention review** (AOTA, 2014). First, the plan is developed using the data gathered in the evaluation process. The intervention plan is influenced by the frames of reference and models of practice used by the occupational therapist, the client's contexts and environments, activity demands, and the goals established in collaboration with the client. Other influences on the intervention plan include care for the health and well-being of the client, the best evidence available, and the domains of occupational practice (AOTA, 2014).

The intervention plan requires identifying specific strategies to help the client achieve desired outcomes (AOTA, 2014). There are five strategic approaches to intervention that an occupational therapist could take in developing the plan (AOTA, 2014):

1. Create or promote
2. Establish or restore
3. Maintain
4. Modify
5. Prevent

Once the strategy and types of intervention are established in the plan, the occupational therapy practitioner works in collaboration with the client to execute the plan during the intervention implementation phase (AOTA, 2014). An important part of the intervention implementation includes ongoing monitoring of the client's progress toward his or her goals. Several kinds of interventions that can be used to help the client achieve established outcomes include (AOTA, 2014):

1. Therapeutic use of occupations and activities
2. Preparatory methods and tasks
3. Education and training
4. Advocacy
5. Group interventions

During the intervention implementation, the intervention must be reviewed to determine whether it is making a difference in the occupational performance of the client (AOTA, 2014). The plan is evaluated and, if necessary, modified to enable the client to most efficiently and effectively achieve the desired outcomes. During the intervention review, a determination is made as to whether or not to continue to provide occupational therapy intervention or to make referrals to other professionals. This substep may include a reevaluation of the client as well as reevaluation of the plan (AOTA, 2014).

The last step in the process is targeting outcomes, the end result of the occupational therapy process (AOTA, 2014). Remember that the overarching outcome of occupational therapy is "achieving health, well-being, and participation in life through engagement in occupation" (AOTA, 2014, p. S4). Occupational therapy practitioners know that each client will define health, well-being, and participation in unique ways in relation to the client's life situation, contexts, and environments.

Throughout the occupational therapy process, the occupational therapist identifies the outcomes and selects the outcome measures (AOTA, 2014). There are eight types of outcomes that concern occupational therapy practitioners:

1. Occupational performance
2. Prevention
3. Health and wellness
4. Quality of life
5. Participation
6. Role-competence
7. Well-being
8. Occupational justice

During the occupational therapy process, the occupational therapist uses the identified outcomes to measure progress and make adjustments to client goals and interventions, and to make recommendations about whether or not to continue occupational therapy services (AOTA, 2014). Outcomes may also influence decisions about discharge disposition for an individual client.

When documenting any phase of the occupational therapy process, using the terminology reflected in *The Framework-III* shows that you are up-to-date and on top of your profession. While it is not necessary to memorize each term within each of the five domains (occupation, client factors, performance skills, performance patterns, contexts and environments) of the domain of occupational therapy, it is useful to understand the differences between the types of items in each aspect. Some clinicians suggest that goals be written only to address occupations; others write goals for performance skills or client factors, depending on the frame of reference the occupational therapy practitioner is using. Some occupational therapy evaluation reports have sections for each of the aspects, so the occupational therapist needs to know what types of terms go into each section.

Exercise 4.1

Using the following key, place the appropriate letter in the blank in front of each phrase.

O = Occupations
P = Performance skills
C = Client factors

1. _____ Combing one's hair
2. _____ Elbow range of motion
3. _____ Wheelchair mobility
4. _____ Making one's needs known
5. _____ Hand strength
6. _____ Career exploration
7. _____ Time management
8. _____ Understanding nonverbal communication
9. _____ Posture
10. _____ Endurance
11. _____ Knitting
12. _____ Balancing a checkbook
13. _____ Making eye contact
14. _____ Balancing on one leg
15. _____ Taking turns during a card game
16. _____ Dressing a wound
17. _____ Texting a friend
18. _____ Changing a diaper
19. _____ Finding items in a hidden picture puzzle
20. _____ Identifying signs of danger

▼ SPECIFIC OCCUPATIONAL THERAPY TERMS ▼

Occupational therapy practitioners often use terms they learn in school. This is usually a good thing. However, sometimes the way in which terms are used changes in official documents of the profession. If a practitioner is unaware of these changes, he or she may be using terms incorrectly in current practice. The following is a list of terms defined by AOTA (AOTA, 2010, p. 1):

Assessment: Specific tools or instruments that are used during the evaluation process.

Client: A person, group, program, organization, or community for whom the occupational therapy practitioner is providing services.

Evaluation: The process of obtaining and interpreting data necessary for intervention. This includes planning for and documenting the evaluation process and results.

Screening: Obtaining and reviewing data relevant to a potential client to determine the need for further evaluation and intervention.

Other professions may use these terms in other ways, and they are not wrong. Each profession has its own standard. For example, in education, assessment is the process and evaluations are the tools. Some facilities may also use terms in certain ways. While it is very important to follow the standards established by your professional organization, it is also important to communicate clearly with co-workers in other professions. If there is any doubt about how a term is being used at a particular facility, ask a department head who has been at the facility for a few years or more. This will be an experienced professional who can advise you on how to best be understood by others at the facility.

SUMMARY

The American Occupational Therapy Association has developed guidelines for the practice of occupational therapy, which in turn influence the words we use in occupational therapy documentation. The *Occupational Therapy Practice Framework-III* is a document that seeks to describe the process of providing occupational therapy services to clients across practice settings and to describe the domains of occupational therapy practice (AOTA, 2014). The process begins with understanding the occupational needs of any client, and then an analysis of the client's occupational performance. Intervention is then planned and implemented in order to assist the client in achieving his or her desired outcomes. The outcome of any occupational therapy intervention is "achieving health, well-being, and participation in life through engagement in occupation" (AOTA, 2014, p. S2). The *Framework-III* describes five domains of occupational therapy practice: (1) occupation, (2) client factors, (3) performance skills, (4) performance patterns, and (5) contexts and environments (AOTA, 2014).

In addition to AOTA, the World Health Organization has developed a taxonomy for describing human function and dysfunction called *International Classification of Function* (ICF) (WHO, 2013). The language of that document is also helpful in choosing words that members of other disciplines will understand. The language used by the ICF was influential in the development of the *Occupational Therapy Practice Framework* (AOTA, 2014).

It is critical to use terminology that is understood and accepted by both others in the profession and those outside the profession. The more consistent occupational therapy personnel are in using terminology, the more likely the documentation is to be understood by others. It is equally critical that you stay current in your use of terminology as the profession evolves and changes.

Using the language of the profession can strengthen one's documentation. Your words carry the weight of the best minds in the profession. In addition, you show that you are current in your understanding of the profession by using the words of the professional association. The importance of staying up-to-date with the profession, with best practice, should never be overlooked.

REFERENCES

American Occupational Therapy Association. (2002). Occupational therapy practice framework: Domain and process. *American Journal of Occupational Therapy, 56*, 609–639.

American Occupational Therapy Association. (2010). Standards of practice for occupational therapy [Supplemental material]. *American Journal of Occupational Therapy, 64,* S106–S111. doi:10.5014/ajot.2010.64S106

American Occupational Therapy Association. (2014). Occupational therapy practice framework: Domain and process (3rd ed). *American Journal of Occupational Therapy, 68*(Suppl. 1), S1-S48. http://dx.doi.org/10.5014/ajot.2014.682006

World Health Organization. (2013). *International classification of functioning disability and health*. Geneva, Switzerland: Author. Retrieved Feb 7, 2013, from http://www.who.int/classifications/icf/en/

Visit **www.pearsonhighered.com/healthprofessionsresources** to access the student resources that accompany this book. Simply select Occupational Therapy from the choice of disciplines. Find this book and you will find the complimentary study tools created for this specific title.

CHAPTER 5

Impact of Models and Frames of Reference

INTRODUCTION

In Chapter 4 we discussed the ways in which the language of the profession is changing. In addition to staying current on terminology, the words occupational therapy practitioners use while summarizing evaluation results, planning intervention, reporting progress, and planning discontinuation will also depend on the model or frame of reference being used for a particular client.

▼ DESCRIPTION OF MODELS AND FRAMES OF REFERENCE ▼

Depending on which textbook you read, the definition of a model and of a frame of reference will vary. Both models and frames of reference are based on theory and help organize knowledge so that it can be used to guide an occupational therapist in determining the cause of dysfunction and ways to assist a client to engage in meaningful occupations.

According to Mosey (as cited in Christiansen & Baum, 1991), a model integrates theoretical assumptions for use in practice. Christiansen and Baum (1991) describe a model as referring to ways of structuring or organizing information that is relevant to practice and for the purpose of guiding thinking.

A frame of reference is closely related to a model but is typically more specific in terms of application of knowledge and information. A frame of reference takes the knowledge we have and organizes it in such a way that it can be applied to working with clients (Christiansen & Baum, 1997). Frames of reference are based on theory and provide direction for evaluating, planning, and implementing intervention, and discontinuing services. According to Mosey (as cited in Christiansen & Baum, 1991), frames of reference are the portions of models that are methodological in focus; they tell the occupational therapist how to use the information in practice.

Think of a frame of reference or model as being the lens through which you see your client. Just as different-colored lenses (i.e., sunglasses) change the way you see your surroundings and what parts of the environment stand out, so do different frames of reference change what parts of the client's situation stand out. For example, a biomechanical frame of reference looks at structural enhancements such as strengthening, decreasing edema, splinting, and range of movement in an injured limb while a task-oriented frame of reference looks at finding goal-directed functional behaviors to encourage use of the affected limb (Kielhofner, 2004; 2009; Trombly Latham, 2008). In this example, the biomechanical approach has a focus on client factors and performance skills while the task-oriented approach looks at performance patterns and performance in areas of occupation (AOTA, 2014).

Some models or frames of reference used by occupational therapy practitioners focus on getting at the root cause of the dysfunction, such as the psychoanalytical or neurodevelopmental frames of reference. Others focus on the level of dysfunction and ways to minimize it, regardless of the cause, such as the cognitive disabilities frame of reference or ecological models. Some use a developmental focus, others an environmental one.

In later chapters, the mechanics of writing goals and completing different types of documents will be discussed. This chapter focuses on identifying different models and frames of reference and how the word choices may vary between them.

▼ HOW MODELS AND FRAMES OF REFERENCE ARE REFLECTED IN DOCUMENTATION ▼

Table 5.1 summarizes different frames of reference used in occupational therapy and hints for how that frame of reference can be reflected in one's documentation. Please note that the summaries of these frames of reference are not intended to be comprehensive or all-inclusive. Because of the vast number of new and developing frames of reference, it would be impossible to cover every one. Memorizing this table will not tell you everything you need to know about each frame of reference.

TABLE 5.1 Influence of Frames of Reference on Documentation

Frame of Reference	Description of Key Concepts	How It Is Reflected in Documentation
Behavioral (Skinner, Pavlov)	A person's behavior is the result of feedback from the environment. Insight and personality are not considered. One can unlearn maladaptive behaviors and learn adaptive ones through the use of techniques such as shaping, teaching, and reinforcement. OT works with others on the team to consistently work toward positive changes in behavior.	Evaluation reports contain detailed observations of behavior, including descriptions of the behavior; frequency of it; and where, when, and under what circumstances the behavior occurs. Progress notes document behavior modification methods used and the results of these interventions. Measurable goals specify the person, the observable behavior expected, and conditions for the behavior such as where, when, frequency, and any cuing that will occur.
Biomechanical	Focus on "the body as a machine." Improving strength, endurance, and structural integrity will lead to improved function. Use splinting, exercise, massage, PAMs, and other physical means of intervention. Once range of motion, strength, edema, and endurance are regained, functional use will follow. Pain, loss of sensation, and poor coordination are not of primary concern.	Evaluation reports focus on performance skills/client factors. Progress notes reflect improvements in range of motion, strength, edema, and endurance. Range of motion, strength, edema, and endurance are easily quantified for goal setting. Functional goals would reflect new activities that increased movement will allow.
Canadian Model of Occupational Performance (Law et al.)	The person is in constant interaction with the environment. Client-centered practice Spirituality gives meaning to occupations.	Evaluation reports focus on activities of daily living, play, spirituality, and work. Progress notes focus on the client's ability and satisfaction in performing meaningful occupations.

Frame of Reference	Description of Key Concepts	How It Is Reflected in Documentation
	Environment influences occupational performance.	Goals relate to ability and satisfaction in the performance of meaningful occupations.
Cognitive-Behavioral Therapy (Bandura; Rotter; Ellis and Beck)	Maladaptive behaviors are the result of cognitive distortions and self-defeating thinking. People have automatic thoughts that they tell themselves internally. "Core schemas" are the thoughts people tell themselves that color the way they perceive themselves and their environment. Clients are taught to repeat positive "self-talk" to alter the core schemas.	Evaluation reports focus on client report of occupational problems and insight into barriers to occupational performance. Progress notes reflect client's report of feelings and thoughts, skills, attitudes, and contexts which lead to changes in behavior. Goals suggest the positive statements the client will repeat to oneself, use of stress management techniques, and identify desired behavioral outcomes.
Cognitive Disabilities (also called Cognition & Activity) (Allen)	Neurological problems lead to limitations in cognitive capacity, which lead to a performance deficit. Cognitive levels are categories of function and dysfunction Occupational therapy cannot change cognitive levels that are the result of brain pathology. Tasks and activities are analyzed for fit with a person's cognitive level; they are adapted to remove obstacles to performance and use a person's available cognitive capacity.	Evaluation reports identify the current cognitive level as supported by functional performance in everyday occupations. Progress notes describe the client's response to adaptations in the task or environment and any changes noted in cognitive level (based on observations). Goals are established to identify desired performance within the context of the client's environment, and relate to palliative, expectant, or supportive treatment.
Contemporary Task-Oriented (Haugen & Mathiowetz)	Focus on the interaction between the characteristics of a person and the contexts in which the person exists. The personal and environmental characteristics have no hierarchy in terms of their influences on performance. The client's perspective is the focus of evaluation and intervention; it is client-centered. Intervention involves practice and experimentation.	Evaluation reports center on the client's unique characteristics, contexts, and motivations. Recording observations is essential in progress notes. Goals relate to functional performance.
Developmental (Piaget, Freud, Erickson, Kohlberg, and many others)	Humans normally develop in a sequential fashion. Each new gain in structure enables a gain in function; each new gain in function enables further development.	Evaluation reports focus on comparing a child's performance to that of a typically developing child of the same chronological age to identify areas in need of intervention.

(Continued)

TABLE 5.1 Continued

Frame of Reference	Description of Key Concepts	How It Is Reflected in Documentation
	Physical, sensory, perceptual, cognitive, social, and emotional development are interconnected and affect the whole person. Stress can cause regression to earlier levels of adaptation. Focus on seven developmental areas: Perceptual–Motor, Cognitive, Drive–Object, Dyadic Interaction, Group Interaction, Self-Identity, and Sexual Identity.	Progress reports show the child has made gains in functional performance of daily occupations. Goals identify desired occupations to enable the child's maximum participation in life situations.
Ecology of Human Performance (Dunn, Brown, & McGuigan)	Ecology is the interaction between a person and contexts (the environment). The person, the context, and task performance interact with and affect one another. Performance is improved by establishing/restoring the person's skills or abilities, altering/ adapting the context or the task to support performance in context, preventing occupational barriers, or creating enriching occupational performance.	Evaluation reports look not only at the person but also at contexts and tasks and the person–context match. Progress reports describe what interventions/alterations have been tried and their results. Goals reflect the person's participation in occupations and performance in context.
Model of Human Occupation (Kielhofner)	Volition, habituation, and performance are interrelated subsystems within a person that regulate choice, organization, and performance. Personal and environmental factors influence choice, organization, and performance. Change is a holistic process. Occupations must be relevant and related to a person's roles, habits, and environment.	Evaluation reports focus on the client's performance in areas of occupation, interests, motivation, habits, and roles. Progress notes focus on the client's choices, habits, and roles during meaningful occupations. Goals relate to performance in meaningful occupations, habits, and roles.
Neurodevelopmental Treatment (NDT) (Bobaths)	Spasticity and hypotonia are the major barriers to normal movement. The trunk and proximal joints need stability to enable limb movement. The brain is plastic and capable of new learning. Work toward inhibiting abnormal reflexes and synergies to enable learning of normal movement. Bilateral focus; use positioning, handling, and sensory stimulation to facilitate normal movement patterns.	Evaluation reports focus on observations of movement patterns and barriers to normal movement. Progress notes need to reflect frequent clinical observations. Goals relate to patterns of movement that enable occupational performance.

Frame of Reference	Description of Key Concepts	How It Is Reflected in Documentation
Occupational Adaptation (Schkade & Schultz)	As clients become more adaptive, their ability to function improves. The ability of clients to adapt can be overwhelmed by stressful life events, including illness, injury, or disabilities. Dysfunction occurs when a client's ability to adapt is challenged so much that performance demand cannot be satisfactorily met. Internal and external factors are continually interact resulting in an occupational response; the observable outcome of the person-environment interaction.	Evaluation reports focus on the environmental demands, internal resources, occupational roles, and occupational adaptation abilities of the client. Progress notes focus on the client's ability to adapt to changing demands. Goals may begin with the client learning adaptive skills, and then evolve into the client using adaptive skills and occupational mastery.
Occupational Behavior (Reilly)	Active participation in tasks can lead to development of mastery and, therefore, permit successful role performance. Focus is on work, play, and self-care. Role fulfillment provides positive feedback to the person and enables that person to go on to new skills, more complex tasks. Occupational therapy intervention moves the client through the continuum of exploration, competence, and achievement.	Evaluation reports focus on work, play, and activities of daily living that are meaningful to the client. Progress notes focus on the client's performance during meaningful occupations. Goals relate to performance in occupations and roles that are meaningful to the client as well as prevention of barriers to occupational performance.
Person–Environment– Occupational Performance (Christiansen & Baum)	Many intrinsic (neurobehavioral, physiological, cognitive, psychological, and spiritual) and extrinsic (social support, social and economic systems, culture and values, built environment and technology, and natural environment) factors contribute to occupational performance. Adaptation is the process used by people to meet challenges in daily living through the use of personal resources. The characteristics of the person, environment, and the nature/meaning of actions, tasks, and roles are considered when trying to understand occupational performance. Focus is on the person's wants and needs rather than on dysfunction.	Evaluation reports reflect the client's assets and limitations in relation to his or her occupational performance as well as the supports and barriers in the environment. Progress reports demonstrate the client's occupational performance within environmental contexts. Short-term goals may relate to intrinsic factors inhibiting occupational performance. Long-term goals may relate to functional performance of daily life tasks and roles.

(Continued)

TABLE 5.1   Continued

Frame of Reference	Description of Key Concepts	How It Is Reflected in Documentation
Proprioceptive Neuromuscular Facilitation (PNF) (Knott & Voss)	Weakness and lack of voluntary control over movements are the main obstacles to normal movement patterns. Frequent repetition and stimulation of the proprioceptors support the learning of new motor abilities. Movements are more often diagonal than linear. Vision, breathing, and verbal commands all play a strong role in movement.	Evaluation reports emphasize observable movement patterns. Progress notes reflect client responses to inhibition and facilitation techniques. Goals relate to the client's movements during activities of daily.
Psychoanalytic (Freud); Object Relations (Fidler)	Intrapsychic (unconscious) conflicts are at the heart of the problem. The major areas of concern are the psychodynamics, level of psychosexual and psychosocial development, and alterations of intrapsychic content. Goal is to resolve these inner conflicts. Use of activity to resolve intrapsychic conflict and reality orientation such as psychodrama, projective art, creative writing and poetry therapy, and guided fantasy.	Evaluation reports focus on the affect of the client, symptoms of psychopathology, and how these interfere with daily life functions. Progress reports often reflect the client's subjective report of feelings as well as observations of client behavior. Goals reflect the client's self-expression of feelings.
Rehabilitative (Compensatory)	Aim is to increase independence by providing environmental adaptations and compensatory strategies Consider client's roles and the tasks the client considers essential for satisfactory performance of those roles.	Evaluation reports emphasize both strengths and areas in need of improvement. Progress notes document what types of adaptations have been tried and the results of each trial. Goals reflect functional outcomes; what the client will do.
Spatiotemporal Adaptation (Gilfoyle, Grady, & Moore)	Movement and activity influence a person's development. Movement is important for physical, psychological, and social development of a child. Development occurs in an ever-widening spiral that represents increasing skills as influenced by experiences with the environment. Emphasis on integration of old behaviors with new ones.	Evaluation reports focus on the movements of the child in relation to environmental demands. Progress reports reflect the increasing complexity of the movement–environment interactions of the child. Goals can be structured to reflect prevention, remediation, and/or adjustment to dysfunction.

TABLE 5.1 Continued

Frame of Reference	Description of Key Concepts	How It Is Reflected in Documentation
Sensory Integration (Ayers)	Sensory integrative dysfunction is a result of a failure of the brain to properly organize and interpret sensory input. There is interaction between brain organization and adaptive behavior. People have an inner drive to participate in sensory motor activities and seek out organizing sensations. Play is self-directed, within an environment carefully set up by the OT to meet that client's needs. Environment provides the opportunities to experience needed sensations in a safe, nonthreatening atmosphere, and includes access to sensory input to all sensory processing systems of the body, including vestibular.	Evaluation reports focus on identifying areas of sensory processing deficits and how these impact participation in everyday life experiences. Progress notes reflect the child's responses to different sensory experiences, qualities of movement, and changes in the client's participation in everyday life experiences. Goals focus on increased duration or repetitions of an activity, the quality of movements during an activity, or on socially acceptable ways of obtaining achieving sensory stimulation.

Sources: Christiansen & Baum (1997); Cole & Tufano (2008); Kielhofner (2004; 2009); Trombley Latham (2008).

The reader is referred to the sources used in developing this chapter for more information on each frame of reference. Having a good understanding of the frame of reference you are using will help you in writing reports and notes and in establishing goals. Often the frame of reference will suggest the use of certain terminology.

There are two primary approaches to occupational therapy that are reflected in the models and frames of reference. One approach is referred to as the top-down approach, and the other is referred to as the bottom-up approach (Weinstock-Zlotnik & Hinijosa, 2004; Trombly Latham, 2008). According to Weinstock-Zlotnik and Hinijosa (2004), using a top-down approach, you would begin by considering the client's performance in areas of occupation and the other aspects of the domain of occupational therapy (client factors, performance skills, performance patterns, activity demands, and contexts and environments) later. The primary concern is the client's ability to engage in meaningful occupations. Trombly Latham (2008) takes a slightly different view of the top-down approach. She suggests that when considering performance in areas of occupation, the client's roles and contexts are a necessary part of the process. Once the occupational therapist has a clear picture of the roles, contexts, and occupations that are meaningful to the client, the causes of the current problems in occupational performance are evaluated, including the specific client factors, performance skills, and performance patterns (Trombly Latham, 2008). The *Occupational Therapy Practice Framework* (3rd ed.) takes a top-down approach by suggesting that the occupational profile be completed first, then the analysis of occupational performance (AOTA, 2014).

An assumption of the bottom-up approach is that if you improve client factors and performance skills (motor, cognitive, sensory perceptual, communication, or emotional regulation skills), then the client's performance in areas of occupation will take care of itself (Weinstock-Zlotnik & Hinijosa, 2004). This approach holds some appeal for practitioners in medical settings where time is limited and pressure from third-party payers to produce measurable results is strong. In these settings, the occupational therapy practitioner may receive a physician order to see a client to increase range of motion following surgery, or increase strength following an injury.

Weinstock-Zlotnik and Hinijosa (2004) argue that bottom-up approaches are useful because of the number of standardized assessment tools available leading to more measurable outcomes. They also argue that top-down approaches are more broad and difficult to measure but provide a stronger professional identity for occupational therapy. In the end, Weinstock-Zlotnik and Hinijosa (2004) suggest that the profession needs both approaches and that using only one or the other approach does a disservice to the profession.

Occupational therapy began by using occupation-based, top-down approaches, then, following the lead of the medical community, became reductionistic, using a more bottom-up approach (Kielhofner, 2009; Weinstock-Zlotnik & Hinijosa, 2004). Coming full circle, the profession of occupational therapy now favors top-down, occupation-based approaches (Kielhofner, 2004; Weinstock-Zlotnik & Hinijosa, 2004). Each of these approaches has generated the formation of models and frames of reference to explain dysfunction and suggest intervention strategies.

Exercise 5.1

For each of the models and frames of reference in Table 5.1, tell whether it is a top-down or bottom-up approach.

1. Behavioral
2. Biomechanical
3. Canadian Model of Occupational Performance
4. Cognitive-Behavioral Therapy
5. Cognitive Disabilities (also called Cognition & Activity)
6. Contemporary Task-Oriented
7. Developmental
8. Ecology of Human Performance
9. Model of Human Occupation
10. Neurodevelopmental Treatment (NDT)
11. Occupational Adaptation
12. Occupational Behavior
13. Person–Environment–Occupational Performance
14. Proprioceptive Neuromuscular Facilitation (PNF)
15. Psychoanalytic (Freud); Object Relations
16. Rehabilitative (Compensatory)
17. Spatiotemporal Adaptation
18. Sensory Integration

People who work together at one facility all tend to use the same model or frame of reference, or the same mix of them. When you start working (or go on fieldwork) at a new place, be sure to ask which models or frames of reference are acceptable to use. Usually, but not always, more than one frame of reference is used at a facility or program. When multiple models or frames of reference are blended together, it is called an eclectic approach. Hopefully, this blending occurs in a thoughtful way, based on the collective experiences of the occupational therapy staff and the types of clients being served in that program or facility.

Exercise 5.2

Are the following goals compatible with the frame of reference cited?

1. In the next 30 days, the client will increase range of motion of shoulder flexion from 40° to 60°. (Bobath)

2. Arwan will eat at least one meal per day, for 5 consecutive days, that contains at least three different textures without screaming, spitting, or turning away by June 15, 2007. (Sensory integration)

3. Robert will consistently brush his teeth twice per day, without cues from his parents, by November 24, 2007. (Model of human occupation)

4. In 1 month, Sonja will independently ride the bus from home to work. (Behavioral)

5. In 6 months, DeNeda will demonstrate the self-care and home-maintenance skills necessary for her to return home to independent living. (Psychoanalytical)

6. In 6 weeks, Christianne will word-process at a rate of 60 words per minute with two or fewer errors. (Cognitive-behavioral therapy)

7. Xia will place eight knobs in a bag, with the use of an adapted jig if necessary, by July 7, 2007. (Cognitive disabilities)

8. Rosita (age 6) will print her name legibly with each letter touching the line by December 12, 2007. (Canadian model of occupational performance)

SUMMARY

Models and frames of reference are ways to organize one's thinking about how to approach a client, and guide the way an occupational therapist evaluates, plans, and implements interventions and determines when a client has achieved desired outcomes. Both models and frames of reference are based on theory.

The model or frame of reference that you choose to work from with a given client needs to be reflected in the way you document about that client. Often the words used in documentation are suggested by the model or frame of reference being used. A model or frame of reference is used to help you select an appropriate evaluation method, set goals, and describe progress. You can use Table 5.1 to help in ensuring that your documentation is reflective of the model or frame of reference being used. Some facilities or programs use multiple models or frames of reference.

REFERENCES

American Occupational Therapy Association. (2014). Occupational therapy practice framework: Domain and process (3rd ed). *American Journal of Occupational Therapy, 68* (Suppl. 1), S1–S48. http://dx.doi.org/10.5014/ajot.2014.682006

Christiansen, C., & Baum, C. (1991). *Occupational therapy: Enabling function and well-being.* Thorofare, NJ: Slack.

Christiansen, C., & Baum, C. (1997). *Occupational therapy: Enabling function and well-being* (2nd ed.). Thorofare, NJ: Slack.

Cole, M. B., & Tufano, R. (2008). Applied theories in occupational therapy: A practical approach. Thorofare, NJ: Slack.

Kielhofner, G. (2004). *Conceptual foundations of occupational therapy* (3rd ed.). Philadelphia, PA: F. A. Davis.

Kielhofner, G. (2009). *Conceptual foundations of occupational therapy* (4th ed.). Philadelphia, PA: F. A. Davis.

Trombly Latham, C. A. (2008). Conceptual foundations for practice. In M. V. Radomski & C.A. Trombly Latham, *Occupational therapy for physical dysfunction* (6th ed., pp. 1–20). Philadelphia, PA: Lippincott Williams & Wilkins.

Weinstock-Zlotnik G. & Hinijosa, J. (2004). Bottom-up or top-down evaluation: Is one better than the other? *American Journal of Occupational Therapy, 58,* 594–599.

Visit **www.pearsonhighered.com/healthprofessionsresources** to access the student resources that accompany this book. Simply select Occupational Therapy from the choice of disciplines. Find this book and you will find the complimentary study tools created for this specific title.

CHAPTER 6

Document with CARE: General Tips for Good Documentation

INTRODUCTION

If you have read the previous chapters, you know that careful wording in documentation is essential. There is a system for double-checking your documentation so that you can be assured that it will be well written. This system is called "Document with CARE" (Sames & Berkeland, 1998). CARE is an abbreviation for:

Clarity: The reader can understand what you are saying.

Accuracy: The documentation reflects what actually happened.

Relevance: The documentation relates to identified needs and purposes.

Exceptions: Any unusual occurrences, noncompliance, or changes are documented.

Let's examine each of these criteria one at a time.

▼ CLARITY ▼

In order for the reader to understand what you have written, it has to be written in clear, concise, unbiased language (Sames & Berkeland, 1998). Abbreviations and jargon need to be kept to a minimum and, when used, must be approved by the facility in which they are used. Grammar and spelling should not interfere with the professional appearance and intended message of the documentation. Usually, simple, shorter sentences are clearer than long ones. In some settings, it is acceptable to use phrases or incomplete sentences to keep the note brief. People who are not familiar with the jargon of the profession must be able to read and understand your notes. These seem like commonsense things, but you would be amazed at some of the documentation that is out there (Sames & Berkeland, 1998).

Remember the discussion about the use of jargon in Chapter 3. Too much jargon makes documentation less clear to people outside the profession, but over simplifying the language may make the documentation sound less than professional. How specific or technical your documentation is depends on the setting, the types of people who are most likely to read your documentation, and the type of service being documented (Sames, 2008). If you are writing an Individualized Family Service Plan (IFSP) for the family of an infant with whom you are working, you would use as little jargon as possible. If you are writing a detailed evaluation report in a teaching hospital, you might use more technical terms and more jargon (Sames, 2008).

> **BOX 6.1**   Statement on an evaluation report of a preschooler
>
> **Not clear:** Traevan's motor development is delayed. He is functioning at 1.5 standard deviations below the mean for his age. He has difficulty with tasks requiring bilateral integration, balance, motor control, and proprioception.
>
> **Clear:** Traevan's test scores indicate that he has movement problems that interfere with his ability to play with other children his age. He has difficulty throwing and kicking a ball, balancing on one leg, doing jumping jacks, and holding and using crayons.

Box 6.1 is an example of clarity in note writing. In this example, the evaluation report is being shared with the child's parents. The information on his test scores are important and can be included in a table that shows his score, the range of scores that would indicate "normal" behavior, and if appropriate, age equivalency scores.

▼ ACCURACY ▼

Your documentation needs to be factually correct (Sames & Berkeland, 1998). Documentation is almost always done chronologically; that is, what happens first is written about first, and then events are recorded in the order in which they happen. Documentation also needs to be consistent with the protocols of the institution or agency involved. Never document about another client by name in your client's record. For example, if Mr. Smith and Mr. Jones play checkers, and you are writing in Mr. Smith's chart, you may say that Mr. Smith played checkers with another client, but do not put Mr. Jones's name in Mr. Smith's note (Sames & Berkeland, 1998).

Another aspect of accuracy is distinguishing between what you observe and what you think it means (Sames & Berkeland, 1998). This will be addressed more completely in Chapter 14. In the meantime, think about the notes in Box 6.2 related to a client that you observe with a plate of food in front of her and a fork in her right hand. She uses her right hand to scoop up the food and begins to raise the food to her mouth. The fork tips and the food falls off. She lowers her fork to the plate and scoops at the food, pushing the food off her plate. She then drops the fork and picks up the food with her fingers. In the bad example, you are interpreting what you saw. You are generalizing a short, one-time observation into applying to every time she eats. There are times when your interpretation is as important as, or more important than, your description, but you must be careful to identify when you are describing and when you are interpreting a client's performance (Sames & Berkeland, 1998).

> **BOX 6.2**   Examples: Objective portion of a note on the chart of a resident in long-term care
>
> **Not accurate:** The client is unable to feed herself with a fork. She gets frustrated and starts using her fingers.
>
> **Accurate:** The client made two attempts to feed herself with a fork, and then proceeded to feed herself with her fingers.

The reader must see, on the basis of what you write, why occupational therapy was initiated, continued, or discontinued (Sames & Berkeland, 1998). In other words, the documentation must demonstrate the need for skilled service. Skilled service means services requiring the expertise of an occupational therapist or an occupational therapy assistant under the supervision of an occupational therapist. The reader needs to see that what you are doing in occupational therapy is something that uses the unique skills and abilities of occupational therapy practitioners. It has to be clear that the client is receiving occupational therapy, not exercise therapy or PAMs therapy.

When the client's chart or file is read from beginning to end, it should be clear that the results of the screening (if there is one), the referral, the evaluation, the intervention planning, the intervention, and the discharge have a common theme. In other words, if an adult with chronic schizophrenia is referred to occupational therapy to learn to live independently, then the evaluation summary should be centered on independent living skills, the intervention plan should address independent living skills, the progress notes should demonstrate work on independent living skills, and the discontinuation summary should also reflect the client's skills in independent living. If a child is referred to you to improve handwriting skills, then the documentation should reflect work on handwriting skills. This does not mean that you cannot document work on any other domain of concern, but other domains are documented only after demonstrating additional needs in those areas. For every problem or need identified, there should be written evidence that the problem or need was addressed or an explanation of why it was left unaddressed (Cathy Brennan, MA, OTR/L, FAOTA, personal communication, June 21, 2006).

Documentation should always be timely (Sames & Berkeland, 1998). This means the documentation, in order to be relevant, needs to be done as close to the time as the event occurred. Generally, evaluation reports are done within a day or two of completing the evaluation; intervention plans are done according to the schedule of the facility (annually, bimonthly, or monthly); progress notes are often done at the close of each visit to occupational therapy; and discontinuation summaries are usually completed within 2 days of discharge. Each facility will have standards related to timeliness. These standards are to be taken seriously, not as general targets, but as deadlines (Sames & Berkeland, 1998).

Other relevant information needs to be available in the client's record. If there are precautions or contraindications that must be observed, they need to be documented (Sames & Berkeland, 1998). It is not necessary to include them on every piece of documentation, as long as they are easy to find in the client's chart. These can be very relevant to the activities and tasks selected during intervention (Sames & Berkeland, 1998).

There can be a tendency to overdocument. Out of fear of lawsuits, fear of forgetting something, or just plain verbosity, some people write very long documents. Time is precious, and time spent documenting is time spent away from clients. Eliminate all but the most necessary information (Sames & Berkeland, 1998). Ask yourself, is this relevant? If you are working with a client on managing a checkbook, is it necessary to document what the client is wearing? Is it necessary to document what the client says about the weather? Is it necessary to document about how the client holds the pen? The answers are no, no, and maybe. You would document only about how the client holds the pen if the act of writing was important to the case. If you were working on managing a checkbook because of cognitive deficits, then how the client holds the pen is not particularly relevant, unless the client used to know what a pen was and how to hold it and today he or she looked at it like it was a new and strange object (Sames & Berkeland, 1998). Box 6.3 shows examples of statements from a discharge summary of a client who has been seen in a mental health partial hospitalization program. The client has bipolar disorder.

▼ EXCEPTIONS ▼

Any unusual occurrences or events need to be documented (Sames & Berkeland, 1998). If a client had suffered a traumatic brain injury, was progressing nicely, then suddenly did not recognize a pen, this would be unusual, and possibly indicate some bleeding on the brain. It would be essential to document this event, as well as inform the client's doctor or nurse verbally about what transpired. This might require immediate medical attention, and it is up to you to see that the people concerned are informed as quickly as possible. It is also up to you to see that this critical event is documented in the chart. You are the one who saw what happened. It should be in your words. The doctor or nurse might also document what you told them, but when they do so, they are documenting secondhand information.

Client noncompliance is also something that should be documented (Sames & Berkeland, 1998). If you have prescribed a home exercise program, and the client reports not following through with it, you need to document that. It might explain why a client is progressing more slowly than you would like.

Since the clients we work with are human, unpredictable things can happen. New problems surface. When you deviate from your original intervention plan, there needs to be a brief explanation of why you are doing something new (Sames & Berkeland, 1998). In other words, you need to provide justification for deviating from the original plan (Cathy Brennan, MA, OTR/L, FAOTA, personal communication, June 21, 2006). Many clients have multiple complications; for example, a person with schizophrenia may have a stroke, a person with rheumatoid arthritis may have diabetes and depression, and a child with Asperger's syndrome may suffer a traumatic amputation. This may mean that the intervention plan you develop may differ from your typical plan of action. A depressed client who rented an apartment could lose her lease and become homeless. This change in the client's environment would likely cause a change in plan.

Box 6.4 is an example of part of a contact note for a person who has not complied with the wearing schedule of his splint, resulting in the development of a wound. The note would go on to explain what action was taken when the wound was discovered.

Figure 6.1 is the Document with CARE checklist. This is a handy, one-page document that you can use to help evaluate your report and note writing.

▼ DOCUMENT WITH CARE ▼

Clarity: The reader can understand what you are saying.

- ❏ Free from jargon
- ❏ Concise
- ❏ Only facility-approved abbreviations
- ❏ Readable/legible
- ❏ Grammar and spelling do not interfere with the professional appearance and the intended message of the note
- ❏ Understandable to all readers

Accuracy: The documentation reflects what actually happened

- ❏ Chronologically, technically, and factually correct
- ❏ Instructions are specific and individualized
- ❏ Reflect the behavior observed, interpretations are labeled as such
- ❏ Consistent use of terminology
- ❏ Adheres to protocol of facility, agency, or school
- ❏ Preserve confidentiality of all involved

Relevance: The documentation relates to identified needs and purposes

- ❏ Clear why OT is initiated, continued, and discontinued
- ❏ Consistency between referral, evaluation, intervention plan, ongoing intervention, discontinuation planning, and follow-up
- ❏ Documentation reflects the skilled service being provided
- ❏ Description of changes in function relates to treatment goals
- ❏ Timely
- ❏ Precautions and contraindications are clearly outlined for the individual
- ❏ Include information necessary for quality management and research projects
- ❏ Eliminate all but necessary information

Exceptions: Any unusual occurrences, non-compliance, or changes are documented

- ❏ Deviations from original intervention plan are justified
- ❏ Deviations from evaluation and intervention protocols are described and explained
- ❏ Client noncompliance is noted
- ❏ Unusual occurrences and events are described
- ❏ Complications and responses are documented

FIGURE 6.1 Document with CARE. *Source: Sames & Berkeland (1998).*

Exercise 6.1

Evaluate the following narrative progress notes using the Document with CARE checklist.

Case 1: This involves a 3-year-old child with cerebral palsy in a preschool setting. Her areas of concern are in hand use, balance, and using sign language.

> Anoushka participated in three 30-minute sessions this week. She participated in group activities, snack, and playground activities each day. She played catch with another child on Monday. She signed "more" during snack. Anoushka loved balancing on the big ball. Wednesday she refused to go down the slide. Plan to continue seeing Anoushka per plan of care.

C:

A:

R:

E:

Case 2: This case involves a teenager in a chemical dependency program.

> Paul attended group as scheduled. He is opening up and talking more. He still does not reveal much about his own feelings, but is identifying feelings in others. When confronted on any issue, he deflects the comments back to the person who made the comment. For example, when a member of the group accused him of being dishonest about the strength of his addiction, he shouted, "As if you people are saints! Your problems are way bigger than mine!" He recognizes that he had enough of a problem to land himself in this program, but he says that he really does not need any intervention; he can quit on his own anytime he wants. He says he is only here because it is better than going to jail.

C:

A:

R:

E:

Case 3: This case involves a 34-year-old man recovering from a massive hand injury from an on-the-job accident. He has had surgical repair of three tendons on the palm of his hand and an amputation of the distal joint of his index finger.

> Ivan has been receiving hard therapy for his injuries for 3 weeks. He is making steady progress. The postsurgical edema is almost gone. He has greater AROM in each finger than at this time last week. Refer to flow sheet for detailed ROM of each joint. Bruising has faded to pale yellow. He is able to squeeze lightweight putty and spread his fingers inside a ring of the same-weight putty. Plan to continue therapy 3x/wk for 45–60 min to work on strengthening of hand and fingers, increased ROM, and functional use of hand and fingers.

C:

A:

R:

E:

Case 4: This case involves a 93-year-old woman recovering from a hip fracture. Up until she fell, she lived independently in an apartment in a large metropolitan area.

Mrs. Nguen was seen today for 30 minutes in the OT clinic. She is partial weight bearing. Although she has been instructed to use her quad cane every time she takes a step, she refuses to use the quad cane in the kitchen. She reports that she prefers to hold on to the counter or a chair back when she is preparing meals in her kitchen, and demonstrated her technique in the OT kitchen. Kim from physical therapy saw her do this and scolded her. Plan to continue 2x/wk for IADLs.

C:

A:

R:

E:

SUMMARY

Documentation is a complex process; there are many things you must consider all at once when writing about a client. The *Document with CARE* checklist is one way to check to see that your documentation is on the right track. It can help you see if you are writing about the right things, and if you are writing them well. CARE stands for clarity, accuracy, relevance, and exceptions. If you document with CARE, you will be a good documenter of occupational therapy practice.

REFERENCES

Sames, K., & Berkeland, R., (1998). *Document with CARE.* Checklist and oral presentation at the Sister Genevieve Cummings Colloquia, June 19, 1998, St. Paul, MN.

Sames, K. (2008). Documentation in practice. In E. Crepeau, E. Cohn, & B. Schell (Eds.) *Willard and Spackman's occupational therapy* (11th ed.). Baltimore, MD: Lippincott Williams & Wilkins.

Visit **www.pearsonhighered.com/healthprofessionsresources** to access the student resources that accompany this book. Simply select Occupational Therapy from the choice of disciplines. Find this book and you will find the complimentary study tools created for this specific title.

SECTION II

CHAPTER 7

Overview of Ethical and Legal Considerations

INTRODUCTION

If an attorney ever asks to see your documentation, it is usually because you, a client/patient, student, or co-worker, are involved in some kind of litigation. Section I of this book talked about general principles for good documentation. In this section, we will talk about ethical and legal considerations in documentation. If the records you write get called into court, the attorneys will likely tell the jury how they would like your writing to be interpreted. Your mistakes might be accidental, but an attorney may not see it that way. Table 7.1 is a list of what your documentation might look like, and how an attorney could interpret it.

TABLE 7.1 Ways an Attorney Could Interpret Documentation

What You Said or Did	What the Attorney Will Say About It
Erasures, cross-outs, or other alterations to original documentation	Provider was unsure of what to say, careless, or incompetent; writer is trying to cover up or hide something; falsification of records
Poor grammar or spelling	Provider is not competent; is careless.
Wrote in the wrong chart	Provider is careless; provider is working too quickly
Using unapproved abbreviations	Provider does not follow the rules; perhaps cuts corners in more ways than one. If another provider takes action based on a note that used unapproved abbreviations and harm comes to the patient, the writer of the note may share in the liability.
Negative statements by one provider toward another provider or toward the facility/administration	Providers not coordinated in care of client; blaming others might indicate decreased quality of care; client is caught in a fight between caregivers; unprofessional behavior. Writer of such a note could be subject to a defamation lawsuit.
Negative statements toward the client	Words like *fat*, *lazy*, *abusive*, *faking*, *stupid*, *silly*, etc., indicate that the provider disliked the client and therefore gave inferior service. Writer of such a note could be subject to a defamation lawsuit.
Gaps in documentation or documentation out of sequence	Provider is careless; problems in staffing, in adequate staff to care for client; writer is hiding something.

Sources: Brous (2009); Fremgen (2006); Scott (2013).

▼ AVOIDING LEGAL ACTION THROUGH DOCUMENTATION ▼

A client's clinical or educational record can be called into court by either or both sides in a legal case (Fremgen, 2006). Some, but not all, errors in documentation may be violations of laws, rules, or regulations. The best defense is to document appropriately and competently every day. Always be sure you are writing in the right chart (Fremgen, 2006). Be sure the client is named on every page of the clinical or educational record; a good electronic record keeping system will do this automatically. If you are using an electronic health record, be sure you are documenting in the correct client's record (Document Defensively, 2008).

Since the clinical or educational record can be called into court, so can the people who write in those records. An occupational therapy practitioner can be called into court as a witness or as the defendant in a malpractice, negligence, defamation, or other lawsuit. The best defense for any occupational therapy practitioner is clear, accurate, relevant, and timely documentation.

When you write that something occurred, you are identifying yourself as a witness in the eyes of an attorney. Only document what you see, hear, touch, or smell. For example, do not document that the patient fell unless you saw the patient fall. Instead, you could say that you found the patient sprawled on the floor and that the patient said she fell.

Documentation should never be derogatory toward the client or a co-worker, or defensive in tone (Fremgen, 2006; Scott, 2013). The health record is not the place to be critical of others; it is unprofessional, is inappropriate, and reflects poorly on you as the writer (Brous, 2009). An attorney could use these derogatory statements to show that improper care was delivered because of conflict on the care team. It could also be used if one healthcare provider sued another over defamation of character (Scott, 2013).

Your documentation needs to be descriptive enough that it accurately reflects what occurred during the occupational therapy session. If you do something, but leave it out of your documentation, a court will determine that it never happened (Nicholson, 2008). Notes that sound repetitive or fail to show the uniqueness of that session may call into question the skill of the provider. According to Nicholson (2008), a growing trend is that plaintiff's (person bringing the lawsuit) attorneys are alleging that documentation with minimal information fails to show the skills of the physical therapist were delivered; therefore, billing for skilled physical therapy is fraudulent. The same could be said for occupational therapy documentation. If the documentation is vague, is nonspecific, and fails to show why the skills of the occupational therapist or occupational therapy assistant under the supervision of an occupational therapist are needed, then the attorney can argue that the service provided was not skilled. If the occupational therapy provider (or employer) is claiming that skilled services were delivered by billing for skilled services, and it is not supported by the documentation, then it might be considered fraudulent billing. Fraud and Abuse are discussed more thoroughly in Chapter 9.

When you give instructions to a client, carefully document those instructions and whether the client or client's caregiver was able to *demonstrate* understanding of the instructions (Scott, 2013). Documenting that the client or caregiver gestured or nodded to indicate understanding is not sufficient to demonstrate understanding (Scott, 2013). The instructions may include activities the client should not do as well as ones the client should do; both must be documented (Scott, 2013). Document any telephone conversations or other correspondence that relates to the client, as well as any actions you take as a result of those conversations or correspondence (Fremgen, 2006).

Errors happen. For handwritten notes, always correct your errors with a single line through the mistake with your initials above or next to the error (AOTA, 2013; Fremgen, 2006; Guido, 2006; Scott, 2013). Then make the correction. Never correct someone else's documentation in a client's record, only your own. Never sign anyone else's documentation, except to cosign in a supervisory situation. Do not leave blank lines or large blank spaces (Guido, 2006; Scott, 2013). Fill the blank areas with a line. Never use correction fluid or erasers. Always use ink in a permanent or official record. In the electronic health record, errors are corrected

- Writing that is squeezed in around other notes
- Changes in the quality of handwriting such as amount of pressure, slant, or uniformity
- Use of different pens in a single note
- Differences in the paper used
- Use of forms that did not exist at the time the care was provided
- An error in the year (date) that is corrected, especially if the correction is from a later year or date to an earlier one.

FIGURE 7.1 Possible Evidence of an Altered Health Record. *Source: Guido (2006).*

by amending documentation following the procedure for the system being used. Figure 7.1 shows what attorneys for patients claiming harm look for as evidence that a health record has been altered. Such evidence may show intent to defraud or cover-up errors.

Documentation that is not timely also presents a potential legal problem for occupational therapy practitioners. The further the time that documentation occurs from the time that the service was actually delivered, the less accurate it may be (Guido, 2006). The diminishing accuracy of documentation can be exploited by an attorney. Always record the date and time of the entry in the client's record; this is automatically recorded in electronic health record systems (Brous, 2009). In addition, if critical information is entered into the health record late, then care may be delivered in the meantime based on the information that is in the record. If the information that is missing would have altered the care, and because of that, suboptimal care was delivered, the person who was late getting the information into the health record could become the target of a lawsuit.

The date and time that the note was entered into the record has to be recorded accurately, even if it is late. You cannot document in advance of the service being delivered even if you are sure of what will happen in the session (Guido, 2006). If documentation is out of sequence because it was done late, it needs be identified as such (Scott, 2013). Better late than never applies to documentation. Figure 7.2 shows an example of how to document a late entry to a health record. Note that the actual time the documentation occurred is listed next to the signature. The format of the note, called SOAP, is discussed in Chapter 17.

Finally, remember to Document with Care (Chapter 6). Be sure to document the reason(s) for any missed evaluation, intervention, or follow-up sessions. Document any unusual occurrences. Be careful to use only abbreviations and acronyms approved by the facility, and avoid the use of slang (Brous, 2009; Scott, 2013).

Late entry for Feb 15, 2014, 1:30 pm

S: "My shoulder still hurts when I try to get dishes down from the cupboard or when I try to take my shirt off over my head. It's my right arm. I have to use it, even when it hurts."

O: Pain-free R shoulder range of motion to 80° flexion and 85° abduction. Myofascial massage provided to rotator cuff area. Client instructed in dressing techniques to prevent lifting of arm overhead. Discussed and practiced strategies for engaging in household tasks without raising R arm above shoulder height.

A: Client is using her arm without limiting use due to pain, but in doing so is not letting the area heal properly. Client needs further instruction and practice in compensatory strategies.

P: Continue per plan of care, with greater emphasis on compensatory strategies.

Su Mi, OTR/L   Feb 16, 2014, 7:45 am

FIGURE 7.2 Late Entry in a Medical Record.

Exercise 7.1

Potential Problems with Documentation

For each potential problem with documentation listed on the left, identify a potential solution or way to prevent the problem in the first place.

Problem	Solution
Illegibility	
Cannot tell which patient the note is about	
Notes written out of sequence	
Pencil or colored ink	
Erasures or white out	
Blank spaces	
Incomplete signatures	
Notes written by students are not cosigned by supervisor	
Poor grammar/spelling	
Poor word choices	
Unknown abbreviations	
Missing documents	
Computer screen with client information displayed left unattended	
Chart left unattended	

▼ COMMON ERRORS IN DOCUMENTATION ▼

Despite all the training and good advice about what constitutes good documentation, in the heat of the moment, it is still likely that occupational therapy practitioners (and other members of the healthcare team) will make errors. A study of occupational therapy documentation in Sweden found that the full occupational therapy process was documented in only 11% of the cases (57) involving intervention they reviewed (Backman, Kåwe, & Björkland, 2008). Evidence that the client's goals were incorporated into the occupational therapy goals was present in 14% of the records reviewed (Backman et al., 2008). Overall, only 21% of the records were complete (Backman et al., 2008). These statistics are alarming, and there is no reason to suspect that documentation in the United States is qualitatively any different than Sweden.

What are the most common errors in clinical documentation? While not a study of occupational therapy practice, a study by Dimond (2005) provides some insight into potential errors that occupational therapy practitioners could make. Figure 7.3 lists some of the most comment documentation errors based on a study of nurses' documentation.

- Unclear documentation; too much jargon
- Failing to document action after a problem was identified
- Gaps and missing documentation
- Misspelled words; poor grammar
- Failing to document unexpected clinical developments
- Failing to document conversations with clients and their families
- Failure to identify the client by name
- Documenting in the wrong client's record
- Use of unapproved abbreviations
- Untimely documentation

FIGURE 7.3 Common Errors in Documentation. *Sources: Dimond (2005); Scott (2013).*

▼ QUALITIES OF GOOD DOCUMENTATION ▼

While the research literature on documentation by occupational therapy practitioners is thin, there is much to be learned by looking at the research literature from other health-care professions. Nursing has produced more research studies on documentation than other health professions. According to Jeffries, Johnson, and Griffith (2010) there are seven essential traits of quality documentation. These can be adapted to occupational therapy practice. A summary of these can be found in Figure 7.4. The first is that consistent with the *Practice Framework* (AOTA, 2014), the documentation is client-centered. The second is that the documentation should demonstrate the interventions that were actually delivered, including client and caregiver education and psychosocial support. Next, the documentation should reflect objective observations, not assumptions. Fourth, the documentation has to be chronological and logical. It has to show the course of interventions as well as the reasoning used to plan and implement the interventions. The fifth essential is that documentation must be written as the care is delivered. Next, the documentation should reflect any variances from the expected and changes in condition, for example if there is new pain or the pain goes away. Finally, all legal requirements must be met. The documentation should be more than a list of activities; it should tell the client's story in a way that would be sufficient if the case was called into court.

- Client-centered
- Demonstrate actual interventions delivered
- Objective observations
- Chronological and logical
- Written as care is delivered
- Reflect variances from expected
- Legal requirements met

FIGURE 7.4 Qualities of Good Documentation. *Source: Jeffries et al. (2010).*

▼ STRUCTURE OF THIS SECTION OF THE BOOK ▼

In this section of the book, we explore the ethical and legal considerations that impact documentation. For the purposes of this book, ethical considerations are defined as those actions that reflect doing the right thing. The principles outlined in the AOTA *Code of Ethics and Ethics Standards* (2010) will be the guide. While situations involving questionable ethics exist in many ways in clinical practice, we focus on those that involve documentation. Examples of these ethical considerations include, but are not limited to, confidentiality, fraud, plagiarism, and retention of records.

Chapter 8 presents considerations in confidentiality and records retention. This includes issues such as how to protect your client's confidentiality and where and for how long to retain client documentation. Specific standards from the AOTA *Code of Ethics and Ethics Standards* (2010) that apply to these issues as well as the Health Insurance Portability and Accountability Act (HIPAA), a federal law designed to protect the rights of recipients of health care services, are discussed.

In Chapter 9, situations that could be construed as fraud are discussed. There is an emphasis on Medicare fraud and abuse, since the government has recently been cracking down on this. You will learn what the penalties are for engaging in fraud. Standards that apply to these situations from the AOTA *Code of Ethics and Ethics Standards* (2010) are described.

The last chapter in this section, Chapter 10, takes us in a slightly different direction. While it is less about documentation and more about writing papers, plagiarism can be considered a form of fraud. As students, you will write numerous papers, and colleges seem to be paying more attention to issues of plagiarism these days. As a clinician, you will put together handouts for in-services, home exercise programs, and general information for your clients. In every case, you must give credit where credit is due. The AOTA *Code of Ethics and Ethics Standards* (2010) standards will be presented along with strategies for avoiding plagiarism.

REFERENCES

American Occupational Therapy Association. (2010). Occupational therapy code of ethics and ethics standards. *American Journal of Occupational Therapy, 64.*

American Occupational Therapy Association. (2013). *Guidelines for documentation of occupational therapy* Retrieved from http://www.aota.org/Practitioners/Official/Guidelines/41257.aspx?FT=.pdf

American Occupational Therapy Association. (2014). Occupational therapy practice framework: Domain and process (3rd ed). *American Journal of Occupational Therapy, 68*(Suppl. 1), S1–S48. http://dx.doi.org/10.5014/ajot.2014.682006

Backman, A., Kåwe, K., & Björkland, A. (2008) Relevance and focal view point in occupational therapists' documentation in patient case records. *Scandinavian Journal of Occupational Therapy, 15,* 212–220.

Brous, E. (2009). Documentation & litigation: Medical records can be the most important evidence presented in legal actions. *Rn, 72*(2), 40–43.

Dimond, B. (2005). Legal aspects of documentation. Exploring common deficiencies that occur in record keeping. *British Journal of Nursing, 14,* 568–570.

Document defensively: Here's how… Reprinted from 2007 HPSO Risk Advisor with permission by Healthcare Providers Service Organization (HPSO), www.hpso.com. (2008). *Dental Assistant, 77*(6), 34.

Guido, G. W. (2006). *Legal and ethical issues in nursing* (4th ed.). Upper Saddle River, NJ: Pearson-Prentice Hall.

Fremgen, B. F. (2006). *Medical law and ethics* (2nd ed.). Upper Saddle River, NJ: Pearson-Prentice Hall.

Jefferies, D., Johnson, M., & Griffiths, R. (2010). A meta-study of the essentials of quality nursing documentation. *International Journal of Nursing Practice, 16*(2), 112–124. doi: 10.1111/j.1440-172X.2009.01815.x

Nicholson, S. K. (2008). *The physical therapist's business practice and legal guide.* Sudbury, MA: Jones and Bartlett.

Scott, R. W. (2013). *Legal aspects of documenting patient care for rehabilitation professionals: A guide for rehabilitation professionals* (4th ed.). Sudbury, MA: Jones and Bartlett.

Visit **www.pearsonhighered.com/healthprofessionsresources** to access the student resources that accompany this book. Simply select Occupational Therapy from the choice of disciplines. Find this book and you will find the complimentary study tools created for this specific title.

CHAPTER 8

Confidentiality and Records Retention

INTRODUCTION

Occupational therapists have access to very personal information about clients. There are rules that have to be followed in order to protect clients' rights to privacy. Confidentiality refers to keeping information to oneself, not releasing information about a client without the written permission of that client. The American Recovery and Reinvestment Act of 2009 (ARRA) added new provisions related to the Health Insurance Portability and Accountability Act (HIPAA) concerning protection of client privacy. These rules describe the kinds of information protected, when written consent is needed, and who may give consent (American Health Information Management Association [AHIMA], 2009). In addition to issues of disclosure of information, in order to further protect confidentiality, how records are stored and who has access to stored records need consideration.

▼ CONFIDENTIALITY ▼

When you write anything that identifies a specific client by name, you are ethically responsible for ensuring that the information remains confidential (AOTA, 2010). This means that you take all reasonable precautions to make sure that only the people who have permission to read the record actually read it. When sending confidential information via the mail, the envelope should be marked "confidential." When sending documents via fax, include a cover sheet marked "confidential," and make sure the person to whom you are sending the fax is there to receive it (Fremgen, 2006). Only send confidential information by e-mail if it is an encrypted program. In other words, no one except those who have written consent of the client or the client's guardian should have access to a client's medical record in any form (electronic or paper).

The client or the client's guardian has the right to see what is written in the clinical or educational record (Fremgen, 2006; United States Department of Health and Human Services [USDHHS], 2002). This is another reason to choose your words carefully, to remain objective and nonjudgmental. Most facilities have specific policies and procedures for allowing clients to read their own records. In some cases, a physician, nurse, or other professional needs to be present to provide immediate answers to any questions that arise, or a physician must also sign a release (Fremgen, 2006). Other facilities will provide photocopies of medical records to the client, although they may charge a fee for the copying (Gartee, 2011). Again, find out the rules at your facility before you share the clinical record with anyone.

The electronic health record has made the accessing of private health information more efficient, but has opened new possibilities for violating the confidentiality of clients (Fremgen, 2006). One way to minimize the potential for breaches of confidentiality is to carefully limit the number of people who have access to individual client information through the use of passwords and other user verification methods. Only those caregivers who have a need to know should be assigned user names and passwords on the electronic health record system. Position computer screens so that no unauthorized people, such as clients or visitors to the clinic can see it (Fremgen, 2006). Never walk away from a computer screen that is displaying confidential information; close out the program or record before even taking a step away from the computer. Some programs may have an automatic log off that turns off the program after a defined period of inactivity, but it is better if you log off yourself (Gartee, 2011). Facilities using electronic record keeping systems will have clearly established policies and procedures to protect the confidentiality of the clients (Shamus & Stern, 2011). These policies must address not only the protection of the record in electronic form, but the backing-up, storage and safe-keeping of discs, tapes, and other electronic media storage devices (Meyer & Schiff, 2004).

▼ ETHICAL RESPONSIBILITY ▼

The American Occupational Therapy Association (2010) has ethical standards that address issues of confidentiality. Occupational therapists are ethically responsible for protecting the confidentiality of all client information regardless of the format of the communication.

> Principle 3: Autonomy and Confidentiality. Occupational therapy personnel shall respect the right of the individual to self-determination.
>
> G. Ensure that confidentiality and the right to privacy are respected and maintained regarding all information obtained about recipients of service, students, research participants, colleagues, or employees. The only exceptions are when a practitioner or staff member believes that an individual is in serious foreseeable or imminent harm. Laws and regulations may require disclosure to appropriate authorities without consent.
>
> H. Maintain the confidentiality of all verbal, written, electronic, augmentative, and nonverbal communications, including compliance with HIPAA regulations.

In addition, Principle 2 also relates to confidentiality.

> Principle 2: Nonmaleficence. Occupational therapy personnel shall intentionally refrain from actions that cause harm.
>
> I. Avoid compromising client rights or well-being based on arbitrary administrative directives by exercising professional judgment and critical analysis.

This means that we avoid compromising the client's right to privacy by disclosing protected health information to anyone who does not have permission to access that information. In addition, Principle 1, item M, requires us to report any breaches of ethics, law, or policy to the appropriate authorities: "M. Report to appropriate authorities any acts in practice, education, and research that appear unethical or illegal" (AOTA, 2010, p.3). If in the course of our fieldwork or practice we have firsthand knowledge of a breach, we have a duty to report it. The National Board for Certification of Occupational Therapy (NBCOT) also requires that occupational therapy practitioners obey laws, including those related to confidentiality. NBCOT Code of Conduct Principle 4 states "Certificants shall comply with laws, regulations, and statutes governing the practice of occupational therapy" (NBCOT, 2011, p. 2).

It is important to note that while AOTA can enforce these ethical standards only with AOTA members, an attorney could present these standards in court as representing prevailing community standards, regardless of whether the occupational therapy practitioner is a member of AOTA or not. The NBCOT Code of Conduct applies to all occupational therapy students who plan to take the NBCOT Certification Exam and to all practitioners who are registered (OTRs) or certified (COTAs) by NBCOT. State licensure laws or practice acts may also include breaches of confidentiality as grounds for disciplinary action.

▼ STATE LAWS ▼

Breaches of confidentiality can invite lawsuits. Many states have laws governing the protection of medical records. It is considered an invasion of privacy to allow unauthorized access to the clinical record or to disclose information about a specific patient/client in any way

(Liang, 2000). Some types of information, such as HIV infection or drug/alcohol addiction, are protected to an even greater degree (Fremgen, 2006; Liang, 2000; Scott, 2013). For example, releasing HIV status of a patient without permission to release that specific information can result in both civil and criminal penalties. A client can make claims of "intentional infliction of emotional distress" (Liang, 2000, p. 51). Check the website for your state Department of Health or Department of Human Services for state regulations on confidentiality and release of information.

▼ HEALTH INSURANCE PORTABILITY AND ACCOUNTABILITY ACT ▼

Occupational therapists are required by law to comply with the Health Insurance Portability and Accountability Act (HIPAA). This law covers many topics, including protections for American workers regarding health insurance, standardization of electronic patient records, and a section on protection of privacy rights of individuals (Bailey & Schwarzberg, 2003; Centers for Medicare and Medicaid Services [CMS], 2002; Fremgen, 2006; Gartee, 2011; Meyer & Schiff, 2004; Shamus & Stern, 2011; Scott, 2013). HIPAA protects all health information "that relates to past, present, or future physical or mental health condition" (Meyer & Schiff, 2004, p. 9). Protected health information must be held in the strictest confidence. Computers, whether desktop, laptop, or handheld, should be password protected for each user, to protect the confidentiality of client information (Fremgen, 2006). Occupational therapists should not discuss with clients in public areas of the facility (especially in hallways, the cafeteria, and in elevators) where they can be overheard. You can imagine what would happen if you were talking to a co-worker in the cafeteria about Mrs. Johnson's rolls of fat getting in the way of her being able to clean herself while her daughter was at the next table listening in on your conversation! Or telling a co-worker how sassy little Timmy is while, unknown to you, his aunt is riding in the elevator with you. Besides being unethical and illegal, it is rude and unprofessional.

Individuals are guaranteed certain rights by the HIPAA privacy rules. They can request an accounting of the people to whom personal health information was disclosed and the dates of the disclosures (Meyer & Schiff, 2004). Individuals have the right to read and copy their health information. They can also request that disclosure of their health information be restricted in some way. While individuals have the right to view their medical record, they do not have an automatic right to access their entire medical record. Psychotherapy notes; information on a criminal, civil, or administrative action or proceeding; and information that "a qualified provider has determined would endanger the life of the individual if he had access to it" (Meyer & Schiff, 2004, p. 23) may be withheld from the individual. A summary of the privacy rules is included in Figure 8.1.

Usually, when a client is seen in an institutional setting (e.g., hospital, nursing home, school), the institution has established policies regarding access to patient/client information. Occupational therapy practitioners must comply with these policies. These may vary somewhat from place to place, but generally all must be consistent with the language and requirements of HIPAA. Staff involved in direct caregiving, supervisors, medical records personnel, billing personnel, and insurance representatives usually are allowed access to a client's record provided it is necessary for "treatment, payment, or health care operations" (Office for Civil Rights [OCR], 2002, p. 8 [§ 164.502 (a)(1)(ii)]).

Individually identifiable health information is protected under the act (Federal Register, 2000; USDHSS, 2002). This includes any means by which a person could be identified, such as by name, social security number, address, phone number, and the like (OCR, 2002). Examples of prohibited activities include using a client's social security number as a client identifier (i.e., case number) on written or electronic documentation, and listing the full name of a client on a schedule hanging on a wall where anyone could see it.

The American Recovery and Reinvestment Act of 2009 (ARRA) further clarified what constitutes a breach of confidentiality (AHIMA, 2009). A breach occurs when anyone who

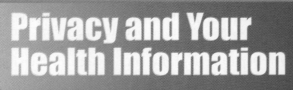

Privacy and Your Health Information

Your Privacy Is Important to All of Us

Most of us feel that our health and medical information is private and should be protected, and we want to know who has this information. Now, Federal law

- Gives you rights over your health information
- Sets rules and limits on who can look at and receive your health information

Your Health Information Is Protected By Federal Law

Who must follow this law?

- Most doctors, nurses, pharmacies, hospitals, clinics, nursing homes, and many other health care providers
- Health insurance companies, HMOs, most employer group health plans
- Certain government programs that pay for health care, such as Medicare and Medicaid

What information is protected?

- Information your doctors, nurses, and other health care providers put in your medical record
- Conversations your doctor has about your care or treatment with nurses and others
- Information about you in your health insurer's computer system
- Billing information about you at your clinic
- Most other health information about you held by those who must follow this law

The Law Gives You Rights Over Your Health Information

Providers and health insurers who are required to follow this law must comply with your right to

- Ask to see and get a copy of your health records
- Have corrections added to your health information
- Receive a notice that tells you how your health information may be used and shared
- Decide if you want to give your permission before your health information can be used or shared for certain purposes, such as for marketing
- Get a report on when and why your health information was shared for certain purposes
- If you believe your rights are being denied or your health information isn't being protected, you can
  - File a complaint with your provider or health insurer
  - File a complaint with the U.S. Government

You should get to know these important rights, which help you protect your health information. You can ask your provider or health insurer questions about your rights. You also can learn more about your rights, including how to file a complaint, from the website at www.hhs.gov/ocr/hipaa/

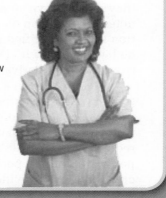

Page 1

FIGURE 8.1 Privacy Summary.

Source: U.S. Department of Health and Human Services, Office for Civil Rights (n.d.).

PRIVACY

The Law Sets Rules and Limits on Who Can Look At and Receive Your Information

To make sure that your information is protected in a way that does not interfere with your health care, your information can be used and shared
- For your treatment and care coordination
- To pay doctors and hospitals for your health care and help run their businesses
- With your family, relatives, friends or others you identify who are involved with your health care or your health care bills, unless you object
- To make sure doctors give good care and nursing homes are clean and safe
- To protect the public's health, such as by reporting when the flu is in your area
- To make required reports to the police, such as reporting gunshot wounds

Your health information cannot be used or shared without your written permission unless this law allows it. For example, without your authorization, your provider generally cannot
- Give your information to your employer
- Use or share your information for marketing or advertising purposes
- Share private notes about your mental health counseling sessions

For More Information

This is a brief summary of your rights and protections under the federal health information privacy law. You can learn more about health information privacy and your rights in a fact sheet called *"Your Health Information Privacy Rights."* You can get this from the website at www.hhs.gov/ocr/hipaa/.

Other privacy rights
Another law provides additional privacy protections to patients of alcohol and drug treatment programs. For more information, go to the website at www.samhsa.gov.

Published by:

U.S. Department of
Health & Human
Services Office for
Civil Rights

The Law Protects the Privacy of Your Health Information

Providers and health insurers who are required to follow this law must keep your information private by
- Teaching the people who work for them how your information may and may not be used and shared
- Taking appropriate and reasonable steps to keep your health information secure

Page 2

FIGURE 8.1 (Continued)

is not authorized to view, use, or disclose any protected health information (AHIMA, 2009; Gartee, 2011). There are three exceptions to this, including unintentional access or use of protected health information, inadvertent disclosure of protected health information, and if the receiver of the impermissible disclosure is believed to not be able to retain or use the information (AHIMA, 2009; Gartee, 2011). If a breach of a person's protected health information occurs, the covered entity must notify the person: the U.S. Secretary of Health and Human Services; and if the breach involves more than 500 individuals, the media (Gartee, 2011).

The penalties for any violation of the privacy provisions are significant. According to the U.S. Department of Health and Human Services, there are two kinds of penalties, each with monetary penalties or imprisonment:

- **Civil penalties.** Health plans, providers, and clearinghouses that violate these standards will be subject to civil liability. Civil money penalties are $100 to $50,000 or more per violation, up to $1,500,000 per person, per year for each requirement or prohibition violated (USDHHS, n.d.).
- **Federal criminal penalties.** A person who knowingly obtains or discloses individually identifiable health information in violation of the Privacy Rule may face a criminal penalty of up to $50,000 and up to one-year imprisonment. The criminal penalties increase to $100,000 and up to five years imprisonment if the wrongful conduct involves false pretenses, and to $250,000 and up to 10 years imprisonment if the wrongful conduct involves the intent to sell, transfer, or use identifiable health information for commercial advantage, personal gain, or malicious harm. The Department of Justice is responsible for criminal prosecutions under the Privacy Rule. (USDHHS, n.d., Enforcement and Penalties for Noncompliance)

Clients must sign a form stating they have been informed of their rights, specifically how the health information will be used, what will be disclosed, and how the client can get access to this information (OCR, 2003). This form, called a HIPAA Privacy Notice, must be written in plain language so that it is readable by most adults, yet meets all the legal requirements of the law (OCR, 2003). The required topics are:

- How the covered entity may use and disclose protected health information about an individual.
- The individual's rights with respect to the information and how the individual may exercise these rights, including how the individual may complain to the covered entity.
- The covered entity's legal duties with respect to the information, including a statement that the covered entity is required by law to maintain the privacy of protected health information.
- Whom individuals can contact for further information about the covered entity's privacy policies (OCR, 2003, para. 3).

In addition to these requirements, the health service provider must include the date the policy took effect and the expiration date. The privacy notice must be posted at the site of health service and posted online at the entity's website (OCR, 2003). It must also be made available to any person who asks to see it. Usually, clients or their guardians are asked to sign and date a document that says they have been provided with the privacy notice.

There are exceptions to this rule. Providers may use and disclose protected health information without written authorization from the individual for treatment; victims of abuse, neglect, or domestic violence; judicial and law enforcement purposes; and health oversight (Meyer & Schiff, 2004). Protected health information may also be released if it has been de-identified. The following information must be removed from the record in order to be considered de-identified:

- Name
- All address information (street as well as e-mail, URL, and IP addresses)
- Day and month of dates (year is acceptable)

- Age, although age group is acceptable
- Telephone and fax numbers
- Social security number
- Medical record and health plan numbers
- Vehicle or device identifiers
- Biometric identifiers
- Facial photographs
- Any other unique information such as identification numbers, characteristics, or codes (Meyer & Schiff, 2004)

For healthcare providers, HIPAA stipulates that both the medical record and billing record of each client be protected (Federal Register, 2000). Under the act, disclosure is defined as "the release, transfer, provision of access to, or divulging in any other manner of information outside the entity holding the information" (Federal Register, 2000, p. 82489). Health information that is necessary for what the act calls "health care operations" does not require written permission of the client before being shared. Examples of healthcare operations include

> quality assessment and improvement activities, reviewing the competence or qualifications and accrediting/licensing of health care professionals and plans, . . . training future health care professionals . . . conducting or arranging for medical review and auditing services and compiling and analyzing information in anticipation of or for use in a civil or criminal legal proceeding (Federal Register, 2000, p. 82490).

If the individually identifiable health information is included in an educational record, it is governed by the Family Education Rights and Privacy Act (Public Law 93-380).

▼ FAMILY EDUCATION RIGHTS AND PRIVACY ACT OF 1974 AND THE INDIVIDUALS WITH DISABILITIES EDUCATION ACT, 2004 REVISION ▼

The Family Education Rights and Privacy Act (FERPA) of 1974 identifies the confidentiality requirements of a student's educational record. It has been revised, as have the regulations that describe how the law should be implemented. The most recent revision of the regulations occurred in 2008, with the final regulations published on December 9, 2008, in the Federal Register (U. S. Department of Education [USDE], 2008). The Individuals with Disabilities Education Act (IDEA), 2004 revision, governs the types of services provided to children with disabilities, and how those services are documented. An educational record includes material written by school district employees and contractors (IDEA Partnerships, 1999; Jackson, 2007). If a student is receiving special education and related services (including occupational therapy), FERPA covers all documents that contain the student's name, address, phone number, parents' names, and any other identifying information. The file may be called a "cumulative file, permanent record, or official educational record" (AOTA, 2003, p. 128). These files contain documents such as the Individual Education Program (IEP) (see Chapter 22), the Individual Family Service Plan (IFSP) (see Chapter 21), and notice and consent forms (see Chapter 20) required by IDEA, as well as grades, samples of student work, and district- or statewide test results.

The Individuals with Disabilities Education Act (IDEA), 2004 revision, also contains language about privacy of information. IDEA has separate sections that address early intervention services (birth through age 2) and school-age (ages 3–21) services. Both sections specifically define identifying information such as the name of the child, parent, or other family member; the address of the child; any identifier such as a social security number; or a list of characteristics or other information that would result in reasonable certainty of the identity of the child (34 C.F.R. § 303.401[a] and 34 C.F.R. § 300.500[b][3]) (USDE, 2007a; 2007b). IDEA further provides for the opportunity for parents to examine the records of their child (34 C.F.R. § 303.402 and 34 C.F.R. § 300.560-576) (USDE, 2007a; 2007b).

Exercise 8.1

Which of the following constitutes a breach of confidentiality?

1. A client was discharged from the hospital yesterday and was admitted to a transitional care facility. The occupational therapist at the transitional care facility calls to get more information about the client than you can usually find in a discharge summary, nitty-gritty things about the personality of the client and the supportiveness of the family. The transitional care facility has permission to get copies of discharge information from the hospital. Based on that, the occupational therapist at the hospital who has worked most closely with the client answers the questions of the occupational therapist at the transitional care facility over the phone.

2. A client at an outpatient clinic has a work-related injury. As a result of participating in the worker's compensation system, this client is assigned a case manager. The case manager comes by the clinic and asks to review the client's record. The client did sign a release for you to share medical records with the insurer.

3. In a busy nursing home therapy room, a schedule is posted on the wall listing each client's full first and last name and room number. The schedule includes intervention sessions for physical and occupational therapy and speech-language pathology. The rehab aide who transports clients to and from their rooms can look at the schedule to see who needs to go where and when.

4. A parent brings a family friend to the IEP team meeting. No one from the school district has ever met this person before. Since the parent brought the friend, the team assumes that constitutes verbal consent and proceeds with the meeting without obtaining written consent to disclose information from the parent.

▼ RECORDS RETENTION ▼

Records, both educational and clinical, are retained for several reasons. One reason is to provide information about what happened in the past that could contribute to the client's present condition. Another reason is to provide comparative data that might enable a practitioner to identify trends toward improved function or loss of function. Records are retained in case legal questions arise after care is discontinued. Finally, we retain records for quality management purposes. By reviewing records of past clients, medical and educational professionals can learn which practices yield the best results.

Each state has laws that govern clinical records retention. Official records for adult patients are usually kept for 5 to 10 years after discharge, although some records may be stored off-site when storage space is limited (Fremgen, 2006; Scott, 2013; Shamus & Stern, 2011). Records for children are kept until the child turns age 21 plus the number of years that state statutes require records to be retained. These are generalities, and some facilities may keep files for as little as 2 years or as long as until the client dies. The American Health Information Management Association (AHIMA) recommends that records be retained for 10 years beyond the last encounter (AHIMA, 2009).

When the required length of time for records retention has elapsed, the records may either continue to be retained or be destroyed. Duplicate records, such as those kept in the occupational therapy department, should not be retained after the client is discontinued unless facility policy requires it. Because of the sensitive information in the records, the term *destroyed* means that the records are shredded and/or burned. Information kept on a disc, tape, or other portable storage devices need to be cut up or otherwise destroyed (Meyer & Schiff, 2004). Simply putting them in the trash or in recycling would violate the client's right to confidentiality, since a good gust of wind could blow them into someone's path, or the trash collector could read them.

SUMMARY

Confidentiality is a major concern of all healthcare providers. As healthcare providers, we are obligated to protect the confidentiality of our clients. This applies to all settings, to all types of documents, and to spoken words as well. A federal law, HIPAA, limits the kind of information that can be shared without written permission and protects clients from public disclosure of any information. FERPA protects the educational records of students. Our clients deserve to have their privacy protected to the furthest extent possible without interfering with intervention.

Records are retained for at least the length of each state's statute of limitations, and often longer. These records are also protected and stored where they will be safe and secure. Access to stored records is limited to only those who absolutely need access to them. Once the statute of limitations has expired, the records may stay in a secure and locked site, or be thoroughly destroyed by burning or shredding. Never toss old records into the garbage.

REFERENCES

American Health Information Management Association. (2009). Analysis of health care confidentiality, privacy, and security provisions of The American Recovery and Reinvestment Act of 2009, Public Law 111-5. Retrieved from http://www.ahima.org/downloads/pdfs/advocacy/AnalysisofARRAPrivacy-fin-3-2009a.pdf

American Occupational Therapy Association. (2003). *Fact sheet: HIPAA privacy rule web links.* Retrieved March 15, 2003, from http://www.aota.org/members/area5/links/LINK07.asp?PLACE=/members/area5/links/link

American Occupational Therapy Association. (2010). Occupational therapy code of ethics and ethical standards. *American Journal of Occupational Therapy, 64,* 639–642.

Centers for Medicare and Medicaid Services. (2002). *HIPAA insurance reform.* Retrieved March 15, 2003, from http://cms.hhs.gov/hipaa/hipaa1/content/more.asp

Federal Register. (2000). *Final privacy rule.* Retrieved March 5, 2003, from http://www.hhs.gov/ocr/hipaa/finalreg.html

Fremgen, B. F. (2006). *Medical law & ethics* (2nd ed.). Upper Saddle River, NJ: Prentice Hall.

Gartee, R. (2011). *Electronic health records: Understanding and using computerized medical records* (2nd ed.). Upper Saddle River, NJ: Pearson Education.

IDEA Partnerships. (1999). *Discover IDEA CD '99* [CD-ROM]. A collaborative project of the IDEA Partnership Projects (through project ASPIIRE at The Council for Exceptional Children) and the Western Regional Resource Center at the University of Oregon.

Jackson, L. L. (Ed) (2007). *Occupational therapy services for children and youth under IDEA* (3rd ed.). Bethesda, MD: American Occupational Therapy Association.

Liang, B. A. (2000). *Health law & policy: A survival guide to medicolegal issues for practitioners.* Woburn, MA: Butterworth-Heinemann.

Meyer, M. J. & Schiff, M. (2004). *HIPAA: The questions you didn't know to ask.* Upper Saddle River, NJ: Pearson Education.

National Board for Certification in Occupational Therapy [NBCOT]. (2011). Retrieved from http://www.nbcot.org/pdf/Candidate-Certificant-Code-of-Conduct.pdf?phpMyAdmin=3710605fd34365e38069ab41a5078545

Office for Civil Rights, United States Department of Health and Human Services. (2002). *Standards for privacy of individually identifiable health information (Unofficial* version) (45 CFR Parts 160 and 164). Retrieved March 17, 2003, from http://www.hhs.gov/ocr/combinedregtext.pdf

Office for Civil Rights, United States Department of Health and Human Services. (2003). Notice of privacy practices for protected health information. Retrieved from http://www.hhs.gov/ocr/privacy/hipaa/understanding/coveredentities/notice.html

Scott, R. W. (2013). *Legal, ethical, and practical aspects of documenting patient care: A guide for rehabilitation professionals* (4th ed.). Burlington, MA: Jones & Bartlett Learning

Shamus, E. & Stern, D. (2011). *Effective documentation for physical therapy professionals* (2nd ed.). New York, NY: McGraw Hill Medical.

United States Department of Education. (2007a). *Federal register May 9, 2007 (34 CFR Part 303).* Retrieved October 10, 2008, from http://edocket.access.gpo.gov/2007/pdf/07-2140.pdf

United States Department of Education. (2007b). *Federal register August 14, 2006 (34 CFR Part 303).* Retrieved May 24, 2007, from http://idea.ed.gov/download/finalregulations.pdf

United States Department of Education. (2008). *34 CFR part 99: Family educational rights and privacy; Final rule.* Retrieved from http://www.ed.gov/legislation/FedRegister/finrule/2008-4/120908a.pdf

United States Department of Health and Human Services. (n.d.). Privacy and your health information. Retrieved from http://www.hhs.gov/ocr/privacy/hipaa/understanding/consumers/consumer_summary.pdf

United States Department of Health and Human Services. (n.d.). Summary of the HIPAA privacy rule. Retrieved from http://www.hhs.gov/ocr/privacy/hipaa/understanding/summary/index.html

United States Department of Health and Human Services. (2002). *Fact sheet: Administrative simplification under HIPAA: National standards for transactions, security and privacy.* Retrieved from http://www.hhs.gov/news/press/2002pres/hipaa.html

---

Visit **www.pearsonhighered.com/healthprofessionsresources** to access the student resources that accompany this book. Simply select Occupational Therapy from the choice of disciplines. Find this book and you will find the complimentary study tools created for this specific title.

CHAPTER 9

Fraud and Abuse

INTRODUCTION

"Fraud is the deliberate concealment of the facts from another person for unlawful or unfair gain" (Fremgen, 2006, p. 125). Fraud can take many forms, but in this book we will be talking only about it in terms of documentation. Falsifying a diagnosis to justify additional tests or procedures and billing for services not provided but documenting as if you did are two examples of fraudulent practices (Pozgar, 2010). Medicare abuse is any action that results in unnecessary costs to Medicare (Medicare Learning Network [MLN], 2012).

▼ MEDICARE FRAUD ▼

According to Kornblau and Burkhardt (2012), Medicare fraud happens when a provider "knowingly or willingly lies to get paid" (p. 34). Medicare abuse happens when a provider gets paid for services provided that were not medically necessary or when Medicare pays for services it should not have. Examples of Medicare fraud and abuse include:

- Submitting a claim for payment for a service that was never delivered
- Submitting false documentation for payment
- Billing for therapy services that were not delivered face-to-face
- Billing for therapy services not provided by a licensed provider (e.g., a student)
- Upcoding: Billing using a therapy code that is reimbursed at a higher rate than the rate for the code for therapy service that was actually delivered
- Participating in a kickback scheme that involves a physician receiving payment for patient referrals

Medicare has strict penalties for fraud. It can cost the practitioner money, jail time, and his or her license to practice occupational therapy. There are both civil and criminal penalties for fraud and abuse (Kornblau & Burkardt, 2012; MLN, 2012). Civil penalties can include fines ranging from $10,000 to $50,000 per false claim as well as damages of three times the amount falsely billed can be assessed (MLN, 2012). Criminal penalties can also include imprisonment in a federal prison (MLN, 2012). Besides these costly consequences, a person participating in fraud can be excluded from ever participating in any federal reimbursement program such as Medicare, Medicaid, Veteran's Affairs, Public Health Service Programs, and other government-funded programs (MLN, 2012). The standard of proof in Medicare fraud cases does not require a specific intent to defraud the government (MLN, 2012). If one acts with "deliberate ignorance" or "reckless disregard," in other words, if one does not know or understand the standards, but should know them, then that could be construed as fraud (MLN, 2012). Obviously, the occupational therapy practitioner is best advised to be truthful and accurate in all documentation in order to avoid claims of fraud.

In July 2006, the Tri-Alliance, a group made up of representatives of the American Occupational Therapy Association, the American Physical Therapy Association, and the American Speech-Language-Hearing Association, took the unusual step of sending a letter to members of all three associations, emphasizing the importance of using the highest standards of ethics and clinical reasoning in documenting the justification for Medicare B therapy cap exceptions (AOTA, 2006). The process of obtaining either automatic or manual exceptions to the cap puts the burden on the clinician to attest that the duration and intensity of the service is reasonable and necessary. The concern that prompted this letter is that the Centers for Medicare and Medicaid Services (CMS) stated "they do not believe a large number of services should exceed the cap" (AOTA, 2006, p. 1), and if postpayment reviews show that exceptions exceeded expectations, that could result in a stricter cap being placed on therapy services. It is critical that "documentation is appropriate to justify additional treatment" (AOTA, 2006, p. 1). While not explicitly stating that there is great potential for Medicare fraud in this process, a warning to clinicians is implied.

Over the last several years, Medicare has stepped up efforts to catch occupational therapy practitioners who attempt to obtain Medicare reimbursement through fraud. If you know that someone else has committed fraud, and you do not report it, you can be charged with conspiracy to commit fraud (Kornblau & Burkhardt, 2012). See Box 9.1 for information on where to report Medicare fraud and abuse.

If you become aware of Medicare fraud or abuse, and you report it, you could receive a reward under the Federal False Claims Act (Kornblau & Burkhardt, 2012). Under this law, you may be eligible for a reward of a 15% to 25% share of the money recovered by the government for damages, civil penalties, and treble damages. To collect the money, you not only have to report the alleged crime, you also have to "substantially assist the U.S. Department of Justice in prosecuting the case" (Kornblau & Burkhardt, 2012, p. 35).

▼ OTHER FORMS OF FRAUD ▼

To avoid allegations of fraud, the occupational therapy practitioner must be knowledgeable of the regulations, must follow those regulations, and must document with sufficient accuracy and honesty. There have been numerous cases where occupational therapy practitioners and others have been accused of fraud because they documented that they provided intervention to a client on a specific date when in fact they did not. Making an honest error on the date of service is one thing; creating fictional progress notes is another. Fraud investigators are trained to know the difference.

Fraud can be more subtle. It can be any documentation that is meant to deceive the reader, especially if payment is sought from any payer for that service (Fremgen, 2006).

BOX 9.1   How to Report Medicare Fraud and Abuse

OIG Hotline - 1-800-HHS-TIPS (1-800-447-8477)
E-mail: HHSTips@oig.hhs.gov

TTY: 1-800-377-4950
Website: http://oig.hhs.gov/fraud/report-fraud/report-fraud-form.asp

Mail: Office of Inspector General
       Department of Health and Human Services
       Attn: Hotline
       PO Box 23489
       Washington, DC 20026

For example, only the time the client spends in contact with the therapist is considered billable time. That means the time an aide spends taking a client to and from the clinic, time spent resting in the therapy room, and time the therapist spends documenting care or on the phone talking to other caregivers are not billable time. It also means that documenting slower progress than is accurate in order to justify keeping a client on one's caseload longer, or faster progress than is accurate to look more effective, is considered fraudulent (Bailey & Schwartzberg, 2003).

Another example of fraud could be intentionally using a billing code that you know will be reimbursed, rather than using a more accurate billing code that may not get reimbursed. I had an occupational therapist once tell me that at her clinic, they were using a new intervention that most insurance companies and the American Academy of Pediatrics considered to be experimental. The clinic manager suggested that rather than name the specific intervention in the notes, which she knew would be a red flag for the payers, clinicians should just document that therapeutic sensory experiences were provided. Rather than billing for an unlisted procedure, they used the billing code for therapeutic activities. Fortunately, that clinic manager left, a new one came in, and the practice of vague and misleading documentation stopped. Instead, the clinic began informing parents that the intervention was considered experimental, that insurance would not cover it, and that parents who were interested in intervention would have to pay for it out of pocket. This is a much more honest approach. Now that the intervention can be mentioned by name, fraudulent billing is no longer a concern, and the occupational therapists can do retrospective chart reviews to determine the effectiveness of the intervention.

▼ ETHICAL STANDARDS ▼

The AOTA *Code of Ethics and Ethical Standards* (2010) specifically states in Principle 6B: "Refrain from using or participating in the use of any form of communication that contains false, fraudulent, deceptive, misleading, or unfair statements or claims." This applies to occupational therapy documentation, advertising and promotional materials, speeches and in-services, or any other form of communication that an occupational therapist might engage in regardless of the setting. In addition, Principle 6D says "Ensure that documentation for reimbursement purposes is done in accordance with applicable laws, guidelines, and regulations" and Principle 6E states "Accept responsibility for any action that reduces the public's trust in occupational therapy" (AOTA, 2010). Engaging in fraud violates the law and is damaging to the reputation of the profession.

For example, an occupational therapist in private practice was accused of adding one billed unit of time (usually 15 minutes of direct service) for every visit that the occupational therapists working for her submitted to her for billing. If the occupational therapists documented in a progress note that the client was seen for a 30-minute session, and marked 30 minutes (two units) on the billing record, the owner of the company would submit the bill for 45 minutes (three units). She did this without the knowledge of the occupational therapists. The occupational therapists found out that this was happening because the family of the client brought a copy of the bill in to the occupational therapist to see why they were being billed for 45-minute visits when they were scheduled for 30-minute visits. The occupational therapists started asking questions and the owner said that she was simply adding a unit to account for the time the therapists spent in documenting services, time on the phone with the client's doctor, cleaning up after sessions, and other miscellaneous clinic expenses. The therapists did some more digging and found that the owner was destroying the progress notes when they were 1-month-old, or as soon as the next intervention plan was written (also a violation of the law). The family reported the fraud to the HMO that was paying for services, and the therapists resigned and then reported the fraud to the state regulatory board. If the allegations proved to be true, the owner could face major penalties and will probably lose her license. Insurance fraud is a federal crime.

Exercise 9.1

Which of the following scenarios constitutes fraud, and which is just carelessness?

1. A therapist dates her notes "Jan. 3, 2014" when in fact the date is January 3, 2015.

2. A therapist writes in her note on Monday that the client was weaker on her right side than on her left. On Wednesday she writes that the client was weaker on her left than on her right. On Friday she writes that although the client is showing improvement in function on her right side, it remains weaker than her left.

3. A therapist bills for hot packs when in fact the client soaked her hand in a bowl of warm water.

4. A therapist bills for a 45-minute session when in fact the client was in the room for 45 minutes, although for 20 of those minutes the client rested while the therapist worked with another client.

5. A therapist realizes that she wrote a progress note in the wrong chart, so she uses white-out to cover up her error.

SUMMARY

Fraud is a form of lying that is absolutely illegal. Fraud happens when an occupational therapist documents in such a way as to create a false perception by the reader about what has actually transpired. Examples of fraud include documenting that you spent more time with a client than you really did, describing progress that is faster or slower than reality, or billing for services not rendered. There can be severe criminal and civil penalties for fraud. AOTA, in the *Code of Ethics* (2010), explicitly prohibits occupational therapists from making false statements. The best advice is to document accurately and be truthful in everything you do.

REFERENCES

American Occupational Therapy Association. (2006). *Letter to occupational therapy practitioners.* Retrieved from http://www.aota.org/~/media/Corporate/Files/Practice/Ethics/trialliance072606.ashx

American Occupational Therapy Association. (2010). Occupational therapy code of ethics and ethical standards. *American Journal of Occupational Therapy, 64,* 639–642.

Bailey, D. M., & Schwartzberg, S. L. (2003). *Ethical and legal dilemmas in occupational therapy.* Philadelphia, PA: F. A. Davis.

Fremgen, B. F. (2006). *Medical law and ethics* (2nd ed.). Upper Saddle River, NJ: Prentice Hall.

Kornblau, B. L. & Burkhardt, A. (2012). *Ethics in rehabilitation: A clinical perspective* (2nd ed.). Thorofare, NJ: Slack.

Medicare Learning Network [MLN]. (2012). *Medicare fraud & abuse: Prevention, detection, and reporting.* Retrieved from http://www.cms.gov/Outreach-and-Education/Medicare-Learning-Network-MLN/MLNProducts/downloads/Fraud_and_Abuse.pdf

Pozgar, G.D. (2010). *Legal and ethical issues for health professionals.* Sudbury, MA: Jones and Bartlett.

Visit **www.pearsonhighered.com/healthprofessionsresources** to access the student resources that accompany this book. Simply select Occupational Therapy from the choice of disciplines. Find this book and you will find the complimentary study tools created for this specific title.

CHAPTER 10

Plagiarism

INTRODUCTION

Plagiarism is a form of cheating and theft that has become very pervasive across the country. The term *plagiarize* is defined as "to steal and pass off (the ideas or words of another) as one's own" (*Merriam-Webster Online,* n.d., *plagiarize*). It includes using someone else's exact words or using someone else's ideas, even if the wording is changed, without giving credit to the originator of the idea or words. Because of the availability of sample intervention plans, student papers, and research papers on the Internet, it is appropriate to discuss plagiarism in the context of a book about documentation. In occupational therapy practice, there are times when an occupational therapist has to put together a report, cite evidence to support practice, or present an in-service with handouts. Each of these situations presents an opportunity for plagiarism.

Plagiarism has a cultural element to it. While some cultures believe that no one can "own" words, in many Western cultures, and American culture in particular, words and ideas are considered to be the intellectual property of the writer or publisher, and cannot be used without giving credit to the author (Lunsford, 2013; On-Line Writing Laboratory [OWL] at Purdue University, 2012).

▼ AMERICAN PSYCHOLOGICAL ASSOCIATION STANDARDS ▼

Since the American Occupational Therapy Association (AOTA) uses the American Psychological Association (APA) standards for writing in the profession, all examples in this book are cited in APA style.

Here is a passage as it appears in the *APA Publication Manual*, Sixth Edition (2010):

> Quotation marks should be used to indicate the exact words of another. *Each time* you paraphrase another author (i.e., summarize a passage or rearrange the order of a sentence and change some of the words), you will need to credit the source in the text (p. 15).

The following is a paraphrase of that same passage in which proper credit is given to the author:

> According to the American Psychological Association (2010), the exact words of another should be enclosed in quotation marks. Rearranging the order of a sentence, summarizing a passage, or changing a few of the words is paraphrasing (APA, 2010). The source needs to be credited each time a source is paraphrased (APA, 2010).

▼ TYPES OF PLAGIARISM ▼

Here is an example of outright plagiarism:

> Quotation marks must be used to indicate the exact words of another, along with a citation of the author, year, and page number. Paraphrasing is rearranging the order of a sentence and changing some of the words or summarizing a passage. Each time a source is paraphrased, you need to give credit to the original author.

In this case, the writer added a few original words, but one cannot tell where any of the ideas come from and whether any of the words are directly taken from a source. Here is the same paragraph with proper citation:

> "Quotation marks must be used to indicate the exact words of another" (APA, 2010, p. 15) along with a citation of the author, year, and page number. Paraphrasing is rearranging the order of a sentence, changing some of the words, or summarizing a passage (APA, 2010). Each time a source is paraphrased, you need to give credit to the original author (APA, 2010).

This paragraph demonstrates a common pitfall that people often fall into: They think that the author of the passage has said what needs to be said in the best possible way, so why paraphrase it? Isn't it safer to quote than to paraphrase? They proceed to write papers that are simply strings of quotes linked with a few transitional phrases in the person's own words. While this may feel like a safe way to go, papers that are strings of quotes are difficult to read; all those quote marks and citations get in the way of the flow of the paper.

Quotes can enhance a paper, but only when used to support the writer's idea (thesis of the paper) by adding a new perspective on it. Too many direct quotes may indicate that the writer does not understand the material well enough to put it in his or her own words. Sometimes writers want to use quotes to show that others agree with them, so they state their opinion and then quote an expert saying essentially the same thing. That makes the quotes redundant and unnecessary.

Another form of plagiarism that can occur happens when students share their work. If you have a friend who took a pediatric occupational therapy course last semester, and you are taking it this semester, your friend might offer you her intervention plans "to look at." If you use them to write your own intervention plans, you are stealing his or her work unless you give credit on your assignment (i.e., "Mary Smith contributed to this assignment"). Most of the time, instructors want you to do your own work, so even if you did give your classmate credit on your assignment, your instructor would probably either make you redo it without help or fail you on that assignment. Using a fellow student's work prevents you from learning and gaining skills needed for the real world. If this was a pattern of behavior, more serious consequences could occur, up to and including expulsion from the program or the school. Disciplinary action can also be taken against the student who did the work herself and then shared it with someone who copied it, because this contributes to the problem of cheating. Clinicians plagiarize when they copy someone else's intervention plan wording. This may be a breach of confidentiality as well. Electronic documentation, which uses standardized phrases that a clinician clicks on to add to the documentation, would not be considered plagiarism.

Many people learn to cheat in middle and high school, and by the time they get to college or the workplace it is so commonplace that they do not see the problem with it. According to a survey administered by Duke University's Center for Academic Integrity, 70% of students admit to cheating in college (McCabe, 2005). In that same survey, nearly 40% admit to cutting and pasting words from an Internet site into their own paper, without citing the source, which is up from 10% in 1995. Just over three quarters of all students surveyed did not think cheating was a serious issue (McCabe, 2005). These are big numbers, and the trend is that they are getting bigger by the decade. Students who cheat in school have been shown to be more likely to cheat in life, for example, cheat on their taxes, lie to customers, or engage in insurance fraud by inflating claims (Novotny, 2011). Survey results like this have gotten the attention of college administrators everywhere, and faculty are examining their academic integrity policies.

I have heard occupational therapy students complain that occupational therapy instructors make too big a deal about plagiarism. Many try to argue that in other majors, instructors do not appear to care if a student plagiarizes. This is a lousy argument. It is not true that other disciplines do not care. However, in a profession where competence and integrity are essential, catching cheaters at an early stage in their careers can help keep the profession respectable. Plagiarizing in school and getting away with it could start one on a slippery slope toward falsifying documentation and engaging in fraud as a clinician.

Related to plagiarism is the concept of copyright infringement. This occurs when someone copies something that someone else has written without getting permission from the creator or publisher (Nolo, 2009). For example, copying journal articles for everyone in the department or on a committee is copyright infringement unless you have written permission from the publisher. Fair use allows a person to use another person's copyrighted works under certain conditions (Nolo, 2009). Under the concept of fair use, you may be able to use someone else's work if you do not profit from its use, you give credit to the originator of the work, and you only use part of the original work; however, there is no guarantee that following these rules will make it fair use (Nolo, 2009). The best advice is to ask before you use anyone else's work.

Often, an occupational therapy department can afford to send only one practitioner to a workshop. When that person comes back from that workshop, he or she copies the handouts for the other members of the department and presents an in-service on it. Unless the practitioner has written permission to copy and distribute those handouts, he or she may be committing copyright infringement (Nolo, 2009). If a clinician copies exercises out of a textbook to give to a client or client's caregiver to use in a home program, it could be considered copyright infringement unless the textbook gives readers permission to copy and distribute material. Copying images from a website like Google or Yahoo images may also violate copyright law. Assume everything is copyrighted and get permission from the copyright holder before using anything from the Internet, unless you see a statement that says it is copyright free.

▼ ETHICAL CONSIDERATIONS ▼

The American Occupational Therapy Association's (AOTA) *Occupational Therapy Code of Ethics and Ethical Standards* (2010) address the issue of plagiarism directly. "Occupational therapy personnel shall give credit and recognition when using the work of others in written, oral, or electronic media" (Principle 6I) and Principle 6J requires occupational therapy personnel to "not plagiarize the work of others" (AOTA, 2010; 2011). Further, Principle 6B additionally reminds occupational therapy personnel to "refrain from using or participating in the use of any form of communication that contains false, fraudulent, deceptive, misleading, or unfair statements or claims." These apply to academic coursework as well as to publications, public presentations, and in-service education, in academic, social, and clinical settings (AOTA, 2011).

The National Board for Certification in Occupational Therapy (2011) has the *Candidate/Certificant Code of Conduct.* The very first principle states:

Principle 1

Certificants shall provide accurate and truthful representations to NBCOT concerning all information related to aspects of the Certification Program, including, but not limited to, the submission of information:

- On the examination and certification renewal applications, and renewal audit form;
- Requested by NBCOT for a disciplinary action situation; or

- Requested by NBCOT concerning allegations related to:
  - Test security violations and/or disclosure of confidential examination material content to unauthorized parties;
  - Misrepresentations by a certificant regarding his/her credential(s) and/or education;
  - The unauthorized use of NBCOT's intellectual property, certification marks, and other copyrighted materials.

Of particular note is the final point related to using NBCOT's intellectual property (NBCOT, 2011). NBCOT's intellectual property includes everything published by NBCOT regardless of format, in other words, in print on paper or on their website.

▼ PREVENTING PLAGIARISM ▼

How can you protect yourself against allegations of plagiarism? The first rule of thumb is that when in doubt, cite a source. If reading something someone else wrote puts a thought in your head and it comes out your fingertips onto the paper (or computer screen), then cite it. Things that are general knowledge, such as using sunscreen can prevent sunburn or that more falls happen to elderly people in the winter in Vermont than in the summer, do not need to be cited. One suggestion is that you can call something common knowledge if you find the same information in five different sources, and each time the author did not document a source for it (OWL, 2012).

To make an allegation of plagiarism against a student, a teacher needs to be pretty sure the work was copied, or at least paraphrased from an identifiable source. New Internet search engines such as Google.com™ and Turnitin.com™ make it easy for instructors to find out if a student has copied someone else's work. The instructor can simply type in a phrase and search the Internet to see if it has been used by someone else on the Internet. If an instructor finds a student has used someone else's work, there can be serious consequences for the student. Some instructors require students to turn in their papers to Turnitin.com™.

> **Exercise 10.1**
>
> Go to your college or university website, find the policy on academic integrity (it might be in the section on the honor code, or code of conduct), and read the policy. Discuss the types of actions that are prohibited in your school (or alma mater), and the types of punishments that could result from a violation of the policy.

To find out what could happen if you got caught cheating or plagiarizing, check out your school's policy on academic integrity, honor code, or plagiarism policy. If you were to get caught using someone else's words when you are a clinician, you would be subject to disciplinary action from your employer, AOTA, the National Board for Certification in Occupational Therapy, and, depending on your state regulations for licensure or registration, disciplinary action from your state regulatory board as well.

This can be scary stuff. It almost makes one afraid to write anything. Chances are that all the good phrases have been taken, that is, "it's all been said before" (author of quote unknown). Bob Newhart had a comedy sketch in which he theorized that if you put a group of monkeys in a room with a typewriter apiece, sooner or later by random efforts they would reproduce all the world's great literature. There are common phrases that everyone uses so that it would be impossible to give credit to any one author. Sometimes two people who have never met can come up with similar word sequences. This cannot be helped.

According to the Georgetown University Honor Council (2002), one way to protect yourself is to allow yourself time to do it right. If you are writing a 12-page paper at 11:59 P.M. the night before it is due at 8:00 A.M., you could inadvertently leave out some quote marks or forget to cite a source. It might seem easier at that point to copy someone else's paper (or buy one off the Internet) than to stay up all night working hard on it. If you find yourself in this kind of situation, it is better to risk a lower grade on the paper (by not being thorough enough, making spelling errors, wandering off topic, etc.) than to risk the disciplinary consequences of an academic integrity violation (Georgetown University Honor Council, 2002). Of course, the best course of action is to not get yourself into this kind of situation in the first place.

Purdue University, On-line Writing Laboratory ([OWL], 2013) offers a printable handout on its web page for avoiding plagiarism. In it there are suggestions for what you can do during the writing process and how your finished product should look. It suggests coding your paper during early drafts with "Q" for quote, and then coding the rest with either an "S" when the material comes from any source, and "ME" when it is your own idea or insight. Others suggest that when you make notes on a reading, anytime you write the words of the author, use quotes around those notes (Lunsford, 2013). OWL further suggests summarizing or paraphrasing from memory, rather than while reading the material. Table 10.1 provides some general guidance on when to quote from, paraphrase, or summarize another writer's words or ideas. Remember that proper citation is required in all of these instances.

Exercise 10.2

Practice paraphrasing the following sentences.

1. "Client-centered therapy requires active participation of the client in the process of evaluation and intervention" (Schwartzberg, 2002, p. 62).

2. "Countersignature of a treatment plan, insurance form, prescription for medication, progress note, or similar document is usually tantamount to declaring oneself responsible, vicariously, for the treatment in question" (Gutheil, as cited in Bailey & Schwartzberg, 2003, p. 91).

3. "To protect confidentiality, medical records should not be released to third parties without the patient's written consent" (Fremgen, 2002, p. 160).

4. "MOHO has received much attention, including criticism, elaboration, application, and empirical testing by occupational therapists throughout the world." (Kielhofner, 2008, p.1)

5. "Wordiness is every bit as irritating and uneconomical as jargon and can impede the ready grasp of ideas" (APA, 2001, p. 35).

6. "The goal of occupational therapy is the development of competence in activities and tasks of one's cherished roles, which promotes a sense of self-efficacy and self-esteem." (Trombly Latham, 2008, p. 3).

Exercise 10.3

Is this plagiarism?

1. You change the verb tense, but otherwise keeping the sentence the same as the original author, but citing the author and year in parentheses at the end of the sentence.

2. You change the order of the sentences in a paragraph and adding one sentence of your own construction to the paragraph, and name the author of the original work as part of one sentence (e.g., According to Garza, such and such).

3. At a conference, the presenter, R. Yount, runs out of handouts, so you ask the presenter to e-mail his or her presentation to you, and then you use it in your own presentation at work. Each slide says © R. Yount, (2006) on the bottom.

4. You write a brilliant paragraph for an evaluation report. You like it so much, you keep pulling it up on the computer whenever you have to write a new evaluation report for a similar client, and change the name, but otherwise use the same wording.

TABLE 10.1 When to Quote, Paraphrase, or Summarize a Source

Type of citation	When to do it	How to do it
Quote	• The wording is so powerful that if you changed it, it would weaken it. • The author is a well-known expert in the field whose opinion you want to emphasize to make a specific point. • The author offers a perspective that is distinctly different from yours, not a restatement of your idea. • The author offers a perspective that is distinctly different that most people's.	• Use quote marks around the words you are quoting for quotes under 40 words, use a block quote format if the quote is over 40 words. • Do not change any of the words, even if they are spelled incorrectly, from the way the original author said it. Use [*sic*] to indicate the error was the original author's. • If you want to shorten the quote to remove extraneous information, use three ellipsis points (. . .) to represent the removed words. • Cite the source, including author's name, year of publication, and page number immediately at the end of the quote.
Paraphrase	• The author's exact words are not as important as the point the author is making.	• If you want to cite the author as part of the same sentence with the summarized material, include the year in parentheses immediately after the author's name. • Alternatively, you can cite both the author and year in parentheses at the end of the sentence. • Paraphrase without looking at the original, but check the original afterward to see if you have accurately captured the author's meaning.
Summarize	• The passages are very long, and not every detail is important to you.	• If you want to cite the author as part of the same sentence with the summarized material, include the year in parentheses immediately after the author's name. • Alternatively, you can cite both the author and year in parentheses at the end of the sentence. • Summarize without looking at the original, but check the original afterward to see if you have accurately captured the author's meaning.

Sources: APA (2010); Lunsford (2013); OWL at Purdue University (2010).

SUMMARY

When you plagiarize, you not only cheat the originator of the material out of his or her proper credit, but also you cheat yourself by not really learning the material. Occasional honest mistakes can usually be tolerated, but repeated instances of the same type of error in citing sources could be used to show a pattern of carelessness that amounts to plagiarism.

A student who plagiarizes can expect to fail the assignment or the course, or be expelled from the program. Blatant and repeated plagiarism can lead to expulsion from a school. Plagiarism done by a professional can result in loss of a job or even a career in occupational therapy. There are ways to prevent plagiarism. Allowing plenty of time to complete written work, learning how to properly cite sources, and summarizing or paraphrasing from memory are a few of the ways that plagiarism can be prevented.

REFERENCES

American Occupational Therapy Association. (2010). Occupational therapy code of ethics and ethical standards. *American Journal of Occupational Therapy, 64*, 639–642.

American Occupational Therapy Association. (2011). Avoiding plagiarism in the electronic age. Retrieved from http://www.aota.org/Practitioners/Ethics/Advisory/51042.aspx?Fl=.pdf

American Psychological Association. (2010). *Publication manual of the American Psychological Association* (6th ed.). Washington, DC: Author.

Bailey, D. M. & Schwartzberg, S. L. (2003). *Ethical and legal dilemmas in occupational therapy* (2nd ed.). Philadelphia: F. A. Davis.

Fremgen, B. F. (2002). *Medical law & ethics.* Upper Saddle River, NJ: Prentice Hall.

Georgetown University Honor Council. (2002). Retrieved May 5, 2002, from http://www.georgetown.edu/honor/plagiarism.html

Kielhofner, G. (2008). Model of human occupation: Theory and application (4th ed.). Philadelphia, PA: Lippincott Williams & Wilkins.

Lunsford, A. (2013). The everyday writer (5th ed.). New York: Bedford/St. Martin's.

McCabe, (2005). *New CAI Research.* Retrieved from http://www.academicintegrity.org/cai_research.asp

Merriam-Webster Online. (n.d.). *Definition of plagiarize.* Retrieved from http://www.m-w.com/dictionary/plagiarizing

National Board for Certification of Occupational Therapy [NBCOT]. (2011). Retrieved from http://www.nbcot.org/pdf/Candidate-Certificant-Code-of-Conduct.pdf?phpMyAdmin=3710605fd34365e38069ab41a5078545

Nolo.com. (2009). The *"fair use" rule: When use of copyrighted material is acceptable.* Retrieved from http://www.nolo.com/article.cfm/pg/1/objectId/C3E49F67-1AA3-4293-9312FE5C119B5806/catId/DAE53B68-7BF5-455A-BC9F3D9C9C1F7513/310/276/ART/

Novotny, A. (2011, June). Beat the cheat. *Monitor on Psychology, 42*, p. 54.

Online Writing Laboratory [OWL] at Purdue University. (2010). Summarizing, paraphrasing, and quoting. Retrieved from https://owl.english.purdue.edu/owl/resource/930/02/

Online Writing Laboratory [OWL] at Purdue University. (2012). *Is it plagiarism yet?* Retrieved from http://owl.english.purdue.edu/owl/resource/589/02/

Schwartzberg, S. (2002) *Interactive reasoning in the practice of occupational therapy.* Upper Saddle River, NJ: Prentice Hall.

Trombly Latham, C. A. (2008). Conceptual foundations for practice. In M. V. Radomski & C. A. Trombly Latham (Eds.) *Occupational therapy for physical dysfunction* (6th ed.; pp 1–20). Philadelphia, PA: Lippincott Williams & Wilkins.

SECTION III

CHAPTER 11

Overview of Clinical Documentation

INTRODUCTION

This section of the book explores the different types of documentation that occupational therapy practitioners write when working with clients whose ability to participate fully in life is diminished or at risk due to physical, psychological, or developmental issues. Typically, in clinical settings, payment for services is sought from third-party payers such as insurance companies, managed care organizations, government programs, or from the clients themselves. When third-party payers get involved in the care process, it adds an additional layer of requirements that occupational therapy practitioners need to address in their documentation. Clinical settings for occupational therapy services may include medical or psychiatric hospitals, clinics, or long-term care settings as well as clients' homes, sheltered workshops, group homes, or other facilities.

▼ CLINICAL DOCUMENTATION ▼

Clinical documentation typically consists of documentation of the client's referral for services, a summary of the evaluation results (including the occupational profile and analysis of occupational performance), intervention plans, documentation of progress, attendance records, discharge summaries, and follow-up documentation (if any). Table 11.1 shows each step of the occupational therapy process and the corresponding documentation for each step. In essence, for each step of the occupational therapy process there is documentation to go with it. Each of these types of documentation is discussed in the chapters in this section.

Regardless of the type of clinical documentation, certain conventions for good documentation must be followed. While there may be differences between the documentation written by an occupational therapist in a hospital in Los Angeles and an occupational therapy assistant in a sheltered workshop in Bangor, Maine, all documentation must be well written, accurate, and clear.

▼ ROLE DELINEATION FOR DOCUMENTATION ▼

In this book, the term "occupational therapy practitioners" refers to both occupational therapists and occupational therapy assistants. The occupational therapist has primary responsibility for assuring that documentation is completed in compliance with standards. The occupational therapy practitioner who provided the services to the client is the person who should document that session's services. If the documentation is written by an occupational therapy assistant, the documentation is often cosigned by the supervising occupational therapist as a way to show that supervision has occurred, and that the occupational therapist has read the documentation. The American Occupational Therapy Association (2013) does not require that an occupational therapist cosign documentation written by an occupational therapy assistant unless it is required by state law, third-party payer, or employer.

TABLE 11.1 Occupational Therapy Process and Clinical Documentation

Steps in the Occupational Therapy Process	Types of Documentation
Client identification	Referral or physician's orders Contact notes
Screening (if required)	Screening reports Contact notes
Initial evaluation	Evaluation reports or evaluation summaries
Intervention planning	Intervention plans (also called a plans of care)
Intervention	Attendance logs Progress flow sheets Progress notes (SOAP, DAP, or narrative) Contact notes Transition plans
Reevaluation (intervention review)	Revised intervention plans
Outcomes **Discontinuation (discharge)**	Discharge summaries
Follow-up	Follow-up notes Contact notes

Sources: AOTA (2013); Moyers & Dale (2007).

It is important to be familiar with state laws and regulations related to occupational therapy practice. The law that describes how occupational therapy practitioners become licensed or registered to practice in that state is often referred to as the *Occupational Therapy Practice Act.* This law will describe the requirements for supervision of occupational therapy assistants including the frequency, type, and how that supervision is documented. Some states not only require a co-signature by the occupational therapist but a log of supervisory visits.

All documentation written by occupational therapy or occupational therapy assistant students need to be cosigned by the student's supervisor. This shows that the supervisor has read the note.

▼ GUIDELINES FOR DOCUMENTATION ▼

The American Occupational Therapy Association (AOTA) sets standards for documentation, *The Guidelines for Documentation of Occupational Therapy* (2013) that lists 15 fundamentals of all occupational therapy documentation. Each fundamental is explained in Figure 11.1, with support from additional sources.

In addition to these standards, there are other common considerations. For example, most handwritten documentation is done in blue or black ink because often the documents must be copied and other colors of ink do not photocopy well (Gately & Borcherding, 2012; Fremgen, 2006; Scott, 2013). Never document in a permanent medical record using a pencil (it is erasable). Some facilities do not allow practitioners to document using erasable pens. Other facilities require the ink to be waterproof (Gately & Borcherding, 2012). Of course, when documentation is done on an electronic health record system, ink color becomes irrelevant.

1. **Client identification:** The client's full name should be mentioned on every page, along with the client's case number, if there is one. The case number may be a medical records number, room/bed number, or other number, whichever is used at a particular facility or program.

2. **Date and time:** Each document should be dated with the day, month, and year. Documentation of occupational therapy sessions (evaluation or intervention) often includes the time of day and sometimes the length of the session. Dates and times are used to show the chronological order of events.

3. **Type:** The type of documentation should be clearly stated, as should the name of the facility/agency and department. For example, the type of document may appear at the top of the page, and the name of the department may be under the signature line.

4. **Signature:** The writer should sign the document using at least his or her first initial and full last name followed by the appropriate professional designation (e.g., OTR, COTA, OT/L, OTA/L, etc.). Using initials only is usually not sufficient. In some cases, such as on an attendance log, the occupational therapist might simply place his or her initials in the space for each day. At the bottom of the page there should be multiple signature lines so that for each set of initials appearing on the page, there is a full name and credentials written out to clearly identify the person who worked with the client. In an electronic health record, the signature will be recorded electronically rather than by hand..

5. **Placement of signature:** Notes should be signed directly at the end of the note; there should be no space between what is written and the signature. This can help prevent someone else from tampering with your documentation. Some facilities have the staff draw a line where there is blank space between the end of a note and the signature (Evidence-Based Nursing Guide, 2009). On an electronic documentation system, once the note is signed, it cannot be altered. If corrections need to be made, they are done as an addendum to the original note.

6. **Co-signature:** As required by state, payer, or employer regulations, occupational therapists co-sign (also called countersigning) the signatures of occupational therapy assistants and students (Gately & Borcherding, 2012). This countersignature signifies that the occupational therapist has read the document and is in agreement with the conclusions drawn by the writer. The person countersigning the note is obligated to make any necessary corrections or addendums to the note before co-signing (Scott, 2013). This also provides documentation of supervision, which may be required by law.

7. **Compliance:** Occupational therapy practitioners comply with all laws, regulations, as well as payer and employer requirements.

8. **Terminology:** All terminology used must be recognized by the facility as acceptable. Official documents of the profession may be used to define terms, or the facility may specify terminology to be used by all professionals at the facility. This includes the term you use to identify the recipient of your services, for example, *patient, client, resident, student* (Gately & Borcherding, 2012).

9. **Abbreviations:** Use only abbreviations approved by the facility. There is usually a list that is used by all disciplines. Some common abbreviations are listed in Chapter 2 of this book. However, just because an abbreviation is listed in this book does not mean that it will be recognized at your facility or in your program.

10. **Corrections:** Follow facility rules for correcting errors. Only correct your own errors (Guido, 2006). The most common method of correcting handwritten notes is to draw a line through the error and initial it. Some suggest writing the word error above the cross-out; but others suggest not doing that (Gately & Borcherding, 2012; Guido, 2006; Nicholson, 2008; Scott, 2013). Never do anything to obliterate erroneous documentation such as use white-out, scribble over an entry, or put tape over it (Gately & Borcherding, 2012; Guido, 2006; Nicholson, 2008; Scott, 2013). If the error occurs on an electronic health record, correct it using an addendum and signed with an electronic signature.

11. **Technology:** Follow professional standards and agency/facility policies and procedures for use of technology in documentation.

12. **Record Disposal:** Follow federal and state laws as well as agency/facility policies and procedures for proper disposal of records.

13. **Confidentiality:** All federal, state, and agency/facility rules and regulations for confidentiality must be obeyed, including the AOTA Code of Ethics and Ethics Standards (2010).

14. **Record Storage:** All federal, state, and agency/facility rules and regulations for storage of records must be obeyed.

15. **Clinical Reasoning and Expertise:** All documentation should demonstrate that the clinical reasoning and expertise of an occupational therapy practitioner is necessary for the safe and effective delivery of care.

FIGURE 11.1 Fundamentals of Documentation

Sources: AOTA (2010, 2013); Gately & Borcherding (2012); Guido (2006); Nicholson (2008); Scott (2013).

Another common consideration is legibility. All handwritten documentation needs to be legible (Fremgen, 2006; Scott, 2013). For some people, this means printing or typing rather than writing in script (Fremgen, 2006; Scott, 2013).

The integrity of the health record is critical. Never write in a clinical record on behalf of another provider, allow another provider to alter your documentation, or document for you (*Evidence-Based Nursing Guide*, 2009; Guido, 2006). Make sure that the chart you are writing in is, in fact, the chart of the client with whom you are working (Document Defensively, 2008). Never document based on hearsay, that is, what another provider tells you occurred, if you did not see it occur (Scott, 2013).

A final common consideration is that your documentation should reflect what the client did, not what you did (Gately & Borcherding, 2012; Kettenbach, 2009). This may require you to reword your note in your head before writing it in the health record. Keep the client the focus of your documentation.

▼ STRUCTURE OF THIS SECTION OF THE BOOK ▼

Chapter 12 provides an overview of the electronic health record. While every electronic health record system is different, there is some basic information that applies to all systems.

Chapter 13 focuses on documentation of the initial contact a clinician has with a client. This includes referrals for intervention, physician's orders, and screenings.

Chapter 14 discusses the ways in which evaluation reports are written. As part of that discussion, the purposes and focus of evaluations, methods of recording evaluation data, interpreting the data, and summarizing the data are presented.

Chapter 15 centers on goal writing. Clinicians may set goals as part of an evaluation report or as part of an intervention plan. Several methods for writing goal statements are offered.

Chapter 16 presents methods for documenting intervention plans. Specific information about documenting progress summaries and intervention methods/strategies are set forth.

Chapter 17 addresses various forms of progress notes. The two most common kinds of progress notes are SOAP and narrative formats. This chapter looks at these and other formats in detail, with practice opportunities for the readers of this text.

Finally, Chapter 18 presents discharge summaries. It offers information on documenting the plan for discontinuation of services and for follow-up if needed.

REFERENCES

American Occupation Therapy Association. (2010). Occupational therapy code of ethics and ethics standards [Supplemental material]. *American Journal of Occupational Therapy, 54,* S17–S26. doi:10.5014/ajot.2010.64S17

American Occupational Therapy Association. (2013). Guidelines for documentation of occupational therapy [Supplemental material]. *American Journal of Occupational Therapy, 67,* S7–S8. doi:10.5014/ajot.2013.67S32

Document defensively: Here's how… (2008). Reprinted from 2007 HPSO Risk Advisor with permission by Healthcare Providers Service Organization (HPSO), www.hpso.com. *Dental Assistant, 77*(6), 34.

Evidence-based nursing guide to legal and professional issues (2009). Philadelphia, PA: Wolters Kluwer/Lippincott Williams & Wilkins.

Fremgen, B.F. (2006). *Medical law and ethics* (2nd ed.). Upper Saddle River, NJ: Prentice Hall.

Gately, C.A. & Borcherding, S. (2012). *Documentation manual for occupational therapy writing SOAP notes* (3rd ed.). Thorofare, NJ: Slack.

Guido, G.W. (2006). Legal and ethical issues in nursing (4th ed.). Upper Saddle River, NJ: Pearson Prentice Hall.

Kettenbach, G. (2009). Writing patient/client notes: Ensuring accuracy in documentation (4th ed.). Philadelphia, PA: F.A. Davis.

Moyers, P.A., & Dale, L.M. (2007). *The guide to occupational therapy practice* (2nd ed.). Bethesda, MD: American Occupational Therapy Association.

Nicholson, S.K. (2008). *The physical therapist's business practice and legal guide.* Boston, MA: Jones and Bartlett.

Scott, R.W. (2013). Legal, ethical, and practical aspects of patient care documentation: A guide for rehabilitation professionals (4th ed.). Boston, MA: Jones and Bartlett.

Visit **www.pearsonhighered.com/healthprofessionsresources** to access the student resources that accompany this book. Simply select Occupational Therapy from the choice of disciplines. Find this book and you will find the complimentary study tools created for this specific title.

CHAPTER 12

Electronic Health Record

INTRODUCTION

It's been reported that in the aftermath of Hurricane Katrina, more than a million Gulf Coast residents found themselves without any access to their medical records, including pharmacy records (Rogers, 2005). This made it much more difficult to provide health-related services to the hurricane survivors that were left in the area with little more than the clothes on their backs. Paper records were blown or washed away. On the other hand, when a major tornado made a direct hit on St. John's Mercy Hospital in Joplin, MO in May, 2011, all patient records remained accessible because the hospital had just completed a conversion from paper to electronic health records (EHRs) (HealthIT.gov, n.d.). Dottie Bringel, the chief nursing officer of the hospital, reported that paper records were flying all over the community, but the EHRs were safe. As patients were sent to other hospitals in the area, staff from St. John's Mercy Hospital were able to forward previous and current medical histories and patient records to those other hospitals within 2 hours of the evacuation of St. John's Mercy Hospital.

Paper files could burn in a fire, be blown away in a tornado or hurricane, or wash away in a hurricane, flood, or tsunami. In those disasters and others, vital medical information recorded on paper can be lost. People who should not have access to a patient's health record could wind up reading the displaced paper health records, destroying the patient's right to privacy and confidentiality. This is one of many reasons why the nation is moving this very private information into electronic format.

Simply stated, the EHR is a computerized system for entering, storing, and retrieving health information related to an individual client. It may be referred to as an EHR, electronic medical record (EMR), electronic patient record, computerized health record, computerized medical record, or computer-based patient record (Carter, 2008). The preferred term today is electronic health record.

EHRs do more than simply provide an alternative to paper charts. They provide a way to retrieve the information so that the data can be used to improve clinical practice; much faster and more efficiently than having someone go through paper charts one at a time. In this way, the EHR is not just a record keeping system; it is a data management system.

▼ HISTORY OF THE ELECTRONIC HEALTH RECORD ▼

The shift from paper to EHRs has been a long time coming. Back in 1991, the Institute of Medicine (IOM) published a report entitled *The Computer-Based Patient Record: An Essential Technology for Healthcare*. In that report, the IOM laid out a vision of what would become the EHR (Gartee, 2011, Shamus & Stern, 2011). By 2003, the IOM began using the term electronic health record in its publications (IOM, 2011). That year, the IOM identified eight core functions of an EHR (see Figure 12.1).

In 2004, President George W. Bush called for the conversion to an EMR for everyone in this country by 2014 (Tieman, 2004). This record would be portable, so it could follow the patient, and contain documentation of the patient's history, including every physician visit, test, and treatment (Tieman, 2004). Many, but not all, hospital and healthcare systems, clinics, and private practitioners have already made the conversion. Not *all* healthcare

- Health information and data
- Result management
- Order management
- Decision support
- Electronic communication and connectivity
- Patient support
- Administrative processes and reporting
- Reporting and population health

FIGURE 12.1 Core Functions of an Electronic Health Record. *Source:* Gartee, 2011.

providers were using EHRs by 2014, but many were. One problem with this is that in the push to get providers using EHRs, little attention was paid to the interconnectivity of the different systems, so while two hospitals may both use EHRs, the two systems may not use the same terminology or functionality and therefore the two hospitals may not be able to share the health data they have on the same patient.

President Obama signed the Health Information Technology for Economic and Clinical Health (HITECH) Act in 2009, as part of the American Recovery and Reinvestment Act (ARRA), sometimes called Public Law 111-5 (AHIMA, 2009; Gartee, 2011). The HITECH Act is actually Title XIII of the ARRA. The HITECH Act provides funding for incentives to get more healthcare providers, especially those who bill Medicare and Medicaid, to use EHRs (AHIMA, 2012). It also directs the Office of the National Coordinator for Health Information Technology (ONC) to develop and adopt standards, specifications, and certification criteria for meaningful use of health information technology (ONC, 2010).

The emphasis for the adoption of EHRs is on hospitals and physician offices; other provider types, such as long-term care, are not a target for now, but will be down the road. According to the Centers for Disease Control and Prevention, as of September 7, 2012, just over 40% of physician offices were using EHRs (CDC, 2012). As of 2012, 35% of hospitals were using at least a basic EHR (Sebelius, 2012). The pace of adoption by hospitals and physician offices is increasing (ONC, 2012).

▼ PURPOSE ADVANTAGES AND DISADVANTAGES ▼

Beyond government funding, there are other good reasons to make the transition to EHRs. The first reason is for patient safety (Gartee, 2011). Problems with legibility of handwritten documentation have contributed too many medical errors, some fatal. In addition, when patients go to multiple healthcare providers, and each provider has his or her own paper system, then the different providers do not know what the other providers have prescribed or provided. This can lead to over-prescription of medications, some of which may have bad interactions, or disjointed care delivery. If all the providers could document on the same system, or at least on systems that can communicate with each other, we could greatly improve the quality of care. Another reason is that all these errors and duplication of services cost money (Gartee, 2011). Estimates are that EHRs systems could save billions of healthcare dollars every year. Electronic systems provide faster access to information, decreasing the cost of staff time spent locating and retrieving paper files, transcribing hard-to-read documents, and improved coding resulting in faster payment (Shamus & Stern, 2011). Finally, more and more consumers use computers on a daily basis, and want to see their lab results and other information from their computers (Gartee, 2011). An EHR system that includes a personal health record application meets consumer demands.

There are many advantages to having an EMR. In addition to improved access to the records, computerized records are easier to read, take less time to locate, decrease the duplication of information, and help streamline the billing processes (Shamus & Stern, 2011). Used properly, the EHR can reduce the amount of paper used and decrease storage space needed. It can improve efficiency by reducing the time spent on paperwork, and reducing errors in coding and billing (Arabit, 2010). The data in the EHR can be used to organize data that can be helpful for tracking staff productivity, identifying referral patterns, marketing management, and quality management (Arabit, 2010; Shamus & Stern, 2011). In large healthcare systems, with multiple providers entering and retrieving client information, electronic systems can alert providers to duplicate physician orders, potential adverse drug reactions, and conflicting medication prescriptions. This can help reduce errors and improve client safety (Arabit, 2010). It makes it easier to access information that can be used to improve practice outcomes (Shamus & Stern, 2011). The EHR can provide an opportunity to increase the awareness and understanding of occupational therapy by other healthcare professions (Arabit, 2010).

Many EHR systems can help improve the management of therapy practices by integrating the clinical record with scheduling and billing components (Shamus & Stern, 2011). Because each client has a unique record number, once that number is entered into the system then all the demographic information about that client can be automatically populated on bills for service. If a payer requests documentation of a client's progress, the office staff can easily access that information to submit with the bill. Some disadvantages include the high cost in time and money for hardware, software, and training; the need to back up the systems in case of power outages and system crashes; and the use of templates which may limit the information that is entered into the record (Arabit, 2010; Shamus & Stern, 2011). Staff may be anxious or resistant to using EHRs, depending on their past experiences with computers (Arabit, 2010; Shamus & Stern, 2011). EHRs require extensive training for which staff expect to be paid. Finally, tech support needs to be available 24/7/365 in order to resolve issues quickly (Arabit, 2010).

There are barriers to the adoption of electronic records across all healthcare providers. The first one is cost. Even basic EHRs systems cost a lot. For some private practices and small rural hospitals, especially those not affiliated with a health system, the cost is prohibitive (ONC, 2012). Another barrier is access to broadband services. Some areas of the country do not have broadband access or if they do, it may be cost prohibitive. Security concerns are another barrier for some healthcare providers. Finally, access to a qualified workforce with the technical skills to support EHRs is a barrier. The HITECH Act tries to reduce these barriers by providing funding and rules to improve funding for the hardware, software, training, and workforce development (ONC, 2012).

While EHRs improve efficiency and safety, they also provide opportunities to raise red flags in the eyes of third-party payers (Shamus & Stern, 2011). Shamus and Stern provide several examples of ways the EHR can put a therapy provider at risk of an audit by a payer:

- Reports that are too short and leave off key information justifying medical necessity
- Use of standardized phrases in note after note, especially if they are the same note for visit after visit
- Physician signature line is on a different page than the rest of the plan of care
- Using only objective measures of impairments without relating these to functional performance
- Generalized goals that are not specific to the client or the client's circumstances

▼ PRACTICAL CONSIDERATIONS ▼

Using the EHR while in the presence of the client presents some interesting challenges. First, clients have concerns over the privacy of the information being entered into the computer (Baker, Reifstech, & Mann, 2003). This is greatly affected by whether or not the client can see the screen. Second, the practitioner tends to guide the conversation with the client to facilitate ease of data entry, rather than letting the client's responses guide the conversation. Finally, if the clinician has to turn away from the client to enter the data, that reduces the time the clinician spends observing or talking with the client, and could lead to errors and unsafe situations (Baker et al., 2003). Let's examine some ways that an occupational therapy practitioner can use the EHR in a way that reduces these concerns.

Screen Position

Clients may be more comfortable if they can see the screen and see what you are entering into the record (Baker et al., 2003). If the screen can be positioned in such a way that both the occupational therapy practitioner and the client can see it, then do so. This is a good way to establish a collaborative relationship with the client. Be aware of any facility policies that may govern whether or not the client or the client's family members can see the EHR at the time of service. If the client is a child or teen, the parent may be in the room. Be sure that in sharing the screen, you do not endanger the child or teen by allowing the parent to see something he or she might be angry about, such as a medication list that includes a birth control drug or a history of physical or sexual abuse (Baker et al., 2003).

Human Positions

The way that the occupational therapy practitioner sits while talking with the client can also impact the sense of collaboration that the client feels (Baker et al., 2003). For example, if the screen is positioned so it hides the face of the occupational therapy practitioner, then it becomes difficult for the occupational therapy practitioner to form a personal connection with the client. If the computer or computer screen is positioned off to one side of the client, the occupational therapy practitioner might have his or her back to the client, again creating a barrier to effective relationship building with the client. The best position is when the occupational therapy practitioner is at a 45–90 degree angle to the client; this facilitates conversation, eye contact, and relationship building (Baker et al., 2003).

User Behavior

Not everyone has an easy relationship with computers. There are some people who are slower to learn to use technology, or have a knack for breaking things. There are other people who talk to inanimate objects, such as computers, as they work. Imagine a client in a room with an occupational therapy practitioner who is having a bad day, is really frustrated with the computer, and then starts mumbling and swearing at the computer. That would be very unprofessional, but it could happen. It would destroy any faith the client had in the EHR system (Baker et al., 2003).

Confidentiality

By their nature, EHRs contain confidential information on a lot of people. EHRs typically are password protected to limit accessibility to that information. It is critical that the users, including occupational therapy practitioners, never leave a screen with client information on it unattended (Baker et al., 2003). In fact, occupational therapy practitioners should never leave a computer logged on no matter what is on the screen. It is not sufficient to simply minimize the screen and step away, even for a few seconds.

A related issue is how easy it is to check anyone's file once an occupational therapy practitioner is logged in to the system. Employees have been fired for unauthorized access of an EHR file. In 2010, a cardiologist was sentenced to jail time for unauthorized access of client records (AMA, 2010). Thirteen employees were fired from a hospital in Los Angeles for looking at Brittany Spears' health record when they were unauthorized to do so (Orenstein, 2008). In Iowa, University of Iowa Medical Center was investigating its employees for looking at the records of University of Iowa football players (Danielson, 2011). In Minnesota, two hospitals from one system fired 32 employees for snooping in the medical records of a group of teenagers who had overdosed at a party (Lauretsen, 2011).

The EHR is set up to track who logs on, when, and which files were accessed by that person. Many facilities have a zero tolerance policy for employees who engage in unauthorized access of EHRs. Not only does this violate facility policy, but it violates HIPAA and the AOTA Code of Ethics and Ethics Standards as well. An occupational therapy practitioner who accesses EHRs that he or she should not could endanger his or her ability to ever practice occupational therapy in the future.

Communication Skills

A study by Baker et al. (2003) provides some insights into the behaviors that result in effective communication between the practitioner and client while using an EHR. Although this study looked at nurse-patient interactions, the findings apply to anyone using an EHR. Baker et al. (2003) identified three clusters of behaviors; connect, collaborate, and close; to describe effective practitioner-client interactions.

Connect refers to the way in which the practitioner greets the client, explains the EHR and confidentiality, and arranges the computer for viewing (Baker et al., 2003). Baker et al. (2003) recommend that the practitioner establish a personal connection with the client before logging in to the EHR. Personal connections happen when the practitioner greets the client by name, makes eye contact, shakes hands, and makes small talk. After that, the practitioner should explain the purpose and use of the EHR. The practitioner then positions both the screen and him- or herself to maximize interaction, or to protect confidentiality if there are others in the room (Baker et al., 2003).

Baker et al.'s (2003) second cluster is collaborate. Collaborate means making the client your partner. Tell the client what you are entering or retrieving in the computer. As a courtesy, ask the client if it is alright with him or her if you type notes while the two of you are talking, and explain why. Remember to make eye contact throughout the dialog. If facility policy allows, show the client any graphs or charts that summarize data about the client over time. Ask the client to share his or her perspective on the data (Baker et al., 2003).

Closing is the final cluster (Baker et al., 2003). As the practitioner logs off the computer, he or she explains that this is to protect the client's confidentiality and to secure the data. At this point, the practitioner could summarize the visit and explain the next steps in the client's care. Finally, according to Baker et al. (2003), leave the room in the same manner in which you entered, that is, making a personal connection to the client.

Exercise 12.1

With a partner, role play the following scenarios using best practices for using the EHR with a client. You need to both introduce yourself and log in to the EHR.

1. You enter a client's room on the orthopedic unit of a large hospital. The EHR is on a desk top computer attached to the wall.
2. You bring a child and her mom back into an intervention room at an outpatient pediatric clinic. There is a laptop computer in the room.
3. You are doing a home visit with an older adult who recently had a stroke. The client's spouse is there too. You use a handheld device for access to the EHR.

▼ HEALTH INFORMATION EXCHANGES ▼

A health information exchange (HIE) takes data from EHRs and puts it into a sharable format (Dhopeshwarkar, Kern, O'Donnell, Edwards, & Kaushal, 2012). An HIE is a system that allows electronic sharing of health information data across providers and settings (HealthIT. gov, 2012a). It supports, for example, interoperability of EHRs that would not otherwise be able to share information. An HIE could collect data on hospital admissions for an entire state. This would allow a state Department of Health to identify trends in illnesses and injuries and better serve the public health. HIEs may include a way for clients to access their health information.

Dhopeshwarkar et al. (2012) asked consumers directly about their preferences for the use of their data on a HIE. In this study, interviewers spoke to 170 consumers in New York and asked them about their preferences for sharing their health information. Eighty-six percent wanted safeguards to protect their health information. The same percent wanted the ability to see who has viewed their information. Half the respondents trust their physician clinic to safeguard their health information, but only 7% trusted hospitals and 7% trusted the government to protect their health information. About one-third of respondents were uncomfortable with having information from their EHR automatically included in an HIE (Dhopeshwarkar et al., 2012). The results of this study provide evidence that consumers want their health information to be protected, but are not very trusting of some healthcare providers to do a good job protecting that information. As practitioners, we need to do what we can to earn the trust of our clients by doing our best to protect their health information.

▼ LOCATING AND ENTERING INFORMATION IN AN EHR ▼

EHRs are databases that organize the data so that it is easy, when using the right terms, to locate the information and add information to the record. Databases depend on users to use consistent terminology. A common system of clinical terminology, a nomenclature, used in EHRs is the Systematized Nomenclature of Medicine-Clinical Terms (SNOMED-CT), which has over 300,000 healthcare concepts organized into 18 hierarchical categories in it (Philar & Carter, 2008). MEDCIN, a product of Medicomp Systems, Inc., is another nomenclature that has over 270,000 healthcare concepts in six broad categories (Gartee, 2011). MEDCIN is designed by physicians for physicians (Medicomp Systems, Inc., 2012). Both systems allow users to enter and retrieve data in a standardized way. With two different systems, each with different nomenclatures, you can see how it would be difficult for the systems to talk to each other.

Every EHR system is organized a little differently. It takes time to learn how to enter data so that it can be retrieved by other users. Once a practitioner learns to use one EHR system, it becomes easier to learn new EHR systems. Each system generally has a toolbar on the top of the screen that contains words or icons for quick access to functions (Gartee, 2011). There may be additional navigation tools along the left side of the screen (Gartee, 2011).

Each EHR system has its own ways of locating and entering information into the EHR. Figure 12.2 shows an example of one system that uses the MEDCIN nomenclature. The data that is entered into these systems and stored there fall into one of three categories (Gartee, 2011). The first data type is digital images. This includes digitized images such as those from x-rays, CAT scans, and MRI images. The second kind is text; words typed into the system or imported from an external source. Finally, there is discrete data. Discrete data are the checklist and other preestablished data. Discrete data is faster for the occupational therapy practitioner to enter, but can also be limiting. Text takes longer to enter and is harder to search when using the EHR to improve practice (Gartee, 2011).

From a practical standpoint, an occupational therapy practitioner will usually enter information into the EHR either at the end of a session with a client, or between sessions. Because there is not a lot of time available for documentation, the notes need to be concise.

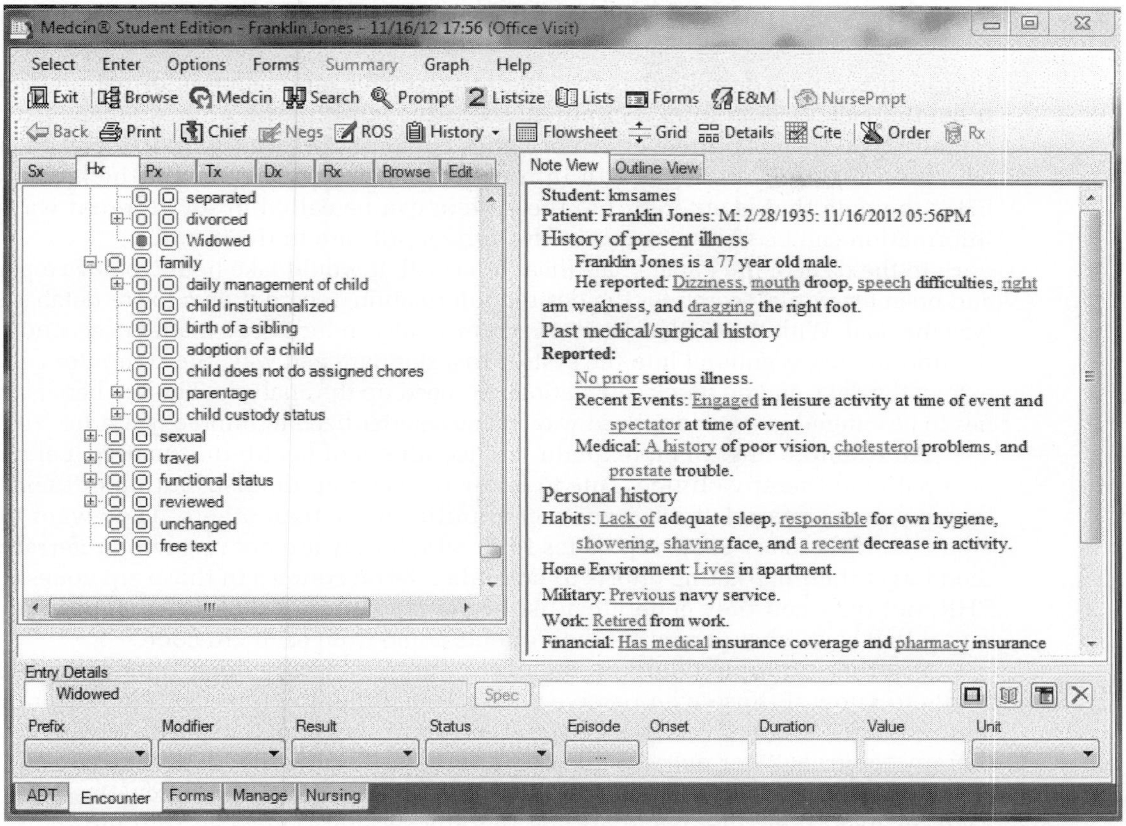

FIGURE 12.2 Screen shot of an electronic health record.

Usually, the documentation system will contain both discrete data and text. In many clinics, the occupational therapy practitioner will use a handheld device such as a smartphone or tablet computer. For larger documents, such as evaluation reports or discharge summaries, the occupational therapist will typically enter them into the system at the end of the day or during times when clients are not scheduled.

▼ MEANINGFUL USE ▼

Meaningful use is the term used to describe the set of standards that govern the use of EHRs established by the Centers for Medicare and Medicaid Services (CMS) Incentive Programs (CMS, 2012). It is not enough to just use an EHR system to document care, the hospital or clinic has to show that it is being used to change the way that information about that care is used to improve care delivery.

Starting in 2011, there are three stages of meaningful use implementation. The first stage is data capturing and sharing, stage two is advanced clinical processes, and stage three is improved outcomes (CMS, 2012). In stage one, there are specific core requirements that must be met, along with at least five objectives selected from a menu of ten possible objectives. In stage two, there are additional core requirements and objectives. By the time all three stages are implemented, CMS expects to see improvements on clinical quality measures. What is important about the implementation of meaningful use is that the EHR system is being used for more than just entering clinical notes; it is being used to improve care to individuals and improve the health outcomes of populations.

▼ INFORMATICS AND QUALITY IMPROVEMENT ▼

Informatics can be described as the obtaining, storing, and using information (Hersh, 2009). It combines concepts from computer, cognitive, and information sciences (Byrne, 2012). Usually, you will hear the word informatics combined with another word, such as biomedical, nursing, consumer or health informatics. Informatics is one of the advantages of an EHR; the data that is entered into the system can be called up in different ways, and that information can be used to improve the delivery of care in the future.

In the days of the paper chart (health record), it would take hours to have a person locate and open every file, search for the desired information, record it on a log or database, then analyze the data. With the EHR, that time is dramatically reduced to a matter of seconds. Assuming the information is entered into the system in a standardized way, the computer can locate and extract the data, and do quick calculations to speed up the analysis. The key here is that the data has to be entered in a standardized way, using standardized terminology (Carter, 2008).

An example might help explain the usefulness of health informatics. Let's say that an occupational therapy clinic wants to know the geographic distribution of their clients; do they get more referrals from some communities more than others. They want this data by zip code. If there are some zip codes from which they are not receiving referrals, they will then target their marketing efforts to possible referral sources in those zip codes. Using their EHR, not only can they generate a list of the zip codes of their clients, but they can get a report that says what percent of their clients come from each zip code.

Another example could be the occupational therapy department in a hospital that wants to know if those who receive occupational therapy intervention within 24 hours of admission for a right CVA have a shorter length of stay than those who receive occupational therapy referrals 25 or more hours after admission. Using the EHR, they can call up all the right CVAs admitted in the last year, their admission dates and times, the dates and times each received their first occupational therapy session. They can find out the percent that received occupational therapy within 24 hours, the percent that received occupational therapy 25 or more hours after admission, and the percent that never received any occupational therapy services, and the average length of stay for each group. If the percent that received occupational therapy within 24 hours is not as high as they would like, they may now have proof that early referrals to occupational therapy reduces lengths of stay. The occupational therapy department can then generate a plan for how to get referrals earlier.

When data is used to improve the delivery of health care, it is called quality improvement. Data can be monitored and when a particular practice is found to result in improved clinical outcomes or reduced costs, or both, that practice can then be replicated improving the clinical outcomes of others.

EHRs improve health outcomes in several ways. One way is by standardizing care. This is done through the use of clinical pathways that require a provider to justify any deviation from what is considered to be best practice. Another way is by creating alerts that identify potential adverse reactions before they occur; for example, by automatically flagging potentially disastrous drug interactions or flashing a warning when a drug is prescribed to a patient who is allergic to that kind of drug (Silow-Carroll, Edwards, & Rodin, 2012). The EHR can prompt providers to follow certain guideline, for example, for infection control, thus reducing infection rates and lowering the cost of care (Silow-Carroll et al., 2012). Once staff become efficient at using the EHR, it can reduce the time spent documenting, and increase the time staff spend with clients (Silow-Carroll et al., 2012). Finally, by reviewing the data provided by the EHR, problem areas can be identified and quality improvement efforts directed toward solving the problem (Silow-Carroll et al., 2012).

SUMMARY

In this chapter, the history, purpose, and rationale of the EHR were discussed.

The EHR is here to stay and its use is spreading rapidly. Digital images, text, and discrete data can be entered in the EHR through desktop or laptop computers, or handheld devices such as tablets or smartphones. Regardless of the type of device used to access the

EHR, there are ways to use it that put clients at ease, and reduce client cooperation and destroy rapport with the client.

In addition to recording and storing clinical records, EHR systems can be used to improve quality of care delivery. Meaningful use assures that the EHR is more than just a repository for the historical record of care. Quality improvement can occur because the EHR can reduce errors, provide outcome data that can be used to improve care delivery, and provide templates for the standardized delivery of care based on the best evidence available.

REFERENCES

American Health Information Management Association [AHIMA]. (2009). *Analysis of healthcare confidentiality, privacy, and security: Provisions of the American Recovery and Reinvestment Act of 2009 PL111-5.* Retrieved from http://library.ahima.org/xpedio/groups/public/documents/ahima/bok1_044016.pdf

American Health Information Management Association [AHIMA]. (2012). *Health care reform and health IT stimulus: ARRA and HITECH.* Retrieved from http://www.ahima.org/advocacy/arrahitech.aspx

American Medical Association [AMA]. (2010). *HIPAA violation leads to jail time.* Retrieved from http://www.ama-assn.org/amednews/2010/06/07/bisb0607.htm

Baker, L.H., Reifsteck, S.W., & Mann, W.R. (2003). Connected: Communication skills for nurses using the electronic medical record. *Nursing Economics, 21,* 85–87.

Byrne, M. (2012). *Informatics 101 module.* Internally published learning module. St. Paul, MN: St. Catherine University.

Carter, J.H. (2008). What is the electronic health record? In J.H. Carter (Ed.), *Electronic health records: A guide for clinicians and administrators* (2nd ed., pp. 3–19). Philadelphia, PA: American College of Physicians Press.

CDC. (2012). QuickStats: Percentage of physicians with electronic Health Record (EHR) Systems That Meet Federal Standards,* by Physician Specialty—Physician Workflow Survey, United States, *2011 Mortality and Morbidity Weekly, 61,* 710. Retrieved from http://www.cdc.gov/mmwr/preview/mmwrhtml/mm6135a4.htm?s_cid=mm6135a4_w

CMS. (2012). *Meaningful use.* Retrieved from http://www.healthit.gov/policy-researchers-implementers/meaningful-use-regulations

Danielson, D. (2011). *Iowa launches investigation into unauthorized access of medical records of football players.* Retrieved from http://www.radioiowa.com/2011/01/28/iowa-launches-investigation-into-unauthorized-access-of-medical-records-of-football-players/

Dhopeshwarkar, R.V., Kern, L.M., O'Donnell, H.C., Edwards, A.M., & Kaushal, R. (2012). Health care consumers' preferences around health information exchange. *Annals of Family Medicine, 10*(5), 428–434. doi:10.1370/afm.1396

Gartee, R. (2007). *Electronic health records: Understanding and using computerized medical records* (2nd ed.). Upper Saddle River, NJ: Pearson Education.

HealthIT.gov. (2012a). *Health information exchange.* Retrieved from http://www.healthit.gov/providers-professionals/health-information-exchange

HealthIT.gov. (2012b). *We can't wait: Obama administration takes new steps to encourage doctors and hospitals to use health information technology to lower costs, improve quality, create jobs.* Retrieved from http://www.healthit.gov/achieving-MU/ONC_Encourage_HealthIT_FS.PDF

HealthIT.gov. (n.d.). *Dottie Bringle RN.* Retrieved from http://www.healthit.gov/profiles/natural-disaster/medical-records

Hersh, W. (2009). A stimulus to define informatics and health information technology. *BMC Medical Informatics & Decision Making, 9*(1), 1–6. doi:10.1186/1472-6947-9-24

HIT. (2012). *Fact sheet: HITECH progress.* Retrieved from http://www.healthit.gov/ achieving-MU/ONC_Encourage_HealthIT_FS.PDF

Institute for Medicine [IOM]. (2011). *Patient safety.* Retrieved from http://www.iom.edu/ Activities/Quality/PatientSafetyHIT/~/media/Files/Report%20Files/2011/Health-IT/ HIT%20and%20Patient%20Safety.pdf

Lauretsen, J. (2011). *Allina fires 32 employees for snooping at patient records.* Retrieved from http://minnesota.cbslocal.com/2011/05/06/allina-fires-32-employees-for-snooping-at-patient-records/

Medicomp Systems, Inc. (2012). *At Medicomp the future is already here.* Retrieved from http://www.medicomp.com/company/ONC. (2010). *Certification and EHR incentives.* Retrieved from http://healthit.hhs.gov/portal/server.pt?CommunityID=3002&spaceID= 48&parentname=&control=SetCommunity&parentid=&in_hi_userid=11673&PageID=0& space=CommunityPage

ONC. (2012). *Update on the adoption of health information technology and related efforts to facilitate the electronic use and exchange of health information: A report to congress.* Retrieved from http://healthit.hhs.gov/portal/server.pt/gateway/ PTARGS_0_0_4383_1239_15610_43/http%3B/wci-pubcontent/publish/onc/public_ communities/p_t/resources_and_public_affairs/reports/reports_portlet/files/ january2012__update_on_hit_adoption_report_to_congress.pdf

Orenstein, C. (2008). *Hospital to punish snooping on Spears: UCLA moves to fire at least 13 for looking at the celebrity's records.* Retrieved from http://articles.latimes.com/2008/ mar/15/local/me-britney15

Rogers, M. (2005). *Hurricanes, health records and you.* Retrieved August 27, 2006 from http://msnbc.msn.com/id/9431650/

Sebelius, K. (2012). HHS Secretary Kathleen Sebelius announces major progress in doctors' hospital use of health information technology. Retrieved from http://www.hhs. gov/news/press/2012pres/02/20120217a.html

Shamus, E. & Stern, D. (2011). *Effective documentation for physical therapy professionals* (2nd ed.). New York, NY: McGraw Hill Medical.

Silow-Carroll, S., Edwards, J.N., & Rodin, D. (2012). *Using electronic health records to improve quality and efficiency: The experiences of leading hospitals.* The Commonwealth Fund, July 2012. Retrieved from http://www.commonwealthfund.org/Publications/ Issue-Briefs/2012/Jul/Using-EHRs-to-Improve-Quality-and-Efficiency.aspx

Tieman, J. (2004). Lurching into the future: Bush sets 2014 goal for EMR's, calls for incentives. *Modern Healthcare, 34*(18), 18.

Visit **www.pearsonhighered.com/healthprofessionsresources** to access the student resources that accompany this book. Simply select Occupational Therapy from the choice of disciplines. Find this book and you will find the complimentary study tools created for this specific title.

CHAPTER 13

Client Identification: Referral and Screening

INTRODUCTION

There are several different ways in which occupational therapy practitioners can discover that they have a new client. Depending on the setting in which the occupational therapy practitioners work, they can find out by phone, fax, a conversation in a hallway, or by a computer alert system (in the EHR). This notification usually comes in the form of a referral or an order.

▼ REFERRALS ▼

A referral is a suggestion from someone that a particular client would benefit from occupational therapy services. Occupational therapists can receive referrals from almost anyone. A parent can call up and refer a child for services. A nurse can refer a client who is struggling to stay in his or her home despite failing health. A chiropractor can refer a client who needs work on body mechanics. A dentist can refer a client with severe jaw pain. A physical therapist, teacher, nursing assistant, or any other person working with someone who has or is at risk of having an occupational performance deficit can make a referral for occupational therapy services. There are no national rules or regulations preventing an occupational therapist from receiving referrals from anyone. However, third-party payers, such as managed care organizations and governmental reimbursement systems, often will not pay for services provided to a client with only a referral, unless the referral comes from a physician. State licensure laws may also govern whether or not referrals are required, and if so, who may write the referral.

▼ ROLE DELINEATION FOR REFERRALS AND ORDERS ▼

The AOTA has established standards for referrals. These can be found in the *Standards of Practice for Occupational Therapy* (2010a) on the AOTA Web site. These standards require that occupational therapists are responsible for receiving and responding to referrals (and orders). *The Standards of Practice* (2010a) also require occupational therapists to refer clients to other practitioners (other occupational therapists with specific expertise or other professionals) when a client needs a provider with expertise beyond his or her own. This is also a standard in the AOTA Code of Ethics (2010b). In order to ensure appropriate referrals or orders, it is incumbent upon both the occupational therapist and the occupational therapy assistant to educate referral sources on the appropriateness of referrals or orders for occupational therapy services (AOTA, 2010a). The AOTA standards do not recommend that occupational therapy assistants receive or respond to referrals or orders (AOTA, 2010a).

▼ ORDERS ▼

An order is a referral written by a physician. It is like a prescription. Just as a pharmacy must fill a prescription written by a licensed physician, an occupational therapist must comply with a physician's order. Many people use the phrase "physician referral" rather than "physician order"; in fact the AOTA (2010a) prefers the term "physician referral." If a client is referred to occupational therapy, often an order from a physician (or nurse practitioner, chiropractor, optometrist, or other legally defined health care professional, depending on state licensure and payer regulations) is required in order to get paid for providing services. There is no national requirement that says occupational therapy practitioners need a physician's order or referral before providing services. Some state licensure laws and some payers require a physician's order for an occupational therapist to see a client.

If an occupational therapist receives a referral for occupational therapy services, and talks to the referral source to find out why the referral was made, the occupational therapist can then contact the physician and ask for an order (or referral). When contacting a busy physician, the occupational therapist needs to have a pretty solid idea of why the client would benefit from occupational therapy evaluation and intervention. Remember SBAR in Chapter 1 of this text? This would be a good situation in which to use SBAR when talking to the physician. In fact, whether or not a busy physician is involved, the occupational therapist and occupational therapy assistant need to clearly understand and articulate why occupational therapy services would be beneficial for every client served by occupational therapy. An occupational therapist who observes a client or does a screening and thinks occupational therapy services would benefit the client can initiate an order by contacting the physician (or other legally defined licensed health care professional) and discussing the ways in which occupational therapy services could benefit the physician's client.

It is up to the occupational therapist, using his or her best clinical judgment, to determine if the referral or order for occupational therapy is appropriate. It is also up to the occupational therapist to determine if additional orders are needed. For example, I have seen orders come through to a rehabilitation department (occupational therapy, physical therapy, and speech-language pathology) for physical therapy for activities of daily living (ADLs). The physical therapy staff hand the order to the occupational therapy department and have the occupational therapists call the doctor to explain that it is occupational therapy that works on ADLs and request that the doctor change the order. Conversely, I have seen orders come through for occupational therapy to provide diversional activities. Generally speaking, third-party payers do not pay for diversional activities, so it behooves the occupational therapist to discuss the situation with the physician and determine if the client has occupational performance issues. The occupational therapist should also consider whether a referral to recreation therapy might be more appropriate for the client than occupational therapy.

Physician orders (referrals) should contain certain information. The order (referral) should specify the full name of the client, the date, and time the order was written, the full name and credentials of the physician (or equivalent according to state law and payer requirements), the reason for the referral (order), and the frequency and the duration of occupational therapy services. Frequency refers to how often the intervention sessions will occur. Duration refers to how long it is expected to take to meet the needs of the client. Some settings also require intensity of intervention to be included in the order. Intensity refers to the length of time for any one session. An order (referral) for occupational therapy services six times a week (frequency) for 3 weeks (duration) of 30-minute sessions twice a day (intensity) would satisfy this part of the requirements. If any of these factors are missing, and they often are, the occupational therapist is responsible for contacting the physician to clarify the orders. Sometimes, the occupational therapist completes the evaluation, then, on the basis of the results of the evaluation, contacts the physician to clarify the frequency, intensity, and duration. These are called clarification orders. Some occupational therapists prefer a vague order, such as a simple "OT to eval and treat" order, feeling that it is up to the occupational therapy professional to determine the best course of action to take. Figure 13.1 shows how a referral might look if it was found in an EHR.

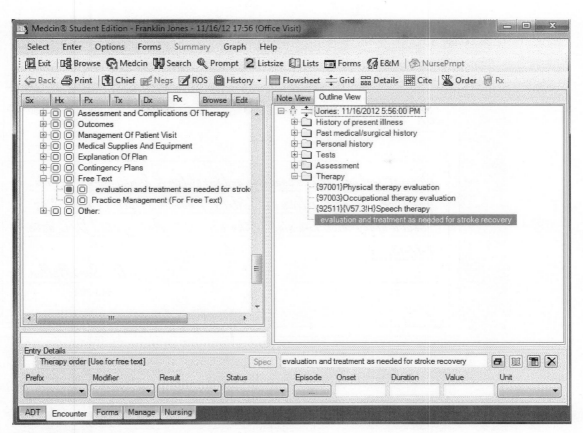

FIGURE 13.1 Order for Occupational Therapy.

An ongoing order is often needed for continued payment for services, especially from third-party payers. Having the client's physician sign the plan of care (intervention plan) serves as ongoing orders. Medicare identifies this process as certification and recertification (CMS, 2008). Medicare requires this recertification every 90 days for anyone receiving outpatient occupational therapy (Part B), and the physician has the right to make any changes to the care plan that the physician deems necessary (Centers for Medicare and Medicaid Services [CMS], 2008).

▼ SCREENINGS ▼

Often, but not always, a screening occurs at the first meeting of occupational therapist and client. A screening is a brief, hands-off check of a client to see if further evaluation or intervention is warranted. It is often based on observations of a client and chart review without the direct intervention of an occupational therapy practitioner. Screenings are generally not reimbursable, but can be a good way to identify potential clients for reimbursable services. In most situations, a screening can be done without a physician referral or order. If there is an order for occupational therapy, a screening may simply be a quick chart review before beginning the full evaluation of the client.

In some settings, the occupational therapist routinely screens potential clients. This is referred to as a type I screening (Collier, 1991). For example, an occupational therapist working in a nursing home might screen all new admissions to the facility, or an occupational therapist in private practice might screen visitors to a local health fair. Then, if the screening demonstrates a need for occupational therapy services, an order can be obtained.

Exercise 13.1

Identify the parts of these referrals:

1.

7-10-08 0803		Gertrude Silverstein #SIL439855GE Room 408B

Occupational therapy to evaluate and treat for R hemisphere CVA bid for 1 wk. Focus on ADLs and IADLs. Provide adaptive equiment as needed along with training in the use of it. Anticipated D/C date 7-17-13.

Dr. Sara Bellar
#5843-392

_____ Date of referral _____ Name of physician
_____ Name of client _____ Frequency
_____ Duration   _____ Intensity

_____ Reason for referral

Is this an adequate referral?   yes   no
Why or why not?

2.

Kyle Beback May 31, 2013

OT to eval and treat

Dr. Don Touchme
#5883-1202

_____ Date of referral _____ Name of physician
_____ Name of client _____ Frequency
_____ Duration   _____ Intensity

_____ Reason for referral

Is this an adequate referral?   yes   no
Why or why not?

ASSESSMENT: Specific tools or instruments that are used during the evaluation process.

EVALUATION: The process of obtaining and interpreting data necessary for intervention. This includes planning for and documenting the evaluation process and results.

RE-EVALUATION: The process of critical analysis of client response to intervention. This analysis enables the therapist to make any necessary changes to intervention plan in collaboration with the client.

SCREENING: Obtaining and reviewing data relevant to a potential client to determine the need for further evaluation and intervention.

FIGURE 13.2 Key AOTA Terms, Defined.

Source: AOTA (2010a, p. S107).

In other settings or at other times, the occupational therapist may only screen after receiving a referral. This is referred to as a type II screening (Collier, 1991).

A screening is not a substitute for an evaluation. Chapter 14 explores evaluations more thoroughly. Evaluations are more thorough and specific than screenings and are reimbursable. It may be tempting at times to use a screening as a substitute for a complete evaluation when time is of the essence. Do not do it. A screening is not adequate for accurately determining a client's strengths and need areas, or for developing goals. See Figure 13.2 for AOTA definition of screening and related terms; see Figure 13.3 for Medicare's definition of screening and related terms. As mentioned in Chapter 4, the word "assessment" means screening in some settings, and is used as a synonym for evaluation in other settings. The AOTA Standards of Practice (2010a) make it clear that the term assessment is not

---

ASSESSMENT is separate from evaluation, and is included in services or procedures (it is not separately payable). The term assessment as used in Medicare manuals related to therapy services is distinguished from language in Current Procedural Terminology (CPT) codes that specify assessment, e.g., 97755, Assistive Technology Assessment, which may be payable). Assessments shall be provided only by clinicians, because assessment requires professional skill to gather data by observation and patient inquiry and may include limited objective testing and measurement to make clinical judgments regarding the patient's condition(s). Assessment determines, for example, changes in the patient's status since the last visit/treatment day and whether the planned procedure or service should be modified. On the basis of these assessment data, the professional may make judgments about progress toward goals and/or determine that a more complete evaluation or reevaluation (see the definitions following this paragraph) is indicated. Routine weekly assessments of expected progression in accordance with the plan are not payable as reevaluations.

CERTIFICATION is the physician's/nonphysician practitioner's (NPP) approval of the plan of care. Certification requires a dated signature on the plan of care or some other document that indicates approval of the plan of care.

EVALUATION is a separately payable comprehensive service provided by a clinician, as defined above, that requires professional skills to make clinical judgments about conditions for which services are indicated based on objective measurements and subjective evaluations of patient performance and functional abilities. Evaluation is warranted, for example, for a new diagnosis or when a condition is treated in a new setting. These evaluative judgments are essential to development of the plan of care, including goals and the selection of interventions.

REEVALUATION provides additional objective information not included in other documentation. Reevaluation is separately payable and is periodically indicated during an episode of care when the professional assessment of a clinician indicates a significant improvement, or decline, or change in the patient's condition or functional status that was not anticipated in the plan of care. Although some state regulations and state practice acts require reevaluation at specific times, for Medicare payment, reevaluations must *also* meet Medicare coverage guidelines. The decision to provide a reevaluation shall be made by a clinician.

FIGURE 13.3 Key Medicare Terms, Defined.

Source: CMS, 2008, pp. 7–9.

interchangeable with screening or evaluation; however, other professions may use the terms differently. Be sure you know how the word is used at your facility/agency and for the reimbursement system used.

According to Collier (1991), there are several general guidelines for when to do screenings:

- Screenings are done only when you believe that the potential problems you will find in your screening can be positively affected by occupational therapy intervention. You do not want to conduct screenings for problems that are beyond occupational therapy's scope of practice. For example, you do not want to screen for problems with articulation of words; a speech-language pathologist would do that.
- Screenings are best done when they are timely, that is, they are done at a time when intervention would be effective. It sounds obvious, but you would not screen for developmental delays in high schoolers; you would screen for delays in preschoolers.
- There must be a reason to believe that the population you are screening will have some people who demonstrate the problem you are screening for. If you are screening a healthy population, you must expect that at least a small percentage of people will ultimately need your services.
- Occupational therapy intervention must be available to help alleviate the problems you identify. It makes no sense to provide screenings where or when there are no services available to work on the problems found.
- Finally, use screening methods that you believe are valid and reliable. This does not mean they need to be standardized, but that your methods are sensitive to finding persons with the problems you are looking for.

There are four possible outcomes of screenings. The first is that the client may, in fact, need occupational therapy intervention. The second is that the client does not need intervention right now, but there is enough concern that it would be worth rescreening in a few months (or whatever time period you think is appropriate). Next is the possibility that the client needs a referral to some other professional. Finally, the client may not need any intervention at all.

▼ ROLE DELINEATION FOR SCREENINGS ▼

The AOTA has established standards for screenings, which can be found in the *Standards of Practice for Occupational Therapy* (AOTA, 2010a). The occupational therapist is responsible for conducting the screening; however, an occupational therapy assistant, under the supervision of an occupational therapist, may contribute to the screening. The occupational therapist is responsible for selecting the proper tools and methods for screening. The AOTA (2009) *Guidelines for Supervision, Roles, and Responsibilities during the Delivery of Occupational Therapy Services* say very clearly that the occupational therapist is responsible for determining the need for occupational therapy services, which is the purpose for doing a screening. Either the occupational therapist or an occupational therapy assistant, under the supervision of an occupational therapist, communicates the results of the screening results and recommendations to other members of the care team, or other appropriate persons (AOTA, 2010a).

▼ CONTACT NOTE ▼

A brief note is usually entered into the health record to acknowledge that the referral/order was received or that the screening took place. This note contains the date and time the referral was received, and when the client is scheduled to begin the evaluation. If you did a screening, the note should also contain the bottom-line results of the screening. Figure 13.4 contains two examples of contact notes for screenings.

1/14/13. 10:35 a.m. Order received today for occupational therapy evaluation and intervention for 3 weeks from Dr. Bush. Jacob Olson is a 21 year old male with tendonitis of R thumb; neck, back, and R arm pain. Client injured his thumb from playing video games, texting, and playing basketball. His thumb is currently immobilized and it is interfering with his daily occupations. Jake reports that he loves video games, and spends much of his non-basketball hours playing them. During a short interview, Jake said that since his thumb has been immobilized, he has watched others play video games, but has not participated himself, and he says he is bored. Jake said he is anxious to get back to basketball because he hopes to play in the NBA after college. He is currently a sports management major. Recommend a complete evaluation of areas of occupation as well as an ergonomic assessment of his work/play spaces.

K. Elemen, MA, OTR/L.

5/2/13. 10:35 a.m. Received referral on 5/1/13 for occupational therapy evaluation and intervention to improve self-care skills. Esse Teeyouvee is a retired librarian who fell on the ice outside her home and broke her L hip and radius. Chart review indicates she has a history of HBP and Afib. Hip precautions noted. She lives in a townhouse with her husband. Her husband was present for the screening. When asked to move her L arm, she showed limitations in ROM. Results of screening show that client would likely benefit from occupational therapy evaluation and intervention in areas of occupation. Evaluation scheduled for this afternoon.

O. Pequeare, OTD, OTR/L.

FIGURE 13.4 Examples of Contact Notes of Screenings.

The AOTA *Guidelines for Documentation of Occupational Therapy* (2013) recommend the content that should be included in documentation of screenings. Figure 13.5 shows the recommended content for contact notes following a screening. Remember that the screening not only includes your interaction with the client but data you review in the client's clinical record or EHR.

Contact notes are also used at other points during the occupational therapy process. The AOTA *Guidelines for Documentation of Occupational Therapy* (2013) recommend that all contacts between the occupational therapist or occupational therapy assistant and the client be documented, including telephone contacts and meetings with others. Missed sessions should be documented using a contact note (AOTA, 2013; Fremgen, 2002). AOTA (2013) guidelines further recommend that the occupational therapy practitioner should document client or caregiver training in a contact note, being sure to include the names of those present for the training and the client's response (if present).

Exercise 13.2

In which of the following situations would it be appropriate to do a screening?

1. A doctor's order comes to the occupational therapy department in an acute care hospital to evaluate a client.
2. You work in a hand therapy clinic. Your caseload has fallen off recently. There is a health fair coming to the strip mall across the street from your clinic. The health fair coordinator suggests that you offer free grip and pinch strength testing.
3. You have a friend who is a building supervisor for a new assisted living facility. She would like you to come once a month to screen all new residents for things like fall prevention and other safety concerns. The facility does not have occupational therapy staff on site. You work in a preschool nearby and have never worked with the elderly before.
4. A nurse asks you to look at a resident of the nursing home at which you work. The resident has been taking longer and longer to eat, and is now the last one to finish even though they serve him first. She asks you to observe the client while he eats lunch and tell her whether you think she should ask the doctor for orders for occupational therapy.

Content	Explanation
Client Information	Name Date of birth/age Gender Diagnoses or conditions Precautions and contraindications known at this time *Note:* Most of this information will be populated into the appropriate places automatically on an EHR
Referral Information	Name of referral source Date of referral Reason for referral Services requested Expected length of service Payer
Brief Occupational Profile	Record as much as you know about: • Reason client is seeking services • Strengths and areas in need of improvement • Contexts and environments supporting or hindering occupational performance • Occupational history • Medical, educational, and/or work history • Client priorities and goals
Assessments Used and Results	Describe how you got your information and what you found.
Recommendation	Professional judgments about next steps (e.g. conduct complete evaluation or not)

FIGURE 13.5 Contents of a Contact Note.
Source: AOTA (2013).

In many clinical settings, a contact note is written for each contact with a client, including each intervention session. These notes include specific intervention participation (type of intervention and client response to the intervention), significant communication to or from a client, modifications made to the environment or tasks, and/or any equipment (assistive or adaptive devices) fabricated or modified (AOTA, 2013). Some settings prefer a specific format such as SOAP, DAP, or narrative format (see Chapter 17).

▼ MEDICARE COMPLIANCE ▼

There are hundreds of potential payers for occupational therapy services. Each insurance company, managed care organization, state Medicaid program, or other state-run program sets its own standards for documentation. As a result, there are no clear national standards that meet the requirements of all these payers. Medicare, as a national insurance program, does set national standards for documentation, although the Medicare Administrative Contractors (MACs) may issue further policies on documentation. Since there are so many payers with individual standards for documentation, and the Medicare standards are often the most stringent of the payer standards, some people recommend using the Medicare standards as the minimum standard for documentation. Certainly in some settings, such as pediatric or some mental health clinics, the Medicare standards may not apply because Medicare is rarely the primary payer. Nonetheless, many payers look to Medicare and follow Medicare's lead for establishing documentation policies.

For the sake of clarity, Medicare defines terms used in its communication with providers. Refer to Figure 13.3 for a review of how Medicare defines the relevant terms. The full set of definitions and rules for outpatient occupational therapy documentation can be found on the Medicare Web site for practitioners (http://www.cms.hhs.gov) and excerpts are included in Appendix B (see website) of this textbook.

Medicare will only pay for services if there is proper documentation that supports the need for the services and justifies payment for those services (CMS, 2008). According to Medicare, Services are medically necessary if the documentation indicates they meet the requirements for medical necessity, including that they are skilled, rehabilitative services, provided by clinicians (or qualified professionals when appropriate) with the approval of a physician/NPP, safe, and effective (i.e., progress indicates that the care is effective in rehabilitation of function) (CMS, 2008, p.23).

In order for Medicare to pay for a service, such as occupational therapy, the service must meet certain requirements. The three main requirements are:

- The client must be under the care of a physician who certifies the plan of care (CMS, 2008, 2012).
- The services provided must require the skills of an occupational therapist or an occupational therapy assistant under the supervision of an occupational therapist. This means that the assessment, evaluation, and intervention require the knowledge, expertise, clinical judgment, decision making, and abilities of occupational therapy practitioners. A skilled occupational therapy practitioner may also be required out of concern for client safety. If an aide can do it, or a family member can do it, then it no longer requires a skilled occupational therapy practitioner, and Medicare will no longer pay for it (CMS, 2008).
- The services are the appropriate for the individual needs of the client. This means that the type of service, the frequency, the intensity, and the duration of the services are specific to the client's condition (CMS, 2008).
- A physician's order or referral is not required, however, in order to be paid, a physician must certify the plan of care (CMS, 2012).
- The certification of the plan of care may be by a physician or non-physician provider (e.g., nurse practitioner or physician assistant) (CMS, 2012).

Documentation for any Medicare client needs to show how the care provided meets all of these criteria. A payer should be able to read your documentation and see that your skills are required, that the care is appropriate, and that a physician has certified the plan of care (CMS, 2008, 2012). A screening can be done without a physician's order or referral, but an evaluation and ongoing intervention required an order/referral from a physician. An order/referral from a physician is evidence of physician involvement in the care of the client.

SUMMARY

The occupational therapist usually makes contact with a client after an order or referral is received for services. The referral can come from any source, including the client or the client's family, other health, social service, or education professionals or physicians. Most payers require either a referral or an order from a physician.

A screening is often the first contact an occupational therapy practitioner has with the client. Sometimes screenings are routinely done for all new admissions to a program or facility. Other times, screenings are conducted at the request of another health, social service, or education professional. Screenings are brief and are generally based on chart review, interview, and observations. A screening helps determine if a full-blown evaluation would be beneficial. A screening can occur before obtaining an order for occupational therapy services, or it can occur after receiving a referral or order.

A contact note is usually written to verify that the occupational therapist has received the referral or order, a screening was done, and to indicate whether further evaluation and/

or intervention will be necessary. In addition, a brief contact note may be written to document every subsequent contact the occupational therapist or occupational therapy assistant has with the client throughout the course of occupational therapy service delivery. The contact note documents communication with the client or client's caregiver as well as a description of the interventions implemented and the client's response to the intervention. Contact notes are also written to document reasons for missed sessions and the content of telephone conversations with the client.

REFERENCES

American Occupational Therapy Association [AOTA]. (2009). *Guidelines for supervision, roles, and responsibilities in the delivery of occupational therapy services.* Retrieved from http://www.aota.org/-/media/Corporate/Files/Secure/Practice/OfficialDocs/Guidelines/Guidelines%20for%20Supervision%20Roles%20and%20Responsibilities.pdf

American Occupational Therapy Association. (2010a). Standards of practice for occupational therapy [Supplemental material]. *American Journal of Occupational Therapy, 64,* S106–S111. doi:10.5014/ajot.2010.64S106

American Occupation Therapy Association. (2010b). Occupational therapy code of ethics—2010 [Supplemental material]. *American Journal of Occupational Therapy, 54,* S17–S26. doi:10.5014/ajot.2010.64S17

American Occupational Therapy Association. (2013). *Guidelines for documentation of occupational therapy.* Retrieved from http://www.aota.org/-/media/corporate/files/secure/practice/officialdocs/guidelines/guidelines%20for%20documentation.pdf

Centers for Medicare and Medicaid Services. (2008). *Pub100-02 Medicare benefit policy: Transmittal 88.* Retrieved May 8, 2008, from http://www.cms.hhs.gov/transmittals/downloads/R88BP.pdf

Centers for Medicare and Medicaid Services. (2012). *Physical, occupational, and speech therapy services.* Retrieved from http://www.cms.gov/Outreach-and-Education/Outreach/OpenDoorForums/Downloads/090512TherapyClaimsSlides.pdf

Collier, T. (1991). The screening process. In W. Dunn (Ed.), *Pediatric occupational therapy: Facilitating effective service provision* (pp. 10–33). Thorofare, NJ: Slack.

Fremgen, B. F. (2002). *Medical law and ethics.* Upper Saddle River, NJ: Prentice Hall.

Visit **www.pearsonhighered.com/healthprofessionsresources** to access the student resources that accompany this book. Simply select Occupational Therapy from the choice of disciplines. Find this book and you will find the complimentary study tools created for this specific title.

CHAPTER 14

Evaluation Reports

INTRODUCTION

The initial evaluation report is one of the most important documents that you will write. All of the other documents (e.g., progress notes, intervention plans, and discharge summaries) are dependent on a clear and valid initial evaluation report. Evaluation reports demonstrate the need for occupational therapy services. If a need for your services is not documented, why should anyone pay for them? Without documentation of an evaluation, it is difficult to identify the client's level of function prior to intervention. In other words, a baseline is needed from which you, other team members, and payers can see progress (Moyers & Dale, 2007).

This chapter focuses on the components of a well-written evaluation report. The evaluation report is dependent on the skills of the occupational therapist in collecting and interpreting data. This book does not cover specific instructions for conducting evaluations, nor will it recommend specific assessment tools. There are many resources available to occupational therapy practitioners that describe selecting and administering the proper assessment tool and interpreting the data gathered. This chapter assumes you have the data and now need to write about it.

▼ ROLE DELINEATION IN THE OCCUPATIONAL THERAPY EVALUATION PROCESS ▼

The occupational therapist is responsible for the occupational therapy evaluation process (American Occupational Therapy Association [AOTA], 2009, 2010). An occupational therapy assistant, under the supervision of an occupational therapist, may contribute to the process. Either an occupational therapist or an occupational therapy assistant may educate the client and others (as appropriate) about evaluation procedures and the reasons for the evaluation.

The occupational therapist determines the most appropriate assessment tools to use (AOTA, 2009, 2010). The occupational therapy practitioner administering the assessment is responsible for following established protocols for administration of standardized tests. The occupational therapist is responsible for summarizing, analyzing, and interpreting the data (AOTA, 2010). He or she also uses that information to develop an appropriate intervention plan based on the client's current functional status. The occupational therapist follows established guidelines for documentation of evaluation results in a time frame and format accepted by the facility/agency, payer requirements, applicable accreditation agency standards, and state and federal laws and regulations. Occupational therapy practitioners also follow confidentiality standards in communicating the results of the evaluation process to others involved in the care of the client. An occupational therapy assistant, under the supervision of an occupational therapist, may contribute to these processes (AOTA, 2010).

Finally, AOTA (2010) standards state that it is the occupational therapist that makes recommendations for evaluation or intervention by other professionals, based on the occupational therapy evaluation results. In practical terms, this means that the occupational therapist has ultimate responsibility for every stage of the evaluation process: directing the evaluation, interpreting the data, and developing the intervention plan (AOTA,

2009). However, an occupational therapy assistant can be a very valuable contributor to the evaluation process. As appropriate to the skill of the occupational therapy assistant and the condition of the client, the occupational therapist can delegate parts of the evaluation process to the occupational therapy assistant (AOTA, 2009, 2010). An occupational therapy assistant must demonstrate service competence when administering any part of the evaluation process, including standardized tests. State licensure laws may contain specific language describing criteria for delegation of duties to an occupational therapy assistant as well as the type and amount of supervision required. It is always prudent to check with your state's licensing authority for specific requirements (AOTA, 2010).

Evaluation is an ongoing process, not a one-time event. All information an occupational therapy practitioner receives, regardless of source, contributes to the evaluation including information provided on the referral and read in the client's chart. As occupational therapy practitioners observe clients during each occupational therapy session, all these observations contain data that can be used during reevaluations. In some settings, where the occupational therapy assistant is the primary deliverer of services, the occupational therapist will be dependent on the occupational therapy assistant to relay the information gathered during interventions for the reevaluation.

▼ CORE CONCEPTS OF EVALUATIONS ▼

Bass-Haugen (2010) identified three main purposes for doing an evaluation: Evaluations are done (1) to describe a client's current level of performance, (2) to select interventions and predict outcomes, and (3) to build theory that supports occupational science and occupational therapy. Most of the time, some kind of occupational therapy intervention will follow the evaluation. As a result, you will need to describe the unique circumstances of your client's situation, predict future function through goal setting, and establish a baseline from which future performance can be measured and compared.

Occasionally, an evaluation is completed and no intervention is needed. In this case, the evaluation serves as documentation of a client's function at that point in time. If another evaluation is completed at a later date, it can be compared to the previous evaluation, to see if functional skills have been gained or lost. If the occupational therapist is functioning in a consultant role, the evaluation may be written with the expectation that others will carry out the intervention. In this case, careful attention to the language of the evaluation report will be needed so that those charged with implementation will understand exactly what needs to be done.

Moyers and Dale (2007) identified the focus of the evaluation process as "the client's engagement in occupations to support participation in the community or in organizations." (p. 22). It would follow, then, that the focus of your evaluation report would be on engagement in occupations rather than on client factors that influence performance. The *Occupational Therapy Practice Framework-III* (AOTA, 2014) suggests that the evaluation process focuses on finding what the client wants to do, needs to do, used to do, and can do; and on identifying those factors that support or inhibit performance.

Both of these perspectives suggest a "top-down" approach to conducting the evaluation. A top-down approach considers occupational roles and performance first and then discerns the factors that contribute to the occupational performance (Stewart, 2001; Weinstock-Zlotnik & Hinojosa, 2004). The specific tasks that a person will need to do or wants to do are considered first; the specific "foundational skills (performance skills, performance patterns, context, activity demands, and client factors) are considered later" (Weinstock-Zlotnik & Hinojosa, 2004, p. 594).

Some models and frames of reference support the top-down approach; however, others support a "bottom-up" approach. In a bottom-up approach, the foundational factors are evaluated first; then occupational performance is addressed (Weinstock-Zlotnik & Hinojosa, 2004). The bottom-up approach calls for an examination of a client's assets and limitations first, under the assumption that, as the limitations are eliminated, reduced, or compensated for, the occupational performance will naturally improve (Weinstock-Zlotnik & Hinojosa, 2004).

TABLE 14.1   Examples of Top-Down and Bottom-Up Models and Frames of Reference

Top-Down	Bottom-Up
Canadian Model of Occupational Performance	Biomechanical
Contemporary Task Oriented	Cognitive Disabilities
Ecology of Human Performance	Neurodevelopmental Treatment
Model of Human Occupation	Proprioceptive Neuromuscular Facilitation
Person Environment Occupational Performance	Sensory Integration

This may be the most reasonable approach to take in some settings, such as in an intensive care unit (ICU) where the patient may not be able to respond verbally, but needs a splint made in order to prevent contractures from developing. Table 14.1 provides examples of top-down and bottom-up models and frames of reference, but it is not intended to be a comprehensive listing.

It is important to base one's evaluation process on a particular model or frame of reference. It gives you a starting point and direction in which to proceed. The model or frame of reference will guide the critical thinking of the occupational therapist in the selection of evaluation methods and assessment tools, as well as the language by which the occupational therapist will describe occupational performance strengths and deficits. Refer to Chapter 5 of this book for further discussion on the influence of models and frames of reference.

Two of the most prominent concepts driving contemporary occupational therapy practice are evidence-based practice and client-centered practice (Hinojosa, Kramer, & Christ, 2010). Evidence-based practice means that, to the extent possible, you must be prepared to show that your interpretation of the data collected and plan for intervention are supported by both the client's needs and research. Being client-centered means that the client is a full partner in the evaluation process (Law, Baum, & Dunn, 2001). As a partner, the client's subjective experiences, as well as the occupational therapist's objective observations and measurements, are both critical to the evaluation process. The establishment of occupational therapy outcomes (goals) is a collaborative effort between the client and occupational therapist. The client's subjective experiences are reflected in the occupational profile, and the objective observations and measurements are reflected in the analysis of occupational performance (AOTA, 2014).

Hinojosa and Kramer (2010) identify several philosophical and theoretical influences on the evaluation process. The first is that the evaluation process is ongoing throughout the service delivery continuum and it is a dynamic and interactive process. It starts with the occupational therapist's first contact with the client. Once the initial evaluation is completed, reevaluation begins. Second, the data collected should "shed light on how to facilitate engagement in personally meaningful activities and occupations that will fulfill life roles" (Hinojosa & Kramer, 2010, p. 25). Next, we know that assessment tools can have biases and so can the people who administer them. Assessment tools can have biases in terms of gender, culture, geographic region, educational level, or socioeconomic status of the test taker. Test administrators, including occupational therapists, can carry expectations, personal prejudices, and preconceived notions into the testing situation. Of course, it is hoped that assessment tools that are selected are as free of bias as possible, and that occupational therapists try to not let biases influence the way they administer the test or interpret it. Next, the client's perspective, as well as that of the client's family and caregivers, is incorporated into the evaluation process. Finally, the evaluation process is based on relevant theories and frames of reference (Hinojosa & Kramer, 2010).

▼ THE EVALUATION PROCESS ▼

The process of evaluation has many steps. These steps are spelled out nicely in the *Guide to Occupational Therapy Practice* by Moyers and Dale (2007) and in the *The Occupational Therapy Practice Framework-III* (AOTA, 2014). Remember that the term evaluation refers to a process, while the term assessment refers to a tool used to gather information for the evaluation (AOTA, 2010). The process of evaluation includes planning the approach, gathering data, interpreting the data, hypothesizing, setting goals, and planning intervention. Moyers and Dale (2007) suggest nine distinct steps in the evaluation process. Figure 14.1 illustrates this process.

The first step is to synthesize the information that is shared during the occupational profile (AOTA, 2014; Moyers & Dale, 2007). This will allow the occupational therapist to focus on the areas of occupation and the contexts in which the occupations occur for the rest of the evaluation process.

Next, the occupational therapist determines the theoretical approach he or she will employ to guide his or her thinking through the rest of the process (AOTA, 2014; Moyers & Dale, 2007). This requires the occupational therapist to use clinical reasoning skills, and evidence-based practice concepts. The theoretical approach or combination of approaches will shape not only the evaluation process, but the interventions and outcomes of occupational therapy as well.

The third step involves observing and documenting the client's performance in the occupations and activities that are important to the client (AOTA, 2014; Moyers & Dale, 2007). In addition to observing the client while engaged in occupations, this step includes reviewing information provided by the occupational therapy assistant or others who have

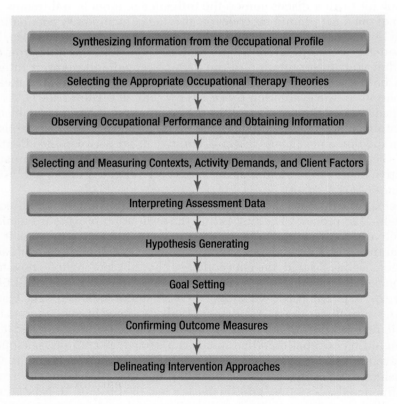

FIGURE 14.1   Steps in the Occupational Therapy Evaluation Process.

observed the client's performance. The focus is on the occupation, the effectiveness of the occupational performance, and the client's satisfaction with the effectiveness of the occupational performance. Time will not allow the occupational therapy practitioners to observe the client engage in every possible occupation that might be of concern, so some prioritization is necessary. Target the ones that are of the greatest concern to the client or the client's caregivers (AOTA, 2014; Moyers & Dale, 2007).

Next, the occupational therapist selects the assessments that will be used (AOTA, 2014; Moyers & Dale, 2007). Either the occupational therapist or occupational therapy assistant, under the supervision of the occupation therapist, then uses the assessments to measure the client factors, contexts, and activity demands. The assessments may be formal tests with specific protocols, or they may be informal, depending on the client's situation and needs.

The fifth step requires the clinical reasoning skills of the occupational therapist. In this step, the assessment data is interpreted so that a clear picture of the supports and barriers to effective occupational performance are identified (AOTA, 2014; Moyers & Dale, 2007). The test manual of a standardized test will provide some guidance for proper interpretation of test results. AOTA (2013) suggests expressing one's confidence in the test results. This can be accomplished by stating whether test scores are consistent with observed behavior. For example, a test may show that a client has poor muscle strength, yet the client is observed using that muscle against gravity during dressing. Or a test could show that a client is not able to follow three-step directions, but during an activity in the occupational therapy room, the client complied perfectly when you asked him to "pick that up, put it on the shelf over there, and then come back and sit in that chair." The results need to be summarized and must relate clearly to the occupational profile (AOTA, 2013).

The next step may blend in with the last one without a clear separation. In this step, the occupational therapist hypothesizes about the client's strengths and weaknesses/need areas in occupational performance (AOTA, 2014; Moyers & Dale, 2007). The weaknesses/need areas will be targeted during intervention planning (next step), and the strengths will be incorporated into the intervention methodology.

In the seventh step, the occupational therapist develops long- and short-term goals for the client to address the weaknesses/needs and the client's desired outcomes (AOTA, 2014; Moyers & Dale, 2007). This happens in collaboration with the client or client's caregivers. The collaboration is a key element in client-centered care.

Next, the outcome measures are confirmed (AOTA, 2014; Moyers & Dale, 2007). The outcome measures are used to determine when therapy will no longer be needed. Outcomes can reflect the client's occupational performance, satisfaction with performance, role competence, adaptation, health and wellness, or quality of life (AOTA, 2014; Moyers & Dale, 2007).

Finally, potential intervention approaches are identified (AOTA, 2014; Moyers & Dale, 2007). These will reflect the theoretical approaches embraced by the occupational therapist and shown to be effective for clients with similar needs. The clinician should be prepared to demonstrate that there is evidence to support his or her planned interventions.

▼ COMPONENTS OF AN EVALUATION REPORT ▼

Evaluations vary in many ways. Some are comprehensive; some are problem specific; some use standardized, formal assessments; some use nonstandardized, informal, activity-based evaluations. There are checklists and self-reporting tools. Documentation of evaluation results may be referred to by different terms: assessment summary report, evaluation summary, evaluation report, evaluation note, or assessment report and plan. In this book, the term "evaluation report" is used.

As with all clinical documentation, certain elements must be present in an evaluation report. Besides the usual identification information (client name, date of birth, gender, and diagnoses), the reason for the referral, when the referral was made and who made the referral, and the type/amount of service requested are also included (AOTA, 2013). Assessment tools used in the evaluation process are listed and references are made to other reports, such as the physician's history and physical examination or client intake forms used by the occupational therapist. Precautions and contraindications that could interfere with or cause problems during occupational therapy evaluation and intervention are clearly stated. Examples of precautions and contraindications are that the client could not find his or her own way out of the building in case of a fire, that the client's blood pressure drops dangerously low when seated at a 90° angle, or that the client is combative. Each of these is something any occupational therapy staff member who works with clients or transports them to the clinic needs to know.

Listing the appropriate diagnoses is not as easy as it sounds. You need to identify which condition (there usually is more than one diagnosis, often identified by the referral source) the occupational therapy interventions are being designed to address. If a client has an upper respiratory infection, diabetes, chemical dependency, and a broken hip, which one is the primary condition you are addressing? The term "diagnosis" is used primarily to satisfy third-party payers. In nonmedical settings, a primary concern or occupational performance deficit may be used instead of a medical diagnosis.

A critical section of the evaluation report is the occupational profile. In this section of the evaluation report, the occupational therapist describes the "client's occupational history and experiences, patterns of daily living, interests, values, and needs" (AOTA, 2014, p. S13). The occupational therapist is trying to understand, from the client's perspective, what the client wants and needs. This requires using a client-centered approach. The occupational therapist needs a solid understanding of the client's past experiences and contexts, current occupational strengths and areas that are problematic, and priorities/desired outcomes (AOTA, 2014). In addition to gaining valuable insight into the unique situation of your client, discussing the client's situation with him or her helps to build rapport and establish a therapeutic relationship necessary for collaboration with the client throughout the occupational therapy process (AOTA, 2014).

In addition to the occupational profile, an essential part of the evaluation is the analysis of occupational performance (AOTA, 2014). In the analysis of occupational performance, the performance skills, performance patterns, client factors, and contexts that affect occupational performance are identified and prioritized. The focus of the analysis of occupational performance is on gathering and interpreting data from assessment tools. It is important to note that the occupational profile and analysis of occupational performance may be performed sequentially or concurrently (AOTA, 2014).

Gathering data for an evaluation occurs primarily in three ways.

1. Observation of occupational performance

2. Interviewing the client and the client's caregivers

3. Selecting, administering, and interpreting assessment tools

Some evaluation reports will also include the initial intervention plan in the form of long- and short-term goals; intervention approaches and methodology; the anticipated frequency, duration, and intensity of occupational therapy services; and recommendations for other services. Goal writing is addressed in Chapter 15, and intervention planning is covered in Chapter 16.

To illustrate the evaluation process, let's pick a client to evaluate.

Case: Jacob Olsen

Jacob "Jake" Olsen is a 20-year-old college basketball star. He is a junior at a major Big Ten school. He has been a starting forward since his freshman year. Since this school has a large athletic department, there are university employees whose only job is to see that the student athletes pass all their courses. Jake loves playing basketball, but not studying for classes, so he appreciates these "tutors." One of the tutors will even write his papers for him since she is paid to type them anyway; she just recycles papers she has typed for other athletes. Jake's other love is computer games. When he is not sleeping, eating, or on the basketball court, he is leaning over his laptop computer (he is a tall man, while the desks are at heights for normal people), playing galactic battle–type games with his thumbs on the controller. Over time the hours and hours he spent bent over and pressing the buttons on the controller with his thumbs and texting with his thumbs have taken their toll on his neck, shoulders, wrist, and thumb. He has pain from his neck to his thumb on his shooting arm. The pain in his thumb has gotten so bad that the athletic trainer advised him to see the team physician. He was diagnosed with "game playing thumb," a combination of tendonitis and osteoarthritis. The physician gives him a thumb support splint to rest the thumb, with strict instructions not to use the thumb for the next couple weeks.

Without basketball or computer games, he is bored. The coach and his fellow teammates are angry with him. He is in constant pain. The pain pills help, but he feels drained of all energy and motivation. His appetite has decreased. The doctor referred him to occupational therapy for pain relief and to "cheer him up," in other words, to keep him motivated.

Using the model of human occupation, the occupational therapist begins collecting data as part of the occupational profile by talking with him. Although she was tempted to give him a lecture on ethics, personal responsibility, and the good of the team, she restrained herself. Instead, she finds out that the areas of occupation that currently concern Jake are that he has nothing to do with his time, no games to play, and keyboarding is impossible with one hand. He wants to get back to his games as soon as possible; he is just itching to do something besides watching TV or going to classes. He wears sweats so dressing is not a problem, and all his meals are prepared for him, so these are not areas of concern.

On the basis of this information, the occupational therapist can select appropriate assessment tools to measure his motor deficits and his play/leisure choices, collect subjective data on his level of pain, and evaluate the ergonomics of his desk and chair. These assessments provide the data for the occupational analysis. She delegates some of the testing to the occupational therapy assistant. On the basis of the data she and the occupational therapy assistant collected, the occupational therapist concludes that the factors affecting his occupational performance are motor skills (poor posture at the computer, repetitive stress on the joints of his thumb), energy (lack of it), dominating routines (computer games dominate his leisure time), and adaptation (anticipating problems, and modifying the environment or his task to accommodate for problems). When he receives the OK from his doctor to begin to move his thumb, occupational therapy will address improving the functional use of this thumb. After she collects and synthesizes this data, she identifies the supports and barriers to his full engagement in the occupations he loves. She identifies his strengths and areas in need of improvement in the analysis of occupational performance. She and Jake then sit down together to write goals and identify a targeted outcome.

▼ WRITING THE REPORT ▼

Evaluation reports can contain objective and subjective information. When reporting subjective findings, record what the client or the client's caregivers said. Objective findings could be test scores, observations, or measurements. It is important to keep the findings separate from your interpretation of those findings.

TABLE 14.2 Descriptive, Interpretive, and Evaluative Statements

Descriptive	Interpretive	Evaluative
She wore a red dress.	She usually wears red dresses.	She wore a beautiful red dress.
He sat down on the edge of the bed and took off his shoes.	He had to sit down on the edge of the bed to take off his shoes.	He was too lazy to bend over and take his shoes off.
He ate everything on the right side of his plate, leaving the food on the left side untouched.	He did not appear to notice the food on the left side of his plate.	He is careless.
She looked over her left shoulder and mumbled, "Get away" six times in the half hour she was in the room. No one was standing behind her.	She seemed to be hallucinating about someone standing too close behind her.	She acted like a crazy person.
She said "please" and "thank you" consistently throughout the session.	She had good manners	She is a very pleasant person.

Descriptive, Interpretive, and Evaluative Statements

In writing, there are descriptive, interpretive, and evaluative statements. Descriptive statements are objective; they describe what you can see, hear, taste, touch, or smell. Interpretive statements are based on observations or data, but draw some inference or conclusion about the observation or data. Evaluative statements pass judgment on something; it is obvious that the person making the statement feels good or bad about it, satisfied or dissatisfied, angry or accepting. Table 14.2 gives examples of the different kinds of statements.

Exercise 14.1

Determine whether each statement is a *description* of an event or person, an *interpretation* of an event or person, or an *evaluation* about an event or person.

1. _____ She ate corn flakes for breakfast.
2. _____ She eats corn flakes for breakfast.
3. _____ She could care less what she eats for breakfast.
4. _____ The client's breath smelled like alcohol.
5. _____ Alyah likes to play with blocks.
6. _____ Jake abuses the system of tutors for scholar-athletes.
7. _____ Jake got a high score of 3,203,485 in Galactoids.
8. _____ Jake usually plays computer games 8–10 hours per day.
9. _____ Jake sat with his body forward at 60°, his elbows resting on his knees.
10. _____ Jake's poor posture contributes to his neck, back, and shoulder pain.
11. _____ Avi refused to make eye contact with this clinician during the evaluation process.
12. _____ Avi is stubborn, yet impulsive.

Reporting Data and Interpreting It

Interpreting data can be tricky. Often people use phrases like "appears" or "seems to." If that is the preferred wording at your facility or program, then use it. Otherwise, stay away from these phrases because they make you sound unsure of yourself. When you are interpreting data/findings, be sure to stay away from evaluative statements.

There is a difference between reporting data and interpreting it. Reporting data means providing objective, factual information, while interpreting data means drawing an inference based on the objective (reported) data. Recording raw test scores or direct observations is reporting data. Taking those raw scores and using the scoring manual to get a t-score or age equivalent is interpreting the data. Drawing conclusions about what you saw is interpreting it.

Exercise 14.2

Using "R" for report and "I" for interpretation, identify which of the following statements are a report of information and which are an interpretation of information.

1. _____ The client completed her meal in 26 minutes.
2. _____ The client did not complete the task of looking up the phone number for "time and temperature" and making the call.
3. _____ The child is functioning at an age equivalent of 3 years, 6 months.
4. _____ Annette completed all tasks at the 3-year, 6-month level.
5. _____ The client has severely limited range of motion in her left arm.
6. _____ Toby has an attention span of about 3 minutes.
7. _____ Rashad scored 21 on the Beck's Depression Inventory, 2nd edition.
8. _____ Bao bites her wrists when she's angry or frustrated.
9. _____ Savion needed assistance to start each task, but once started, he finished without additional cuing from staff.
10. _____ Juana used the "two bunny ears" method of tying her shoes.
11. _____ Jake has 30 degrees of flexion in his first right metacarpal joint.
12. _____ Jake's thumb movements are limited by pain.

When you are interpreting the data and paving the way for your plan, it is important to keep the principles of efficiency and effectiveness in mind (Law et al., 2001). Since the evaluation report may be used by payers to determine if the services will be paid for, you need to make convincing arguments that occupational therapy intervention is necessary to improve the quality of life for your client. Using Jake as an example, one argument could be that poor posture will contribute to lifelong recurring joint injuries and pain. Teaching him ways to arrange his furniture and computer could prevent future injuries. In clinical settings, you often have to show that your services are medically necessary, which may be defined differently by different payers. You can make your arguments more convincing by demonstrating that there is support in the literature for your conclusions (interpretations) and your plan for intervention. We call that evidence-based practice. You also have to demonstrate that what you plan to do with the client is uniquely based on occupational therapy principles, and not something that could be done through the use of other disciplines in place of occupational therapy.

Exercise 14.3

Given the data provided, write a brief interpretation of that data.

1. *Findings:* Client drooled throughout the meal. He coughed and gagged with water and juice, but not with applesauce, mashed potatoes, or Jell-O. When he chewed, he frequently opened his mouth and protruded his tongue with food on it. Sometimes food fell off his tongue back onto his plate. He was provided with eating utensils, but he did not use them. Client scooped food with both hands, putting large quantities into his mouth at one time. He swallowed five times during the entire meal.

   Interpretation:

2. *Findings:* Active range of motion is within normal limits on the right side, but the left shoulder moved 80° in flexion and 70° in abduction (normal is 180° in both directions). Client moved her elbow between 80° flexion and 40° extension (normal is 0–150°). She had no active movement of the forearm, wrist, or fingers. Passive range of motion is within normal limits in all joints and directions.

Interpretation:

3. *Findings:* During the interview, Goran turned away from the interviewer every 1–2 minutes and spoke over his shoulder in unintelligible words, sometimes laughing out loud. He responded to questions with short phrases. He made eye contact with the interviewer for no more than 2 seconds at a time, 3 times during the 10-minute interview. When asked where he lived, he said, "Here." When asked what kind of work he wanted to do, he said, "Guava." He said he "made the Internet" and that "they stole it" from him. His clothes were dirty, his hair uncombed, and his fingernails appeared bitten off, ragged, and dirty. His breath was sour and he gave off a foul body odor.

Interpretation:

Suggested Evaluation Report Format

Appendix D (see website) contains sample evaluation report formats. Notice that there are four sections to the evaluation report: background information, findings, interpretation, and plan. You can remember these parts with the mnemonic "BiFIP." The first section (Bi) is for background information. It provides the context for the rest of the report. This is where you record the information you gather for the occupational profile (AOTA, 2014). The second section (F) is for reporting the findings. This is where objective data is reported using descriptive language. This is the place to record the analysis of occupational performance (AOTA, 2014). In as few words as possible, explain the client's current level of performance. It is not necessary to list the client's level of function for every possible activity of daily living (ADL) if only a few areas are affected by his or her current condition. Refer back to Chapter 4 for explanations of each item listed on the format. Next is the interpretation section (I), sometimes referred to as the analysis portion. You want to use interpretive statements in this section to help the reader make sense of your findings. Finally, there is the plan (P) section. This is where you set goals in collaboration with your client, and determine the methodology you will employ to help your client meet those goals. The ultimate goal of occupational therapy intervention, according to AOTA (2014), is "supporting health and participation in life through engagement in occupation" (p. 626). In writing goals, you will need to specifically state which area or areas of occupation the client will participate in. In collaboration with your client, establish concrete, measurable, timely goals. Goal writing will be covered in Chapter 15. Intervention planning will be discussed in Chapter 16.

The BiFIP format is one of several possible formats for writing evaluation reports. A format simply provides a structure for presenting information in an organized fashion. Sections will vary in length according to the amount of information you have to present. Sometimes the structure is invisible; the report is written in a narrative format with a different paragraph for each section. Figure 14.2 shows a completed evaluation report for Jake Olsen.

If you are using an EHR, you will have the format for the evaluation report built into the system; in that case just follow the format. It may or may not follow BiFIP. EHRs usually have space for entering narrative information, some drop-down boxes for common phrases, and some check boxes for routine items. Because each system is different, it is important to get trained on the particular system used in each facility.

OCCUPATIONAL THERAPY EVALUATION REPORT AND INITIAL INTERVENTION PLAN

BACKGROUND INFORMATION

Date of report: 1-15-14   **Client's name or initials:** Jacob Olsen

Date of birth &/or age: 6-25-93   **Date of referral:** 1-14-14

Primary intervention diagnosis/concern: Tendonitis of Ⓡthumb; neck, back, and Ⓡarm pain

Secondary diagnosis/concern: Depression

Precautions/contraindications: Thumb immobilized until 1-28-14

Reason for referral to OT: Immobilization of thumb interferes with daily life tasks

Therapist: Ina Second, MA, OTR/L

Assessments performed:
- ☐ 9-Hole Peg Test
- ☑ ADL Observation
- ☐ Allen Cognitive Level (ACL)
- ☐ Berg Balance Scale (BBS)
- ☐ Canadian Occupational Performance Measure (COPM)
- ☐ Cognitive Assessment of Minnesota (CAM)
- ☐ Cognitive Performance Test (CPT)
- ☑ Ergonomic Assessment
- ☐ Fall Risk Assessment
- ☐ Functional Capacity Testing
- ☐ IADL Observation
- ☑ Jebson Hand Function Test
- ☐ Manual Muscle Test
- ☐ Motor Free Visual Perception Test—Revised (MFVPT-R)
- ☐ Occupational Performance History Interview—Second Version (OPHI-II)
- ☑ Patient Interview
- ☐ Role Checklist
- ☑ ROM
- ☑ Routine Task Inventory
- ☑ Sensory testing
- ☑ Other: UMOT Interest Inventory
- ☐ Other: _____

FINDINGS

Occupational Profile: Jake is a 20-year-old college athlete. In addition to playing varsity basketball, Jake reports that he loves video games, and spends much of his non-basketball hours playing them. Since his thumb has been immobilized, he has watched others play video games, but has not participated himself, and he says he is bored. According to Jake, he is anxious to get back to basketball because he hopes to play in the NBA after college. He is currently a sports management major.

Occupational Analysis:

Areas of occupation: Jake wears sweats so he does not have to deal with fasteners. His meals are prepared for him and he eats in the dorm cafeteria. He performs grooming and hygiene tasks with his non-dominant hand, but reports it takes longer to do than when he did them with his right hand. He is keyboarding with his left hand, although he is very slow. He reports being bored, having no energy and not eating or sleeping well.

FIGURE 14.2 Evaluation Report for Jake Olsen.

Areas of occupation:	Not tested	Dependent	Max Assist	Mod Assist	Min Assist	Adaptation	Independent
Bathing	☐	☐	☐	☐	☐	☐	☑
Toileting	☐	☐	☐	☐	☐	☐	☑
Eating	☐	☐	☐	☐	☐	☐	☑
Feeding	☐	☐	☐	☐	☐	☐	☑
Dressing	☐	☐	☐	☐	☐	☑	☐
Functional Mobility	☐	☐	☐	☐	☐	☐	☑
Grooming	☐	☐	☐	☐	☐	☐	☑
Safety	☐	☐	☐	☐	☐	☐	☑
Handwriting or keyboarding	☐	☐	☐	☐	☑	☐	☐
Meal prep	☑	☐	☐	☐	☐	☐	☐
Play (video games)	☐	☐	☑	☐	☐	☐	☐
Other (describe)		☐	☐	☐	☐	☐	☐

Performance skills: An ergonomic evaluation of Jake's desk and computer set up shows that his joint alignment is poor and the hunched posture puts extra pressure on neck, shoulders, and back. He sat hunched down with his knees hitting the underside of the desk. He looked down more often than he looked ahead or at a person. At three points during the evaluation his eyes got watery but he did not cry. Cognitive, communication, and visual sensory perception skills were not tested. Video gaming and texting require repetitive motions, especially of his thumbs.

Performance skills:	Not tested	Limited or inefficient	Competent	Proficient	Comments:
Posture	☐	☑	☐	☐	Poor joint alignment
Balance	☑	☐	☐	☐	
Fine motor coordination	☐	☑	☐	☐	
Gross motor coordination	☑	☐	☐	☐	
Visual motor integration	☑	☐	☐	☐	
Following directions	☐	☐	☐	☑	
Emotional regulation	☐	☐	☑	☐	
Cognitive skills	☑	☐	☐	☐	
Communication and social skills	☑	☐	☐	☐	
Other (describe)		☐	☐	☐	

Performance patterns: Jake sits in one position, hunched in a chair, for hours at a time. Activities are concentrated on a few selected tasks for long periods of time. TV or watches friends play video games for 8–10 hours per day, which he says is more than he did when he was practicing with the team. He spends 1 hour a day on the stationary bike while watching TV to keep his legs in shape for basketball.

FIGURE 14.2 (Continued)

Client factors: Jake reports pain throughout his dominant hand and arm, limiting his use of that limb. He is wearing a thumb immobilizer splint, preventing him from forming a fist or holding things in that hand. He reports some pain in his left thumb, but not severe enough to limit use of it. The pain in his right thumb sometimes wakes him up at night. Sensory testing reveals some tingling in his thumbs on both hands, and some tingling in the fingers of his right hand. No deficits in hot/cold, sharp/dull, or two-point sensation. Energy and drive are currently below what they were before the injury. Other cognitive and sensory factors are normal.

Body Functions:	Not tested	Absent	Impaired	Adequate	Comments:
Attention	☐	☐	☑	☐	Reports inability to focus
Distractibility	☐	☐	☑	☐	
Memory	☑	☐	☐	☐	
Sequencing	☑	☐	☐	☐	
Initiative	☐	☐	☑	☐	Reports low energy and drive
Sight	☑	☐	☐	☐	
Hearing	☑	☐	☐	☐	
Smell	☑	☐	☐	☐	
Taste	☑	☐	☐	☐	
Touch	☐	☐	☑	☐	Tingling in B thumbs; worse on R.
Vestibular	☑	☐	☐	☐	
Kinesthetic	☐	☐	☐	☑	
Proprioception	☐	☐	☐	☑	
Temperature	☐	☐	☐	☑	
Pain	☐	☐	☐	☑	
Muscle tone	☐	☐	☐	☑	
Reflexes	☑	☐	☐	☐	
Endurance	☑	☐	☐	☐	
Joint stability	☑	☐	☐	☐	
Bilateral integration	☐	☐	☐	☑	
Praxis	☐	☐	☐	☑	
Other (describe)	☐	☐	☐	☐	

Body structure:	Deformity	Movement Limitation	Normal	Comments:
Head	☐	☐	☑	
Neck	☐	☑	☐	Pain with movements to left
Shoulders	☐	☑	☐	☑ R ☐ L ☐ B Pain
Elbows	☐	☑	☐	☑ R ☐ L ☐ B Pain
Forearms	☐	☑	☐	☑ R ☐ L ☐ B Pain
Wrists	☐	☑	☐	☑ R ☐ L ☐ B Pain
Hands	☐	☑	☐	☐ R ☐ L ☑ B Pain
Trunk	☐	☐	☑	
Hips	☐	☐	☑	☐ R ☐ L ☐ B
Knees	☐	☐	☑	☐ R ☐ L ☐ B
Legs	☐	☐	☑	☐ R ☐ L ☐ B
Ankles	☐	☐	☑	☐ R ☐ L ☐ B
Feet	☐	☐	☑	☐ R ☐ L ☐ B
Other (describe)	☐	☐	☐	

FIGURE 14.2 (Continued)

ROM	DIP flexion	DIP extension	PIP flexion	MCP flexion	MCP extension	Abduction
R thumb	0	0		0	0	0
L thumb	90	10		60	10	70
R index	30	10	80	60	25	10
L index	70	10	100	90	30	20
R middle	30	0	80	70	25	10
L middle	70	0	100	90	30	20
R ring	30	0	80	70	20	10
L ring	70	0	90	90	25	20
R little	30	0	80	80	25	10
L little	70	0	100	90	30	20

Contexts: Desk and chair not fitted to proper working heights for a person as tall as Jake (6'11"). Laptop computer screen too low; Jake has to look down too far to see it. Jake spends most of his time in the gym or his room.

INTERPRETATION

Strengths and areas in need of intervention: Jake is motivated to return to playing basketball. He is in very good physical condition, with the exception of his right arm and hand, with excellent muscle tone and gross coordination consistent with a top athlete. Cognition and sensory integration are intact.

Jake needs to learn principles of ergonomics so that he can adjust future environments to fit his body while maintaining proper body alignment. He needs to consider adding a broader array of leisure activities to his repertoire. He needs to increase his energy level and engagement in occupations.

Supports and Hindrances to Occupational Performance: Jake does not feel supported by his team or coaches, but does feel pressured to recover quickly. His friends on campus are all gamers and want him to get back to gaming. He loves gaming. Peer pressure may be a hindrance to his recovery. His family is supportive but they live 3 hours away by car. His desire to avoid injuries like this in the future is highly motivating.

Prioritization of Need Areas:

1. Ergonomics
2. Life balance
3. Function of thumb after immobilization

PLAN

Mutually agreed-on long-term goals:	Mutually agreed-on short-term goals:	Recommended intervention methods and approaches:
Jake will return to the basketball team in 6 weeks.	Jake will engage in 3 hours per day of physical activity, not using his right hand, by Feb 1, 2014	Coordinate with team athletic trainer regarding exercise opportunities.
	By Feb 1, 2014, Jake will try three alternatives to gaming on which he could spend his time that do not require repetitive motions of his thumbs.	Try different activities Education on repetitive motion injuries

FIGURE 14.2 (Continued)

Mutually agreed-on long-term goals:	Mutually agreed-on short-term goals:	Recommended intervention methods and approaches:
Jake will make needed adaptations to his physical environment to support his successful occupational participation by Feb. 28, 2014.	By Jan 22, 2014, Jake will identify six occupations during which his posture is poor.	Education on body alignment and posture Self-awareness activities
	By Feb 1, 2014, Jake will identify three adaptations he could make to his physical environment to support good posture while engaging in occupations.	Education on ergonomic principles and types of adaptations that are possible

Expected frequency, duration, and intensity: 3x/wk for 6 weeks, 45-min. sessions
Location of intervention: OT clinic at U of M Medical Center, possible "home visit" to Jake's dorm room.
Anticipated D/C environment: Dorm, gym, and basketball court
Service providers: Ina Second MS, OTR/L and Justa Minute, COTA/L

Ina Second, MS, OTR/L   _1-15-14_
Signature   Date

FIGURE 14.2 (Continued)

Exercise 14.4

For the following case, write an evaluation report. You may make up supplemental information, but the information you add must be consistent with the case.

Donna is a 23-year-old mother of five, who has been admitted to the locked unit for a 72-hour hold. She was brought in by police. She was found on a bridge over a major river, allegedly throwing her oldest child (6 years old) over the railing and preparing to throw the rest over. She said she planned to jump in after them; none of them could swim. She was despondent and said she did not want to live anymore. The child was rescued by bystanders and all the children were sent to stay with other family members. Tomorrow her case will be heard by a judge, who will hold a commitment hearing.

Donna recently lost her job as a receptionist at a car dealer's, which she had held for 3 months. Prior to that, she had a series of jobs, none of which lasted more than 6 months. She did not graduate from high school, but did complete her GED. Her children are ages 6 (girl), 5 (boy), 3 (boy), 21 months (girl), and 5 months (boy). She is not married. She has a history of chemical dependency, and twice completed inpatient treatment programs. When she was arrested, she tested positive for crack cocaine, and a small amount was found in her coat pocket. She was arrested twice for prostitution and served short (30- to 90-day) sentences.

When you interview her, she does not make eye contact, slurs her speech, gives very short answers, and expresses no interest in returning to independent living. She sees no future for herself. She has not been eating; she has no appetite. She sleeps a little, she says, because they give her "the good stuff." She tears up as she talks about her children. She admits that she has spanked them, sometimes repeatedly, when they "won't leave her alone," but she insists that she loves them with all her heart. She says that it's not her fault that she didn't finish high school, she got pregnant in the summer before sophomore year by a man she met at her cousin's house. He disappeared when he heard she was pregnant, so there was no child support. She stated no man wants to support her or her kids—there are too many of them. She said there are no good jobs for someone like her, so she will never be able to support herself and her kids.

You administer a Beck Depression Inventory, 2nd ed., and she scores a 48, indicating severe depression. You attempt to administer a Kohlman Evaluation of Living Skills, but she says she doesn't feel like doing anything. She tells you that nothing interests her. She says she doesn't do anything with her leisure time except go to bars or watch TV. She does not think she needs help learning child-rearing strategies, nutrition, job-seeking skills, or leisure activities.

Reevaluation

Evaluation is an ongoing process. While the focus of this chapter has been on documenting an initial evaluation, there is an element of evaluation that occurs throughout the intervention process. At every intervention session, the occupational therapy practitioner makes observations, collects information about changes in the client's circumstances and performance, and sometimes makes adjustments in the intervention methodology. If the intervention is going to occur over several weeks or more, periodic reevaluations are conducted.

Reevaluation may be formal or informal. Informal reevaluation occurs every time the occupational therapist revises the intervention plan (see Chapter 16). A formal reevaluation may involve repeating previous testing so that changes in performance can be measured and documented. Often formal reevaluation occurs when a client is close to being discharged or at regular intervals, such as yearly for a child with developmental delays.

Nielson (1998) suggests that reevaluation is a three-step process: data collection, reflection, and decision making. Data collection involves gathering subjective and objective information relative to the targeted outcomes identified by the client and clinician. Reflection is a thought process centered on the client's current status, changes in status since the last evaluation, and a judgment on the effectiveness of the current intervention plan. In the decision-making step, the occupational therapist decides whether the current intervention plan is sufficient, whether it should be changed in some way, or whether the client is ready to be discontinued from occupational therapy services (Nielson, 1998).

Medicare Compliance

Medicare requires documentation of an evaluation that demonstrates the necessity for occupational therapy services. The necessity for occupational therapy services is documented through "objective findings and subjective patient self-reporting" (Centers for Medicare and Medicaid Services [CMS], 2008). Under Medicare, only the occupational therapist may conduct the initial evaluation, reevaluation, and ongoing assessment, but may include objective measures or observations made by an occupational therapy assistant. Medicare wants to assure that the occupational therapist is actively involved in the evaluation and ongoing intervention of the client; that he or she does not simply rely on the input of others (CMS, 2008).

In the evaluation report Medicare requires that the clinician document the client's condition and complexities, and the impact these have on the client's prognosis and/or plan of intervention (CMS, 2008). A medical diagnosis established by a physician or a treatment diagnosis identified by the occupational therapist should be part of the evaluation report. For the occupational therapy evaluation under Part B (outpatient), Medicare recommends using the Patient Inquiry by Focus on Therapeutic Outcomes (FOTO) or the Activity Measure—Post Acute Care (AM-PAC) as outcome measures. If one of these two measurement systems is not used, then other commercially available outcome measurement instruments, validated tests and measurements (evidence based), or "other measurable progress towards identified goals for functioning in the home environment at the conclusion of this therapy episode of care" (CMS, 2008, p. 30) may be used. Examples of other commercially available assessment tools include the Canadian Occupational Performance Measure, the Kohlman Evaluation of Living Skills, the Short Form 36 Health Survey, or the Routine Task Inventory. In addition, there should be documentation that supports the illness severity or complexity, identification of other health services the client is receiving for the condition being addressed in the evaluation/intervention plan and/or durable medical equipment needs, the type of medication the client is currently taking, any factors that complicate care or impact severity, and any documentation of medical care prior to the current condition. The occupational therapist must document the client's answer to the question (or why the client cannot answer the question) "At the present time, would you say that your health is excellent, very good, fair, or poor?" (CMS, 2008, p. 28). There also needs to be documentation that indicates the client's social support, such as where the client lives or intends to live at the conclusion of occupational therapy services, who the client lives with or intends to live with, whether this intervention will return the client to the pre-morbid living environment, and whether this intervention will reduce the level of assistance in ADLs or IADLs. The occupational therapist must use his or her clinical judgment to describe the client's current function status. Finally, the occupational therapist must make a determination whether intervention is needed or not needed. If intervention is needed, the occupational therapist must provide an expected time frame and a plan of care (CMS, 2008).

Depending on the setting, the occupational therapist may contribute to the completion of specific forms that are used to determine whether or not the client will continue to qualify for Medicare coverage. For example, in long-term care settings, the Minimum Data Set (MDS) 3.0 is used, and in home health, the Outcome and Assessment Information Set (OASIS) is used. The information that occupational therapists contribute to these Medicare documents are informed by data gathered in the evaluation and reevaluation process.

SUMMARY

The evaluation report is a critically important document. When another team member or a payer reads your evaluation report, he or she should have a clear picture of how the client is functioning and what the hope is for change. The report will justify the need for occupational therapy involvement in this case. All the rest of the work you do with that client hinges on an evaluation report that shows a strong need for your services, clearly states where the client is starting from, and establishes a doable plan.

In the evaluation report, describe your findings/data and then interpret them. Without findings, an interpretation is meaningless. The interpretation cannot stand alone; there must be data/findings to back it up. There is a difference between descriptive, interpretive, and evaluative statements. In the findings section, only descriptive statements should be used. In the interpretation sections, interpretive statements are used. Evaluative statements have no place in evaluation reports. Be absolutely sure you distinguish between reporting information and interpreting it. Follow all the guidelines for general documentation as well as professional standards for evaluation reports.

The occupational therapist is responsible for conducting and documenting the evaluation process. An occupational therapy assistant may contribute to the process. The occupational therapist is also responsible for making referrals to other professionals if the client has needs that are better met by another professional.

There are many formats for reporting evaluation results. Medicare has a form that is available in both electronic and paper formats. Other vendors sell documentation systems that include evaluation formats. The format presented in this chapter is a paper-based format called "BiFIP," which stands for background information, findings, interpretation, and plan. The AOTA describes the evaluation process in *The Occupational Therapy Practice Framework* (2014). The evaluation process is client-centered.

Reevaluation occurs periodically throughout the course of occupational therapy service delivery. It may be formal or informal. It should contain subjective input from the client and client's caregivers as well as objective data gathered through observation and testing. The reevaluation helps the occupational therapist determine whether the current intervention plan is sufficient, needs adjustment, or if the client is ready to be discontinued from occupational therapy services.

REFERENCES

American Occupational Therapy Association. (2009). Guidelines for supervision, roles, and responsibilities during the delivery of occupational therapy services. Retrieved from http://www.aota.org/-/media/corporate/files/secure/practice/officialdocs/guidelines/guidelines%20for%20supervision%20roles%20and%20responsibilities.pdf

American Occupational Therapy Association. (2010). Standards of practice for occupational therapy. *American Journal of Occupational Therapy,* 64, S106–S111. doi:10.5014/ajot.2010.64S106

American Occupational Therapy Association. (2013). *Guidelines for documentation of occupational therapy.* Retrieved from http://www.aota.org/-/media/corporate/files/secure/practice/officialdocs/guidelines/guidelines%20for%20documentation.pdf

American Occupational Therapy Association. (2014). Occupational therapy practice framework: Domain and process (3rd ed). *American Journal of Occupational Therapy, 68*(Suppl. 1), S1-S48. http://dx.doi.org/10.5014/ajot.2014.682006

Bass-Haugen, J. (2010). Assessment identification and selection. In J. Hinojosa & Kramer (Eds.), *Evaluation: Obtaining and interpreting data* (3rd ed., pp. 21–40). Bethesda, MD: American Occupational Therapy Association.

Centers for Medicare and Medicaid Services. (2008). *Pub100-02 Medicare benefit policy: Transmittal 88.* Retrieved May 8, 2008, from http://www.cms.hhs.gov/transmittals/downloads/R88BP.pdf

Hinojosa, J., & Kramer, P. (2010). Philosophical and theoretical influences on evaluation. In J. Hinojosa & Kramer (Eds.), *Evaluation: Obtaining and interpreting data* (3rd ed., pp. 21–40). Bethesda, MD: American Occupational Therapy Association.

Hinojosa, J., Kramer, P., & Crist, P. (2010). Evaluation: Where do we begin? In J. Hinojosa & Kramer (Eds.), *Evaluation: Obtaining and interpreting data* (3rd ed., pp. 21–40). Bethesda, MD: American Occupational Therapy Association.

Law, M., Baum, C., & Dunn, W. (2001). *Measuring occupational performance: Supporting best practice in occupational therapy.* Thorofare, NJ: Slack.

Moyers, P. A., & Dale, L. M. (2007). *The guide to occupational therapy practice.* Bethesda, MD: American Occupational Therapy Association.

Nielson, C. (1998). Reevaluation. In J. Hinojosa & P. Kramer (Eds.), *Evaluation: Obtaining and interpreting data.* Bethesda, MD: American Occupational Therapy Association.

Stewart, K. B. (2001). Purposes, processes, and methods of evaluation. In J. Case-Smith (Ed.), *Occupational therapy for children* (4th ed., pp. 190–213). St. Louis, MO: Mosby.

Weinstock-Zlotnik, G., & Hinojosa, J. (2004). Bottom-up or top-down evaluation: Is one better than the other? *American Journal of Occupational Therapy 58,* 594–599.

CHAPTER 15

Goal Writing

INTRODUCTION

Setting appropriate goals, ones that can be measured and are realistic, can help you demonstrate that you did indeed help your client. The trick is to set the goals so that the client can meet them. The goals cannot be so easy that they are not meaningful, yet not so hard that they cannot be accomplished in the time you have to work together. In other words, they have to represent a just-right challenge.

Goal writing is an essential step in both the evaluation and intervention processes. Goals are often first established as part of the evaluation process, and then revised as part of the intervention process. Goals guide the direction of interventions. They help occupational therapy practitioners determine the effectiveness of their interventions. If a client is meeting goals, the intervention is likely to be appropriate. If a client is not meeting established goals, perhaps a different approach or intervention method should be tried.

▼ ROLE DELINEATION IN GOAL WRITING ▼

Goals are established in collaboration with the client, or if the client is unable to collaborate, the client's caregiver or guardian (American Occupational Therapy Association [AOTA], 2014). Primary responsibility for the development of intervention plans and goal setting rests with the occupational therapist; however, occupational therapy assistants may contribute to the process (AOTA, 2010). The *AOTA Occupational Therapy Standards of Practice* (2010) further state that "an occupational therapist has overall responsibility for the development, documentation, and implementation of the occupational therapy intervention based on the evaluation, client goals, current best evidence, and clinical reasoning" (AOTA, 2010, Standard III.1).

▼ GOAL DIRECTIONS ▼

The models or frames of reference you used in determining your evaluation strategies are used to help you frame your goals (see Chapters 5 and 14). For example, if you are using the biomechanical frame of reference, the goal would address client factors while a goal formulated under the Canadian model of occupational performance would address areas of occupational performance. The type of setting in which you are working will impact the wording of the goals you write, and your employer may prefer that certain words are used or avoided (see Chapter 3).

In writing goal statements, there are a limited number of directions the goals can go. *The Framework-III* suggests the ultimate outcome of occupational therapy intervention is "Achieving health, well-being, and participation in life through engagement in occupation" (AOTA, 2014, p. S4). To achieve that outcome, the intervention approaches that you can take with your client are geared toward assisting "clients in reaching a state of physical, mental, and social well-being; identifying and realizing aspirations; satisfying needs; and changing or coping with the environment" (p. S14). *The Framework-III* further presents the following intervention approaches: create or promote, establish or restore, maintain, modify, or prevent. These intervention approaches can be used to help determine the direction a

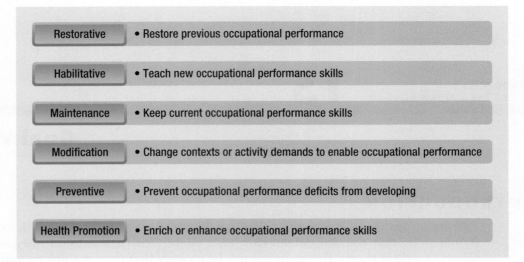

FIGURE 15.1 Goal Directions.
Sources: AOTA (2014); Moyers & Dale (2007).

goal will take (AOTA, 2014). Moyers and Dale (2007) describe six kinds of outcomes: occupational performance, client satisfaction, role competence, adaptation, health and wellness, and quality of life. Based on a synthesis of these two documents, goal directions can be summarized as restorative, habilitative, maintenance, modification, preventive, and health promotion. Figure 15.1 summarizes the types of goal directions.

Restorative Goals

Restorative goals (rehabilitative or remediative) are used when you have a client who used to be able to do something, but now cannot (AOTA, 2014). This usually happens when there has been an illness or injury. Occupational therapy practitioners working in hospitals, rehabilitation facilities, nursing homes, outpatient clinics, home health, or psychiatric facilities typically write restorative goals. These goals are written to reflect a desired change in function.

Examples of restorative goals include:

- By discharge, client will feed herself three meals a day independently.
- By July 15, 2014, client will state three strengths about herself with no more than one prompt.
- The client will return to work as a carpenter, consistently using good body mechanics, by August 1, 2014.

Habilitative Goals

Goals that teach new skills are often called habilitative goals. Habilitation refers to teaching skills that the client never had, typically because of delayed development. This is different from rehabilitation, which seeks to restore a lost function or to help a client relearn a lost skill. Habilitative goals are often used with children whose development is delayed, or when teaching new skills to adults with developmental disabilities.

Examples of habilitative goals include:

- Eric will write his name legibly on all his school papers by June 10, 2014.
- Pahoa will consistently package the correct number of products, using adaptive jigs if needed, in the sheltered workshop by September 1, 2014.
- Emmalee will demonstrate increased mobility by independently moving from prone on the floor to standing by November 3, 2014.

Maintenance Goals

Maintenance goals seek to keep a client at his or her current level of function despite disease processes that normally would cause deterioration of function (AOTA, 2014). These goals would be written in long-term care or outpatient settings when a client has a progressive or deteriorating condition. Sometimes, maintenance goals are written when the client's condition is so complex that only someone with the specialized knowledge and skills of an occupational therapy practitioner can carry out the intervention. For example, a client with severe contractions may require occupational therapy intervention to open up the hand so that nursing can clean the client's palm and prevent skin breakdown.

One concern about maintenance goals is that many third-party payers will not pay for them. The payers often only want to pay as long as progress is being made. A maintenance goal may be seen as an indication that progress is no longer being made.

Examples of maintenance goals include:

- Client will maintain independence in dressing for the next 3 months.
- Client will actively participate in a current events group eight times in the next 30 days.
- For the next 6 months, the client will continue to live in her own home with minimal assistance of home health aide.

Modification Goals

Modification goals (also called compensation or adaptation goals) seek to change the contexts or activity demands rather than change the skills and abilities of the client (AOTA, 2014). In other words, instead of increasing the strength and range of motion of an elderly client, address adapting the environment or tools used to complete the task. These goals are difficult to write in the sense that they can sound prescriptive and limiting. The trick is to be general enough to allow you to experiment and see what products work best, yet specific enough that you have some direction.

Examples of modification goals include:

- By August 12, 2014, Pyter will open boxes, cans, and bags with the use of adaptive equipment as needed so that he can independently prepare meals at home.
- By discharge, client's home will be modified to allow wheelchair access both inside and outside the house.
- In 3 months, the client will return to work with workplace modifications as needed to allow completion of essential functions of the job.

Preventive Goals

Preventive goals are written to assist persons who are at risk of developing occupational performance problems (AOTA, 2014). The person may or may not be completely healthy at the time the goal is written. A preventive goal may be written when the potential exists for a client to get hurt, such as through a repetitive motion injury or self-injurious behavior.

Examples of preventive goals include:

- By discharge, client will consistently demonstrate proper body mechanics while lifting.
- By next session, Reed will list five strategies for removing himself from situations that tempt him to engage in the use of cocaine.
- By next week, Chenyse will identify three people she can call for help when she begins to feel depressed or overwhelmed.

Health Promotion

Goals that relate to health promotion are written for clients who may not have a disability, but are more about enrichment or enhancement of occupational performance (AOTA, 2014). Health promotion goals may apply to an individual, group, community, or organization. In these settings, there is usually no attempt to correct a performance deficit; rather, the emphasis is on enhancing the contexts and activities to enable maximum participation in life (AOTA, 2014).

Examples of health promotion goals include:

- By the end of this class, parents will demonstrate minimal competency in infant massage.
- Playground surfaces will be replaced to provide a safer play environment for children by May 25, 2015.
- Within the next 3 months, create raised gardens at the community center so that wheelchair-bound gardeners can access their own garden plot.

▼ GOAL SPECIFICS ▼

Goals are also written for varying amounts of time. Long-term goals are overarching goals that guide the intervention to a conclusion. Often, long-term goals are the goals that, when met, will determine the time to discontinue therapy. Some facilities call them discharge goals or outcome goals. If a client is expected to receive services for more than one year, then the long-term goal might reflect the progress expected by the end of a year.

Short-term goals are written for specific periods of time, and change from time to time, leading up to the achievement of the long-term goal. In some settings, short-term goals are called objectives (Richardson & Shultz-Krohn, 2001). For example, if the long-term goal is to become independent in dressing, the first short-term goal might address dressing in clothes that have no fasteners, such as sweats. The next short-term goal might include zippers or Velcro®. The next might include buttons, snaps, hooks, or ties. The last one might include outerwear (especially in cold climates) such as parkas, mittens, boots, hats, and scarves.

In acute care settings where clients are seen for a short time, the occupational therapy staff may not distinguish between short- and long-term goals. There are just goals. It is not necessary to separate goals by length of time when the occupational therapy practitioner is only going to work with the client for a few sessions. Some facilities or programs may not separate long- and short-term goals if the clients are seen for 30 days or less, but some do, so be sure to find out what the facility's standard practice is before you start setting goals.

The way in which you refer to your client in the goal statement will vary by facility or program. In some facilities, the preferred phrase is "the client." In others, it is "the patient," "the resident," or "the participant." Some programs prefer that you use the client's first or last name. The best advice is to either ask your supervisor what his or her preference is, or read the goals written by others in the department.

There are several formats for writing goals, but all of them require the use of action words (verbs). Actions are things you can see or hear. Box 15.1 is a list of some verbs (there are more than those on this list, but these give you an idea) that can be used in goal writing. Of course, a lot depends on how you use the word. For example, when you use the verb *focus* in reference to vision rehab, you can see if the client is focusing on an object. If you use *focus* in reference to thought processes, can you see that?

Verbs that are not action-oriented would rarely, if ever, be used in occupational therapy goals. These are listed in Box 15.2.

Except for maintenance goals, most goals need to describe change, and how that change will be measured. Box 15.3 shows examples of ways to measure change. However, depending on the unique wants, needs, and circumstances of each client, there are many other ways to document change as well. For example, attainment of health status, level of prevention of dysfunction, and client perception of life satisfaction, role performance, or quality of life may be measured qualitatively rather than quantitatively.

BOX 15.1 Action Verbs

Accesses	Creates	Keeps	Raises
Accomplishes	Crochets	Knits	Reaches
Accommodates	Crushes	Knots	Reads
Achieves	Cuts	Labels	Rebuilds
Acquires	Dances	Leads	Records
Acts	Demonstrates	Leaves	Reduces
Adapts	Develops	Lies	Reestablishes
Adheres	Digs	Lifts	Regards
Adjusts	Diminishes	Lists	Rejoins
Agrees	Discriminates	Listens	Relates
Aligns	Discusses	Locates	Remarks
Allows	Displays	Locks	Reminds
Applies	Distributes	Loosens	Removes
Approaches	Does	Maintains	Repairs
Arranges	Doffs	Makes	Repeats
Asks	Dons	Manages	Requests
Asserts	Draws	Masters	Researches
Assists	Dresses	Meets	Responds
Attempts	Drinks	Modulates	Rests
Attends	Drives	Moves	Restores
Avoids	Dries	Navigates	Resumes
Bakes	Eats	Notices	Returns
Balances	Employs	Obeys	Reverses
Bathes	Endures	Obtains	Reviews
Becomes	Engages	Opens	Revises
Behaves	Establishes	Organizes	Rinses
Bends	Explores	Paces	Rises
Breathes	Expresses	Paints	Rolls
Brushes	Extends	Participates	Rotates
Builds	Facilitates	Pauses	Rows
Buttons	Fastens	Pays	Rubs
Buys	Feeds	Pedals	Runs
Calculates	Finishes	Performs	Says
Calls	Focuses	Picks	Scrubs
Changes	Folds	Places	Secures
Chooses	Follows	Plans	Seeks
Chops	Gains	Plays	Selects
Clasps	Gathers	Positions	Sends
Cleans	Gazes	Posts	Sequences
Clears	Generalizes	Practices	Serves
Closes	Gets	Prepares	Sets
Collaborates	Gives	Presses	Sews
Collects	Grips	Prevents	Shares
Comes	Grooms	Prints	Shaves
Communicates	Goes	Prioritizes	Shops
Completes	Handles	Procures	Shows
Complies	Has	Promotes	Showers
Conforms	Heeds	Propels	Shuts
Confronts	Heeds	Provides	Signs
Connects	Identifies	Pulls	Simulates
Contacts	Improves	Punches	Sings
Continues	Initiates	Purchases	Sits
Contributes	Inquires	Pursues	Skis
Converses	Irons	Pushes	Sleeps
Cooperates	Interacts	Puts	Slides
Coordinates	Is	Questions	Snaps
Corrects	Jumps	Quits	Socializes

Solves	Stitches	Throws	Vocalizes
Sorts	Stops	Tightens	Volunteers
Speaks	Straightens	Toilets	Walks
Specifies	Succeeds	Touches	Washes
Spreads	Sucks	Tracks	Watches
Stabilizes	Supports	Transfers	Wears
Stands	Sustains	Transports	Wipes
Starts	Talks	Tries	Withdraws
Strengthens	Taps	Types	Works
Stretches	Tastes	Unwraps	Wraps
States	Takes	Uses	Writes
Stays	Tends	Utilizes	Zips
Stirs	Terminates	Verifies	

BOX 15.2 Verbs to Avoid

Commits	Feels	Loves	Resolves
Considers	Forgives	Perceives	Respects
Contemplates	Hears	Prefers	Sees
Decides	Imagines	Processes	Senses
Desires	Infers	Realizes	Smells
Determines	Interprets	Recognizes	Sympathizes
Empathizes	Knows	Reflects	Thinks
Enjoys	Learns	Remembers	Wants
Expects	Likes	Represses	

BOX 15.3 Ways to Measure Change

Frequency or Consistency

- Percentage (number of successes divided by the number of opportunities for success)
- "x" out of "y" trials
- Consistently

Duration

- Time, such as number of seconds or minutes of sustained activity
- Number of repetitions

Assistance

- Maximum (assistance with 75% or more of task)
- Moderate (assistance with 25–74% of task)
- Minimum (assistance with 1–24% of task)
- Standby
- Setup
- Adaptive equipment
- Verbal cuing/prompts
- Physical cuing
- Independently

Quality of Performance

- Number of errors
- Accuracy
- Amount of aberrant task behavior (i.e., tremors, off-task behavior)
- Amount of pain perceived by client
- Adherence to safety precautions

Level of Complexity

- Amount of instruction
- Number of steps in the process
- Cognitive level
- Multitasking

Participation (may require additional measure)

- Attend
- Engage
- Initiate
- Transition
- Interaction
- Adapt to environmental signals or social cues
- Obtain needed tools and equipment

Other (may require additional measure)

- Express feelings
- Specific task completion
- Variety of environments in which desired behavior will occur
- Level of cooperation
- Complete steps of a task

Source: Moyers & Dale (2007).

▼ FORMATS FOR GOAL WRITING ▼

There are many systems for formulating goals. In this chapter, I share four of these with you. I do not propose that any one system is better than the others; they are all just different. It is good to be familiar with more than one system, as you never know which system your supervisor will prefer. Figure 15.2 provides a summary of the different goal writing systems. It is not necessary that the goal be written to reflect the format in the acronym represented by the name of the format. Sometimes, for the sake of clarity and good grammar, the order may be changed as long as all the elements are there.

▼ ABCD ▼

Kettenbach (2009) uses the "ABCD" method: **A**udience, **B**ehavior, **C**ondition, and **D**egree. The *audience* represents the person who will do the behavior. The *behavior* is what the audience will do. The *condition* describes the circumstances around the behavior. The *degree* describes how well the behavior must be done to meet the goal.

Usually, the *audience* (or actor) is the client (Kettenbach, 2009). Since occupational therapy practice is client centered, this makes sense. Occasionally you might write a goal for a

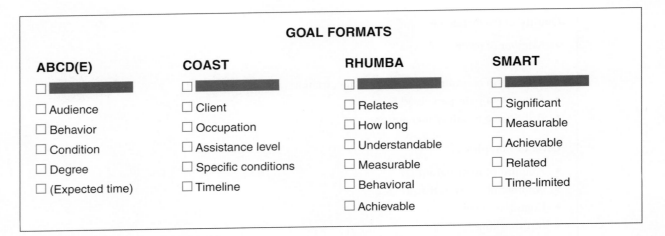

GOAL FORMATS

ABCD(E)	COAST	RHUMBA	SMART
☐ ▬▬▬▬	☐ ▬▬▬▬	☐ ▬▬▬▬	☐ ▬▬▬▬
☐ Audience	☐ Client	☐ Relates	☐ Significant
☐ Behavior	☐ Occupation	☐ How long	☐ Measurable
☐ Condition	☐ Assistance level	☐ Understandable	☐ Achievable
☐ Degree	☐ Specific conditions	☐ Measurable	☐ Related
☐ (Expected time)	☐ Timeline	☐ Behavioral	☐ Time-limited
		☐ Achievable	

FIGURE 15.2   Goal Formats.

Sources: CSC, 2001; Gately & Borcherding, 2012; Kettenbach, 2009; Quinn & Gordan, 2003; University of Victoria Counseling Services, 1996.

caregiver, but you should never write a goal for what you, the occupational therapist, will do (Kettenbach, 2009). What you plan to do, the methodology, belongs in the plan, not in the goal.

A *behavior* is usually something you can see or hear the person doing or saying. Examples of behaviors include reaching, dressing, carrying, demonstrating, expressing, eating, or crocheting. Behaviors represent an action and thus are stated as verbs (Kettenbach, 2009). However, not all verbs represent action. Refer to the word lists earlier in this chapter.

Conditions, circumstances that support the behavior, help to clarify the goal (Kettenbach, 2009). Conditions can represent something in the environment that is necessary for the behavior to occur (Richardson & Schultz-Krohn, 2001). For example, in the goal "The client will independently dress herself in clothes that have no fasteners," *clothes that have no fasteners* is the condition. The client needs access to clothes that do not have fasteners (elastic-waist pants, pull-over tops) in order to meet the goal. Conditions can also be the amount of cuing or assistance needed.

The *degree* is the measurable part of the goal (Kettenbach, 2009). It tells the reader how many, what percent, what degree, or other distinguishing characteristic of the behavior. The degree has to be realistic, functional, and identify a specific time frame. Realistic means that you can reasonably expect the client to achieve the goal in the time frame you establish. Functional means the goal describes an area of occupational performance. The time frame is when you realistically expect the goal to be met. This is dependent on the condition of the client, the frequency and duration of occupational therapy, and your professional knowledge and experience with similar types of clients.

A variation of the ABCD format is ABCDE, which is advocated by Quinn and Gordon (2003). They use the same audience, behavior, condition, and degree as does Kettenbach (2009). The "E" stands for **E**xpected time. The expected time part of a goal is an estimate of the length of time it will take to meet the goal, for example, within a week or within a month (Quinn & Gordon, 2003).

Exercise 15.1

Identify the parts of the goal that correspond to the letters ABCD:

1. The client will prepare a complete meal (meat, vegetable, starch, and beverage) independently on three consecutive days. *(Client has osteoarthritis and diabetic neuropathy in her upper extremities.)*

   A:

   B:

C:

D:

2. The patient will bathe herself using adaptive equipment, if needed, in less than 15 minutes. *(Client has a right hemiparesis.)*

A:

B:

C:

D:

3. Bobby will independently retrieve the tools necessary to complete his project in three of the next five sessions. *(Client has chronic schizophrenia and is seen in a day program.)*

A:

B:

C:

D:

▼ COAST ▼

Gateley and Borcherding (2012) developed the COAST format of goal writing. This format is the only one to specifically mention occupation as an element of the goal.

C stands for client (Gateley & Borcherding, 2012). Using COAST, the goal is written to specify what the client will do. According to the AOTA (2014), the client may be a person, organization, or population.

O is for occupation (Gateley & Borcherding, 2012). Since the goal is being written as part of an occupational therapy program, the goal needs to reflect the occupation the client will perform.

A represents the assistance level required in order for the client to perform the desired occupation (Gateley & Borcherding, 2012). Assistance can be physical, verbal, or gestural.

S corresponds to the specific conditions that need to be in place for the client to meet the goal (Gateley & Borcherding, 2012). Conditions can include modifications to the environment, equipment, or technique (Gateley & Borcherding, 2012).

Finally, *T* signifies the timeline for achieving the goal (Gateley & Borcherding, 2012). The timeline should be reasonable and achievable.

Exercise 15.2

Identify (label) the parts of these goals that correspond to the letters in COAST.

1. Varsha will tie her shoe with one verbal cue using the bunny ears method within 1 month.

C:

O:

A:

S:

T:

2. Ndomo will prepare a meal for his dog, following the task checklist, independently, within one week.

C:

O:

A:

S:

T:

3. The client will independently send a text using the speech to text function on his smartphone by July 19, 2014.

C:

O:

A:

S:

T:

4. By November 28, 2014, Monte will propel his wheelchair from his home to the grocery store and back, with no more than one prompt.

C:

O:

A:

S:

T:

▼ RHUMBA (RUMBA) ▼

A third method for writing goals is RHUMBA (College of St. Catherine [CSC], 2001) or RUMBA (McClain, 1991; Perinchief, 1998). According to Perinchief (1998), the American Occupational Therapy Association (AOTA) developed RUMBA in the 1970s. A *rhumba* (also spelled *rumba*) is an Afro-Cuban dance that is especially rhythmic and complex (New World Encyclopedia, 2008). In goal setting, the client represents the music, the goals must "dance" to the client's tune, and each of the parts of the goal must "rhumba" with each other (CSC, 2001). As with the other systems for goal writing, each letter in the word "rhumba" stands for something.

Relevant/**R**elates: *The goal/outcome must relate to something, be relevant.*
How Long: *Specify when the goal/outcome will be met.*
Understandable: *Anyone reading it must know what it means.*
Measurable: *There must be a way to know when the goal is met.*
Behavioral: *The goal/outcome must be something that is seen or heard.*
Achievable: *It must be realistic and doable.* (CSC, 2001, p. 1).

Let's examine each of these in more detail.

The "R" can stand for **relevant** (McClain, 1991; Perinchief, 1998). If a goal is relevant, it answers the question "So what?" Does achieving this goal really matter? Will it make a difference in the client's life? Think about what matters more, that the client can bend her elbow 40°; farther or that she can now feed herself? Here are some examples of meaningless goals adapted from CSC's *Goal Writing: Documenting Outcomes* (2001):

1. I will take 94E to 90S, averaging 70 mph and 30 mpg, on Saturday, driving for approximately 7 hours, in my red '02 MX6, by myself, taking enough luggage for 3 days and food for the trip, stopping no more than 3 times.

   So what? What is the point of all of this? Where are you going? Is how you do it more important than getting there? What needs to be stated is the expected outcome, not the method for getting there.

2. Patient will count coins of varying denominations and combinations of up to $.77 with 65% accuracy on 3 of 5 tries each day for 7 of 10 days within 30 days.

   So what? How will this make a significant difference in a client's life? What happens if the patient counts $.77 with 60% accuracy on 4 of 5 tries for 6 of the next 10 days? Is the goal met? Will the next goal be $.78? How will you keep track of all this data? I do not understand this goal; it is too complicated.

The "R" can also mean *relates* (CSC, 2001). The long- and short-term goals must relate to an area of occupation (keep it functional); they must relate to each other, and they must relate to identified wants and needs of the client (the client's music) (CSC, 2001). In other words, there must be a clear relationship between the areas of occupation identified during the evaluation process as being in need of intervention, the goal statements themselves, and the intervention strategies used to help meet the goals. For example, if in your evaluation you determine that the client needs to learn to hold a crayon using a three-point grasp, then the goals need to say something about holding a crayon, and the intervention needs to involve crayons. It would be inappropriate to identify the need to hold a crayon, set a goal to improve hand use (too vague), and then suggest intervention strategies using jungle gyms, large balls, and finger painting.

How long is a realistic estimate of the time you expect it will take to reach the goal (CSC, 2001). For long-term goals, it usually means when the client will be discontinued, which may be a specific date or an estimate such as 6 months or a year. For short-term goals, it could be a number of visits, a specific date, or, if you write a new intervention plan, every 30 days, you can assume the short-term goals are meant to be met in 30 days. Since how you state the time frame will vary by the setting in which you are working, always check with your supervisor to see what the standard is in that setting. I have seen some goals that simply state that a client will do something on 3 consecutive days, and then the goal will be met. Well, that is not really putting a time limit on a goal. The client could do the task on 3 consecutive days next week, or 6 months from now. If I am paying for occupational therapy services, I want to know whether to expect the client to meet the goal in 2 weeks or 2 months. If a client needs to do something 3 days in a row, that may be OK as a measurement, but it does not tell me when to expect the goal to be met.

Understandable involves several dimensions. In order for the reader to understand the goal, it has to make sense to the reader, which means using easily understood, grammatically correct, and accurately spelled language free from jargon and using only acceptable abbreviations. Use an active voice rather than a passive voice. This means you say that the client will do something rather than that something will be done; that is, "The client will change her socks," rather than "The socks will be changed by the client." Again, check a grammar guide for more information on active voice. Finally, consider avoiding noncommittal language. Examples of noncommittal language include phrases like "will appear" or "will be able to."

You want the client to do something, not just look like she can do it. There is a difference between actually doing something and being able to do something. If you say the client will be able to feed himself, it does not necessarily mean he will do it. Maybe the nurse does it for him, even though he could do it if they let him. If you say the client will feed himself, it means he will do it himself. The goal has to be so clearly stated that anyone stepping in for you if you are sick will know, beyond a shadow of a doubt, what your plan was for providing services to a client.

If you look at the two example goals from earlier in this section you will see that, in addition to not being relevant, they are also not understandable. The goals contain so many clauses and conditions that it is impossible to know what the focus of the goal really is. I can't even tell how to measure the second example.

Measurable is usually expressed as a quantitative statement that identifies how you will know when the goal is met (CSC, 2001). A goal is not met just because the time frame has elapsed. There has to be a measurement of function. You can measure progress as well as maintenance of function. Examples of measurements include frequency, accuracy, level of efficiency, consistency, grade, degree, speed, level of independence, or duration (CSC, 2001; McClain, 1991; Perinchief, 1998).

The *behavioral* component is the same as it was in the ABCD system. The behavior has to be observed, not inferred. It can be reflected as an action verb (see lists earlier in the chapter). By observed, I mean something you can see the client do or hear the client say (Perinchief, 1998). Since you cannot see or hear how a client feels or knows something, these would not be behaviors you would include in goal statements. You can hear a client express his feelings, but you can never be completely sure that because someone says he feels something he actually feels it. You can see if a client can demonstrate a behavior, but that may or may not mean she understands it.

Achievable means that the goal is reasonable and likely to be met in the time frame established (CSC, 2001; McClain, 1991; Perinchief, 1998). It is reasonable given the condition of the client, the frequency and duration of projected occupational therapy sessions, and the contexts of the client and the environment. It is not overly ambitious or too easy.

Exercise 15.3

Identify the parts of the goal that correspond to the letters RHUMBA:

1. By January 2, 2014, the client will accurately cut and paste eight individual letters using the mouse with his left hand in 5 minutes or less. *(Client had a stroke affecting his dominant (right) hand and wants to become proficient at using a mouse with his nondominant (left) hand.)*

   R:

   H:

   U:

   M:

   B:

   A: *You do not have enough information to answer this, but I assure you it is achievable.*

2. By June 26, 2013, the client will consistently catch himself each time he begins to make self-defeating/self-derogatory statements. *(Client is experiencing major depression and has committed himself to an inpatient psychiatric program following a failed suicide attempt.)*

   R:

   H:

   U:

M:

B:

A: *You do not have enough information to answer this, but it seems achievable.*

3. By the end of the year, Kylie will independently maintain a sitting position without support for 10 minutes, so that she can participate more actively in the world around her. *(Client is a 9-month-old near-SIDS baby seen in her home.)*

R:

H:

U:

M:

B:

A: *You do not have enough information to answer this, but it is achievable.*

▼ SMART ▼

The last system for goal writing is writing SMART goals. There are many versions of SMART goals as well. Angier (1995) says SMART goals mean goals that are specific, measurable, action-oriented, realistic, and timely. The University of Victoria Counseling Services (1996) uses SMART as an acronym for specific, measurable, acceptable, realistic, and time frame. Paul J. Meyer (2002) describes SMART as standing for specific, measurable, attainable, realistic, and tangible. In this book, SMART stands for significant (and simple), measurable, achievable, related, and time-limited.

Significant means that achieving this goal will make a significant difference in this person's life. This implies that you know your client's strengths and need areas so well that you know what will matter most to her (or him); in fact, your goals would ideally be developed in collaboration with her (or him), ensuring significance. By remembering to keep it simple you are more likely to achieve the goal, and it will be easier to understand.

Measurable, as in RHUMBA, means that you have a clear target to aim for, and that you will know when the client gets there (CSC, 2001). The client will dress herself with no more than one verbal cue. The client will feed himself a whole meal in less than 30 minutes. Timothy will check his daily schedule every hour. These are incomplete goals, but I mention them here to emphasize the measurement component of goal writing. One common error I have seen in goal writing is goals that say the client will improve at something without stating how big the improvement must be. For example, the client will improve her accuracy at measuring dry ingredients. How much improvement is enough to say that goal was met?

Achievable also has the same meaning as it does in RHUMBA. It must be reasonable that the client could achieve this goal in the time allotted for it (CSC, 2001). Realistically, not every client will achieve every goal. When you first start out writing goals, you may have to guess a little at how much the client can achieve in your time frame. As you gain experience, your guesses will become more accurate.

Related, in SMART as in RHUMBA, means that the goal clearly has a connection to the client's occupational needs as stated in the evaluation report (CSC, 2001). Long- and short-term goals relate to each other.

Finally, *time-limited* means the goal has a chronological end point (CSC, 2001). You know when to evaluate whether the goal is met. If the long-term goal is met, then it is time to discontinue services. If the short-term goal is met, then it is time to set a new short-term goal that gets the client closer to the long-term goal. If the short-term goal is not met at the designated time, then perhaps that goal needs to be either modified or continued.

Exercise 15.4

Identify the parts of the goal that correspond to the letters SMART:

1. By next week, client will demonstrate proper lifting techniques on 80% of opportunities for lifting boxes weighing 10 lbs. or more. *(Client had a back injury and is now being seen in a work-hardening program.)*

   S:

   M:

   A: *Seems achievable given what we know.*

   R:

   T:

2. By April 22, 2014, Nellie will feed herself with a fork or spoon, spilling two or fewer times per meal. *(Nellie is in a long-term care facility with diagnoses of rheumatoid arthritis, COPD, and macular degeneration.)*

   S:

   M:

   A: *I think it is achievable in the time frame given.*

   R:

   T:

3. Mandy will cut out basic shapes with scissors within 1/4" of the line consistently by the end of the school year. *(Mandy is in first grade and has fine motor deficits that make her stand out from her classmates.)*

   S:

   M:

   A: *It is achievable.*

   R:

   T:

Exercise 15.5

Write a goal statement for the following cases using the format listed.

1. **ABCD:** This client has recently had tendon transfer surgery on his dominant hand. The surgeon wants you to make a splint and teach the client how to don and doff the splint. The hand will be immobilized for a week.

2. **COAST:** This 2-year-old child was recently adopted from Albania. She is behind on her development. She does not speak or understand English. She came to occupational therapy on a referral from the foreign adoption clinic at the University Hospital. Her adoptive parents would like to improve her eye contact with them and her interactions with toys.

3. **COAST:** This client was admitted yesterday after an episode of mania in which she got little sleep, shopped till she dropped, and then engaged in wild parties involving sex, drugs, and rock 'n' roll. She is loud, often saying and doing things that embarrass other clients, and is in constant motion. Her husband admitted her to get her back on an appropriate medication routine.

4. **RHUMBA:** This client is 6 years old. She has cerebral palsy. She is in occupational therapy to learn to use a new electric wheelchair.

5. **SMART:** This client was badly burned in a house fire. She has had numerous skin grafts. She is past the extreme pain phase, and now rates her pain level as very bad. In occupational therapy, she is working on increasing her reach and grasp with both arms while wearing compression garments.

6. **ABCDE:** This elderly client was recently discharged from the hospital following surgery to remove a brain tumor. She is being seen in her home to increase her endurance and begin to do her own self-cares.

7. **COAST:** This teenager is recovering from a gunshot wound to the head. He has mobility impairments on the left side of his body, impulsivity, visual perceptual deficits, and is relearning all his ADLs.

8. **ABCD:** This homeless man needs to work on skills related to budgeting. He has a full-time minimum wage job.

9. **RHUMBA:** This man has schizophrenia and lives in a group home in the community. He is receiving occupational therapy at a sheltered workshop for organizing his work space and staying on task.

10. **SMART:** This 4-year-old child was recently diagnosed with autism. He will only wear soft clothes, avoids certain textures of food, bumps into objects and people, and bites his wrist when he becomes excited.

Exercise 15.6

What is wrong with each goal? Tell which criteria you used to answer this question (ABCD, COAST, RHUMBA, or SMART).

1. Tiffany will be evaluated for a new wheelchair within the next 30 days.

2. By next week, Dylan will feed himself with minimal assist, 3×/d, for 50% of the meal, using adaptive utensils, with extra time allowed, and a pureed diet.

3. Darnell will complete his resume and send it to three potential employers.

4. Hector will bring his memory book to therapy every day for the next week.

5. Hui will express satisfaction with the quality of her work at least three times.

SUMMARY

Goal writing is tricky business. You have to think about what the client wants or needs, what is a reasonable amount of time needed to meet the goal, how you will measure it, and assorted other conditions, depending on the format you use for goal writing. Four separate formats for goal writing were presented: ABCD, COAST, RHUMBA, and SMART. While there are subtle differences between them, they all result in well-written goals.

Goal writing is a collaborative process involving the occupational therapist and the client or client's surrogate (i.e., parent or guardian). An occupational therapy assistant contributes to this process.

Goals are written to help a client improve occupational performance, learn to do a new task, maintain function, modify or adapt contexts to enable performance, prevent occupational performance problems, or promote health (AOTA, 2014). The verbs used to show the action of the goal will vary by the direction of the goal, but all verbs used should be active rather than passive in nature. Word selection is also important in describing change and the measurement of change.

The ultimate goal in occupational therapy is "*Achieving health, well-being, and partici-pation in life though engagement in occupation*" (AOTA, 2014, p. S4). For each client, the occupations the client wants or needs to engage in will be different. Long-term goals are writ-ten to describe the final outcome of occupational therapy intervention and are sometimes called discharge or discontinuation goals. Short-term goals are usually written for a specific period of time, often monthly, but may be written for a week, biweekly, or bimonthly. Long-term goals generally stay the same throughout occupational therapy service delivery, unless the client's life circumstances change. Short-term goals change or are revised often.

Goal writing is an essential part of both the evaluation and intervention processes. Goals give you a yardstick by which you can measure the effectiveness of the intervention approaches and methods used with a given client.

REFERENCES

Angier, M. (1995). *Setting S-M-A-R-T goals.* Retrieved December 20, 2002, from http://www. positiveath.net/ideasMA20_p.htm

American Occupational Therapy Association. (2010). Standards of practice for occupational therapy. *American Journal of Occupational Therapy, 64,* S106–S111. doi:10.5014/ ajot.2010.64S106

American Occupational Therapy Association. (2014). Occupational therapy practice frame-work: Domain and process (3rd ed). *American Journal of Occupational Therapy, 68*(Suppl. 1), S1-S48. http://dx.doi.org/10.5014/ajot.2014.682006

College of St. Catherine. (2001). *Goal writing: Documenting outcomes* [Handout]. St. Paul, MN: Author.

Gateley, C. A., & Borcherding, S. (2012). *Documentation manual for occupational therapy: Writing SOAP notes.* Thorofare, NJ: Slack.

Kettenbach, G. (2009). *Writing patient/client notes: Ensuring accuracy in documentation* (4th ed.). Philadelphia, PA: F. A. Davis.

McClain, L. H. (1991). Documentation. In W. Dunn (Ed.), *Pediatric occupational therapy* (pp. 213–244). Thorofare, NJ: Slack.

Meyer, P. J. (2002). *Creating S.M.A.R.T goals.* Retrieved from http://achievement.com/smart.html

Moyers, P. A., & Dale, L. M. (2007). *The guide to occupational therapy practice* (2nd ed.). Bethesda, MD: American Occupational Therapy Association.

New World Encyclopedia. (2008). Rumba. Retrieved from http://www.newworldencyclope-dia.org/entry/Rumba

Perinchief, J. M. (1998). Management of occupational therapy services. In M. E. Neistadt & E. B. Crepeau (Eds.), *Willard and Spackman's occupational therapy* (9th ed., pp. 772–790). Philadelphia: Lippincott.

Quinn, L., & Gordon, J. (2003). *Functional outcomes: Documentation for rehabilitation.* St. Louis, MO: Elsevier.

Richardson, P. K., & Schultz-Krohn, W. (2001). Planning and implementing services. In J. Case-Smith (ed.), *Occupational therapy for children* (4th ed., pp. 246–264). St. Louis, MO: Mosby.

University of Victoria Counseling Services. (1996). *Learning skills program: Smart goals.* Retrieved December 20, 2002, from http://www.coun.uvic.ca/learn/program/hndouts/ smartgoals.html

Visit **www.pearsonhighered.com/healthprofessionsresources** to access the student resources that accompany this book. Simply select Occupational Therapy from the choice of disciplines. Find this book and you will find the complimentary study tools created for this specific title.

CHAPTER 16

Intervention Plans

INTRODUCTION

The intervention plan is where the occupational therapist articulates expected outcomes and how they will be achieved. It is based on the results of the evaluation and the wants and needs of the client or surrogate (i.e., parent or guardian) (American Occupation Therapy Association [AOTA], 2010a). The development and revision of the intervention plan are a collaborative effort between the occupational therapist, the occupational therapy assistant, and the client (AOTA, 2010a). Medicare uses the term *plan of care* rather than intervention plan (Centers for Medicare and Medicaid Services [CMS], 2008). You may also hear the terms *care plan*, *treatment plan*, or *plan of treatment* used interchangeably with intervention plan. Regardless of what you call it, the intervention plan tells the occupational therapy practitioners what they are going to do to help the client.

Establishing goals and determining intervention strategies that will be effective, and that third-party payers will pay for, is critical to the ongoing viability of your practice in occupational therapy. If you do not get paid for what you do, you will not be able to make a living at being an occupational therapy practitioner. To be paid for your services, you have to show that the intervention made a difference in your client's life. That is what motivates us to become occupational therapy professionals in the first place—we want to help make people's lives better.

▼ ROLE DELINEATION IN INTERVENTION PLANNING ▼

The occupational therapist is responsible for developing and documenting the intervention plan, and complying with the time frames, formats, and standards required by the facility/agency, accrediting bodies, and payers (AOTA, 2009, 2010a). An occupational therapy assistant collaborates with the occupational therapist to develop the intervention plan. The occupational therapist or occupational therapy assistant under the supervision of the occupational therapist reviews the intervention plan, the rationale for the plan, and the risks and benefits of the plan with the client and appropriate others (AOTA, 2010a). When necessary, the occupational therapist revises the plan of care and documents the revised goals, changes in the client's condition or situation, and the client's performance; the occupational therapy assistant may contribute to the revised intervention plan (AOTA, 2010a).

The intervention planning process makes the client an active partner in the process. As in the evaluation process, it is client-centered. It also requires close interaction between the occupational therapist and the occupational therapy assistant. In some settings, the occupational therapy assistant is the professional who is at the facility day in and day out, while the occupational therapist makes periodic supervision visits to the facility to conduct evaluations, develop and revise intervention plans, and prepare discharge plans and summaries. This is most likely to occur in settings where the clients are fairly stable, and the occupational therapy assistant is experienced and has demonstrated service competence in a wide variety of clinical skills. In situations like this, the occupational therapy assistant has more regular contact with the clients and can provide extremely valuable input to the occupational therapist regarding the skills and abilities of the client as they relate to occupational performance.

Medicare requires that all services are delivered under a plan of care (CMS, 2008, 2012). In addition, Medicare requires certification and recertification of the need for treatment by a physician or nonphysician practitioner (NPP). An NPP is a physician assistant, clinical nurse specialist, or nurse practitioner who is authorized by state law to certify or supervise therapy services. Medicare does not allow chiropractors or dentists to order, certify, recertify, or supervise therapy (CMS, 2008, 2012).

The plan of care must be established before any occupational therapy services can be provided (AOTA, 2008; CMS, 2008, 2012). The word *established* implies that it is written or dictated by either a physician or NPP, or the occupational therapist who will provide the services. Medicare allows the interventions to begin before the plan is written only if the occupational therapist who established the plan is providing or supervising the occupational therapy interventions. This means that the evaluation and initial intervention can occur on the same day (CMS, 2008, 2012). As stated earlier in this book, the closer to the actual event (evaluation or intervention) that the documentation of it occurs, the more accurate and trustworthy it will be. In other words, even though Medicare allows interventions to begin before the plan is written, it is crucial to get the plan in writing as soon as possible.

According to Medicare, the plan of care needs to include at least the client's diagnoses; long-term treatment goals; and the type, amount, duration, and frequency of the occupational therapy services (CMS, 2008, 2012). The plan needs to reflect the results of the evaluation. Medicare wants the plan to be the most efficient and effective means of treating the client's needs. Occupational therapy is considered reasonable and necessary when it is expected that the therapy will result in significant improvement in the patient's level of function within a reasonable time (AOTA, 2008). The long-term goals are written for the entire episode of care (number of calendar days from the start of care to the end of care) in that setting. Unless otherwise specified in the plan of care, Medicare assumes that interventions will be provided one time per day (CMS, 2008).

Certification and recertification indicate that the client is under the care of a physician or NPP, and that the physician or NPP approves the plan of care (CMS, 2008, 2012). A physician or NPP must certify the occupational therapy plan of care in order for Medicare to pay for the occupational therapy services delivered to a specific client. The certification/recertification occurs when the physician or NPP signs the plan of care, writes a physician's progress note or orders occupational therapy interventions. The initial plan of care must be certified (signed) by the physician or NPP as soon as possible, or within 30 days of the start of care (CMS, 2012). After initial physician or NPP certification, a recertification is required at least every 90 days, or sooner if there is a need to change the plan of care (CMS, 2012).

Optional, but recommended elements of a Medicare plan of care include short-term goals and specific treatment interventions, procedures, modalities, or techniques (CMS, 2008). Brennan and Robinson (2006) stress that these should always be included because they show why the specialized skills of an occupational therapist or occupational therapy assistant under the supervision of an occupational therapist are needed.

Medicare requires that the plan of care demonstrate that the "expertise, knowledge, clinical judgment, decision making, and abilities of a therapist" are required (CMS, 2012, p. 23). This means that an unsupervised assistant, other qualified personnel, caretaker, or patient could not provide this service. To demonstrate this, the occupational therapist needs to document any changes made to the plan of care, based on the occupational therapist's clinical judgment (CMS, 2012).

A standard that Medicare applies to all therapy services is that the services are "reasonable and necessary" (CMS, 2012). This means that the occupational therapy services meet standards of medical practice, are specific and effective in treating the condition, are of a level of complexity or sophistication, or the care can only be provided by a skilled occupational therapist or occupational therapy assistant under the supervision of an occupational therapist, or the client's condition requires the skills of an occupational therapist. In addition, the amount, frequency and duration of intervention must be considered reasonable under accepted professional standards of practice (CMS, 2012). Medicare has historically applied a standard of demonstrable improvement for coverage of occupational therapy services in skilled nursing facilities and home health care (Yamkovenko, 2012). This meant that the occupational therapist had to show that the client's ability to perform ADLs was improving at a reasonable pace. Recently, two courts just ruled that Medicare was being too strict in its interpretation of that standard (Yamkovenko, 2012). This legal interpretation implies that even if the person's condition is not changing, or is deteriorating, occupational therapy services may be covered if they prevent deterioration. It would allow maintenance therapy, not just restorative therapy, at least under Part A Medicare. As of the time this book went to press, only skilled nursing and home health were impacted by this court decision.

Brennan and Robinson (2006) identify common pitfalls in documenting the plan of care that could lead to payment denials by Medicare. If the intervention does not have a sufficient level of complexity to justify the intervention by an occupational therapy practitioner, payment can be denied for the services provided. Medicare expects that the intervention plan will change to reflect changes in the client's level of function; if the plan does not change or the client's level of function does not change, that could be grounds for a Medicare denial of coverage. The outcome goals have to be based on some kind of baseline measure; failure to do so could result in a Medicare denial. Finally, while standardized test scores are helpful in determining outcomes, outcomes tied to a specific test score are meaningless because a test score is not the same as functional performance in an area of occupation (Brennan & Robinson, 2006).

Exercise 16.1

1. Go to the Medicare website at www.cms.hhs.gov
2. Find the following publications:
   a. Pub 100-02 Medicare Benefit Policy, Transmittal 88, Sections 220 and 230
   b. Pub 100-08 Program Integrity Manual, Chapter 13—Local Coverage Determinations 13.5.1
   c. Program Memorandum Transmittal AB-01-56
   d. Medicare Claims Processing Manual, Chapter 5, Section 20 (Pub 100-4)
3. Down load them to your computer.
4. In each publication, find the information that pertains to the documentation of the delivery of occupational therapy services. What limits does Medicare set?

▼ CONCEPTS FOR INTERVENTION PLANNING ▼

To help your client make progress toward his or her desired outcomes, you must select intervention strategies that will lead your client in the same direction as the mutually-agreed-upon goal(s). This requires knowledge of both the skills and abilities of your client and the qualities of the activities (occupations) so that there is a match between what the activity has to offer and what the client needs. For example, if a client has difficulty with problem solving, you need an activity that requires some problem solving, but at a level that is just a bit above where the client is currently functioning. In this case, perhaps problems that require abstract thought, such as story problems in math or exercises of the "2-minute mysteries" type, would be too hard. Instead, an activity that involves real-life situations with rules to follow, such as getting from one place to another within the building or using a substitutions list at the back of a cookbook, would be a better place to start.

An intervention plan is not engraved in stone; it is subject to change as the client's condition and contexts change. If the occupational therapist believes that a change in the goals or intervention strategies, including the frequency, intensity, or duration of intervention sessions, is needed, he or she writes up a new intervention plan. If the client is a

Medicare Part B (outpatient) recipient, the Medicare forms require a physician signature every 90 days, so changing the frequency or duration on that form carries the weight of a doctor's order (CMS, 2008, 2012). Factors to consider when changing the frequency or duration include the client's potential to benefit from services, the degree of dysfunction, outcomes research on clients with similar conditions and interventions, potential for caregiver follow-through, and possible complications that could change the client's rate of progress (Moyers & Dale, 2007).

Intervention plans are established as soon as the occupational therapist determines that the client needs intervention and may be reviewed every 30 days, 60 days, quarterly, or semiannually (twice a year), depending on the setting, the needs of the client, and the demands of the payer.

The intervention plan must consider not only the client's goals, skills, abilities, and deficits, but also the client's values, beliefs, current and desired state of health and well-being, contexts and environments of the client and the setting in which the intervention will occur, and activity demands (AOTA, 2014). In addition, the occupational therapist must use the best available evidence in determining the best course of action for the interventions.

▼ PARTS OF AN INTERVENTION PLAN ▼

The BiFIP format that was used in Chapter 14 can also be used to format an intervention plan. The background information, findings, interpretation, and plan sections may contain similar, yet different, content from an evaluation report.

The first intervention plan you write for any one client might be part of the evaluation report, or it may be a stand-alone document, depending on the policies of the facility at which you work. If it is part of the evaluation report, then there is no need to repeat identification/background information. However, if it is a stand-alone document, then you will need to include the same kind of identification information that you included on your evaluation report (AOTA, 2013):

- Client name, gender, and date of birth
- Date of the document (may be part of the signature) and the type of document; name of agency/facility and department
- Intervention diagnosis/condition and other diagnoses/conditions
- Precautions and contraindications

An electronic health record system may automatically insert this information once the client's name or client ID number is entered.

The next section of an ongoing intervention plan is findings. On an intervention plan, the findings section is for reporting a brief summary of progress since the last intervention plan was written, within the client's current context. Describe progress or lack thereof using the language of the *Occupational Therapy Practice Framework-III* (AOTA, 2014), addressing the client's performance in areas of occupation, and the performance patterns and skills, contexts, client factors, and activity demands that impact the client's occupational performance. Remember that in this section, you are reporting data, not interpreting it (see Chapter 14).

There is a difference between reporting on the current status of a client and reporting the progress made by that client (McQuire, 1997). According to McQuire, a status report tells what a person can do now with no comparison to prior performance, while a progress report contains some comparative statements. If you want to convince a payer or a referral source that you have provided a worthwhile service, you must choose your words carefully so they show progress. (There will be more information on this in the next section of this chapter.)

The third section of an intervention plan is for recording your interpretation of the findings. This is where you record any barriers or challenges to attaining the short-and long-term goals, and identify the client's current strengths and supports.

The fourth section of the intervention plan is for spelling out what you hope to accomplish in the next review period, adjustments to the short-term goals, intervention strategies, or the duration, frequency, and intensity of intervention sessions can be made. AOTA (2013) specifically states that the short-term goals must be "...directly related to the client's ability and need to engage in desired occupations" (p. 5).

Along with revising goals, you must determine appropriate intervention strategies and methods given the client's current condition and contexts (AOTA, 2013). For example, you will determine if a particular client is a good candidate for using adaptive equipment, or whether teaching the client an adaptive technique would be better. In the course of your occupational therapy education, you will learn many strategies for interventions.

AOTA (2013, 2014) distinguishes between intervention approaches and types of intervention. The intervention approaches are (AOTA, 2013, 2014):

- Create or promote
- Establish or restore
- Maintain
- Modify
- Prevent

Types of intervention are the "consultation, education process, advocacy, and/or the therapeutic use of occupations or activities" (AOTA, 2013, p. 5).

The people reading your intervention plans (other facility staff, physicians, third-party payers, quality management personnel, lawyers, etc.) must be able to see the logical thinking that went into your plan. They have to see that if you set a long-term goal to improve someone's dressing skills, then the short-term goals and methods of intervention must also directly relate to dressing. Not everyone who reads your intervention plan will understand the link between improving dexterity and improving dressing, so if your intervention plan calls for stringing 14-inch beads, it will not make logical sense. If, however, your intervention plan calls for learning to don and doff certain articles of clothing with certain types of fasteners, it will make logical sense. (More about this later in this chapter.)

AOTA (2013) suggests that the service delivery mechanisms and plans for discharge be included in this section. Service delivery mechanisms include such details as who will provide the services, where the services will be provided, and the frequency and duration of services. The plan for discharge includes criteria for discontinuing occupational therapy services, discharge disposition (where the client will be discharged to), and the need for follow-up care. AOTA (2013) also suggests that the tools that will be used to determine outcomes be identified.

The last part of the intervention plan is for signatures. Every intervention plan needs to be signed by an occupational therapist. The *AOTA Guidelines for Documentation of Occupational Therapy Practice* (2013) suggests including the name and position of each person responsible for overseeing the implementation of the plan. Each time you sign a document, always include the date it was written in the signature line. If you are using an EHR, your signature and the date will appear automatically.

▼ SUMMARIZING PROGRESS ▼

Generally, you will write an intervention plan for a client every 30–90 days. Between intervention plan revisions, you will write progress notes (see Chapter 17). On your initial intervention plan, you will not be able to summarize progress, but on subsequent intervention plans you will. It is helpful to go back over the progress notes written over the last month (or whatever the interval between plans is in your setting) while you summarize changes since the last intervention plan was written.

It is important to give the reader an accurate picture of progress. Inaccurately reporting progress so that it appears faster or slower than reality is fraud (see Chapter 9). Do not do it. As stated in the AOTA *Code of Ethics*, occupational therapy practitioners "Refrain from using or participating in the use of any form of communication that contains false, fraudulent, deceptive, misleading, or unfair statements or claims" (2010b, Principle 6.B). In addition, Principle 6.D. says "Ensure that documentation for reimbursement purposes is done in accordance with applicable laws, guidelines, and regulations" (AOTA, 2010b).

So how do you describe progress accurately? Choose your words carefully. Understand how others interpret words. Some words are "loaded," that is, some readers will twist them in ways you never intended (see Chapter 2). When you write, "Continues to have difficulty with _____," a payer might interpret it as "not making progress." In reality, the client has made progress, but not as fast as you had hoped. Think about the difference between these words:

Attends	Participates
Understands	Complies or demonstrates
Approachable	Sociable

In each of these pairs, the word on the right is more active. If you write that a client attended occupational therapy sessions, a reader could interpret that as the client came into the room, but did not do anything. If you write that the client participated in the occupational therapy session, it implies that the client engaged in the process. Someone can nod and say she understands, but unless you see them do it, are you sure she can do it? *Approachable* implies that you can go up to this person and initiate conversation. *Sociable* implies that this person is equally comfortable approaching others and being approached by others. Box 16.1 contains a list of words that convey progress or change.

When you summarize progress over time, the focus needs to be on engagement in occupation. Describe the new occupations the client does now that he or she could not do last month (or whatever your time frame is). The World Health Organization's ICF document (see Chapter 4) contains a comprehensive list of activities that might be helpful to you as you think about function (WHO, 2002). Focusing on function means making sure you address what the client does, not the underlying skills and abilities. For example, if a client is now able to reach to the top shelf in the kitchen and bring down what she needs from that shelf without assistance, that is focusing on function. If, instead, you report that the client has increased range of motion to 170° in shoulder flexion, you are not reporting on function. Reporting increased range of motion is nicely measurable, but just because someone can move his arm farther does not necessarily mean he uses it to do anything that his functional performance has improved. Another example would be describing ways a client demonstrates improved self-esteem rather than stating the client scores 26% higher on a test of self-esteem. Perhaps the client is now checking her appearance in the mirror before leaving her room, or she is expressing confidence in her skills.

How do you demonstrate progress? By choosing words that show change as much as possible while still being honest. On an intervention plan, it is not necessary to describe everything the client did over the past month; hit only the highlights, only ones that directly relate to the goals you set last month. To do otherwise would result in a lengthier document than you want to write and than anyone wants to read. Evaluation reports can be long, but intervention plans usually have limited space for recording progress.

What do you write if there has not been the progress you had hoped for? Explain what barriers to progress were encountered. There is probably a reasonable explanation for the lack of expected progress; maybe there was a medical complication or change in life circumstance that got in the way. Whatever the explanation, keep it simple and short. Explain how you will modify your intervention plan to encourage greater progress.

In some places, the payers allow maintenance therapy. In maintenance therapy, a client has a condition that is likely to cause functional deterioration. Occupational therapy intervention can delay or prevent this deterioration. If this is the case, showing progress is not expected; maintaining function is good. Do not try to describe progress when maintenance is the goal.

BOX 16.1 Descriptive Words for Progress Notes

Describing Physical Behavior

Adapts
Against gravity
Assistance
Athetoid
Awkward
Barely
Bouncy
Careful
Clumsy
Compensate
Complains
Completely
Consistent
Coordinated
Crooked
Creates
Crepitus
Delayed
Deliberately
Dependent
Difficulty
Easily
Effort
Effortless
Endurance
Energetically
Even
Exertion
Gently
Gracefully
Guarded
Haphazardly
Heavily
Hesitantly
Holds
Imitates
Inconsistent
Independent
Jerky/jerkily
Less
Limits
Maintains
Minimum
Mildly
Moderate
Modifies
More
Precise

Rapid
Regressed
Rigid
Roughly
Shaky
Slow
Smoothly
Softly
Spastic
Steady
Stimulating
Strength
Swiftly
Tentative
Thoroughly
Tires
Uneven
Violently
Withdraws
With ease
Writhe

Describing Social Behavior

Acceptable
Adapts
Aggressive
Agitated
Alert
Angry
Antagonistic
Anxious
Apathetic
Approachable
Appropriate
Argumentative
Argues
Asks
Attentive
Aware
Behaves
Boisterous
Bored
Careful
Changeable
Cheerful
Childish
Complacent
Complains
Complies

Confident
Confused
Consistent
Contributes
Consults
Converses
Cooperative
Curious
Decides
Demanding
Demands
Demonstrates
Dependable
Destructive
Diligent
Distractible
Drowsy
Easily upset
Elated
Empathetic
Encouraging
Engaging
Enjoys
Enthusiastic
Establishes
Euphoric
Evasive
Even disposition
Excessive
Excitable
Explores
Explodes
Expresses
Fearful
Flat affect
Flexible
Flexibility
Follows
Friendly
Fussy
Gathers
Giddy
Guarded
Hostile
Hyperactive
Immature
Impolite
Impulsive
Inappropriate touching
Inappropriate

laughter
Inattentive
Incessantly
Inconsistent
Initiates
Intrusive
Involved
Irritable
Lethargic
Limits
Listens
Manipulative
Moody
Narcissistic
Observes
Obsessive
Overdependent
Pacing
Passive–aggressive
Permissive
Pleasant
Polite
Preoccupied
Proud
Quarrelsome
Receptive
Reliable
Reserved
Respectful
Responsible
Responsible
Restless
Reticent
Rigid
Satisfied
Seductive
Self-confidence
Sensitive
Shallow
Shy
Sluggish
Sociable
Socialize
Suspicious
Tenacious
Tense
Terse
Tolerant
Trepidation
Unaffected
Unassuming

(Continued)

BOX 16.1   Continued

Uncomfortable
Unpopular
Unrealistic
Vacillates
Volunteers
Withdrawn

**Describing
Cognition**
Adapts
Alert
Attentive
Aware
Clarifies
Concentrates
Conscious
Consults
Decisive
Demonstrates
Determines
Distinguishes
Distractible
Explores
Fidgety
Follows
Follows routine
Follows rules
Forgetful
Formulates
Identifies
Impatient
Inattentive
Inquisitive
Intellectually
curious
Interprets
Is Realistic
Knowledgeable
Learns from
mistakes

Needs reminders
Obtains
Organizes
Perseverate
Perfectionistic
Prepares
Prioritizes
Problem-solves
Reads
Refuses
Relaxed
Reliable
Retains
Seclusive
Selects
Thoughtful
Thoughtless
Writes

**Describing
Participation**
Attends
Contributes
Conversation
Diligent
Engages
Expresses
Eye contact
Industrious
Initiates
Participates
Quiet
Reserved
Responds
Responsive
Sociable
Solitary
Talkative
Team player
Terminates

**Describing
Appearance
and Touch**
Appropriate
Ashen
Bewildered
Blush
Body odor
Bored
Clean
Clenches teeth
Colors clash
Concerned
Damp
Dirty
Disheveled
Disordered
Disrepair
Drooling
Ecstatic
Erect posture
Excessive layers
Eyes get big
Fastidious
Flushed
Furrowed brows
Fussy
Glared
Goosebumps
Grimaces
Hot (temperature)
Ill-fitting
Mannerism
Monotone
Neat
Pale
Poised
Presents
Puffy
Raises eyebrow

Scarred
Shiny
Shivered
Sloppy
Slouched posture
Smiles
Sneer
Sweaty
Teary
Tired
Torn clothes
Unaware
Uncombed
Unkempt
Worn out

**Describing
Speech**
Babbles
Clear
Disarticulates
Echolalia
Expresses
Expressive
Flat
Gibberish
Grunts
Lisps
Mispronounces
Monotonous
Mumbles
Pressured
Rambles
Rapid
Repetitive
Slow
Slurred
Word
substitutions

▼ DOCUMENTING INTERVENTION STRATEGIES ▼

Once you and the client have reviewed progress to date and revised short-term goals toward which to work (the outcome or long-term goal is not likely to change, although under some circumstances it might), your thoughts can turn toward intervention strategies to use to help the client meet those goals. The section of the intervention plan where the intervention strategies are listed may be called "interventions," "strategies," "approaches," "methods," or some combination of these words. This is the section where you have to tell the reader what you plan to do to help the client meet his or her goals. To distinguish this from the intervention approaches described earlier, the term "strategies" will be used here.

Strategies can include specific techniques for intervention that are suggested by the model or frame of reference you are using (see Chapter 5), the manner in which you approach the client, general principles for intervention, types of adaptive aids/assistive technology, or task/environmental modifications that will be tried (AOTA, 2013). It also includes whether the client would be best served in an individual or group session (Moyers & Dale, 2007).

As you develop intervention plans, remember that problem identification (evaluation results), goal setting, and intervention strategies all have to relate directly to each other. One way to ensure this interrelationship is to use a frame of reference to guide your thinking. Specific intervention techniques are usually explained by the frame of reference you are using. If you refer back to Chapter 6, you can see how knowledge of a frame of reference can direct your thinking about how to approach the client and the problem. For example, if you were using a biomechanical approach with a client who has had a stroke, your strategies would reflect splinting and range of motion exercises. If instead you were using a contemporary task-oriented approach, you would have the client practice functional activities that are meaningful to the client. If you were using a cognitive disabilities or cognition and activity approach, you would focus on ways to adapt techniques or the environment to enable task performance.

The way you approach the client should be specified in your intervention strategies section. This can have several meanings. It could mean that you identify whether you approach the client at eye level, whether you approach the client like you are the expert or a partner in recovery, or whether you approach the client at bedside or in the clinic. Will you follow the client's suggestions or will you be making suggestions? Will you be firm or flexible? Some of this will depend not only on the frame of reference, but also on the age and condition of the client and the philosophy of the program that is serving the client. For example, the program philosophy may emphasize clients taking an active role in their recovery, and all staff need to actively listen to what the client is saying, letting the client direct the activities he or she tries. Another program may have rigid rules to follow, and the client must obey staff directions.

Other information to record in the strategies section of the intervention plan includes the types of assistive technology, adaptive equipment, or task/environmental modifications the client will try and what home programs or training will be provided to the client or client's caregivers. Since your strategies are simply descriptions of what you will try during the plan period, you can suggest many options. If you put the specific type of equipment in the goal statement, you get locked into using that equipment. If the goal says that the client will do something with or without adaptive equipment, you are freer to experiment. Then in the strategy section, you can list several possibilities for different types of equipment or different techniques.

In addition to establishing goals and intervention strategies, the plan section includes the occupational therapist's recommendations on the frequency, duration, and intensity of occupational therapy intervention sessions (AOTA, 2013). Along with this information, intervention plans specify the location of intervention sessions (e.g., bedside, clinic, and client's home) and the anticipated environment to which the client will be discharged (AOTA, 2013).

When you first start out writing intervention plans and client goals, it is not uncommon for your professor or supervisor to ask that you specifically state your rationale for the goals you set and the intervention strategies you suggest. This is actually a good way to start out because it forces you to articulate why you made the choices you did. In most clinical settings, your rationale will be implied; there will not be time or space to spell out your rationale on every intervention plan. To help you think about your rationale, consider the following questions:

- Why did you choose the goals you wrote down?
- How do they relate to the client's needs?
- How do your intervention strategies relate to each goal?
- What frame of reference (or model of practice) guided your thinking?
- Were there goals or strategies that you considered, but chose not to record? If so, why?

Exercise 16.2

For the following goals, suggest three activities that the client could engage in to help reach his or her goals, and then state your rationale for the suggested activities.

1. Client: 2-year-old female with Down syndrome whose lack of coordination and low muscle tone interfere with her ability to engage in age-appropriate play activities.

   Goal: The client will successfully participate in three age-appropriate play activities by 6 months from now.

   Three suggested activities:

   Rationale:

2. Client: 54-year-old man with a traumatic amputation of his right arm just below the elbow.

   Goal: In the next 30 days, Mr. Smith will spontaneously begin to use artificial arm with hook to pick up solid objects.

   Three suggested activities:

   Rationale:

3. Client: 72-year-old woman with a total hip replacement.

   Goal: Ellie will dress herself independently, with or without the use of adaptive equipment, by April 10, 2014.

   Three suggested activities:

   Rationale:

4. Client: 28-year-old woman with postpartum depression.

   Goal: Naomi will initiate conversations with three people outside her family in the next 2 weeks.

   Three suggested activities:

   Rationale:

▼ SAMPLE INTERVENTION PLANS ▼

Sample intervention forms are also provided in Appendix D (see website). Figure 16.1 shows an intervention plan for Jacob Olson, the basketball player from Chapter 14. This plan was written 30 days after his intervention started. Figure 16.2 contains three sample, simplified intervention plans (based on plans developed by occupational therapy students at the College of St. Catherine). They have been modified and simplified, with only one long-term goal and two short-term goals listed, whereas in reality there may be more goals than that. However, I will caution you to avoid setting too many goals in one plan. I have seen plans with eight

OCCUPATIONAL THERAPY INTERVENTION PLAN

BACKGROUND INFORMATION

Date of report: 2-15-14   **Client's name:** Jacob Olsen

DOB: 6-25-93   **Date of referral:** 1-14-14

Primary intervention diagnosis/concern: tendonitis of R thumb; neck, back, and R arm pain

Secondary diagnosis/concern: depression

Precautions/contraindications: thumb immobilized until 1-28-14

Reason for referral to OT: Immobilization of thumb interferes with daily life tasks

Therapist: Ina Second, MS, OTR/L

FINDINGS

Occupational profile: Jake is a 20-year-old college athlete. In addition to playing varsity basketball, Jake reports that he loves video games, and spends much of his non-basketball hours playing them. According to Jake, he is anxious to get back to basketball because he hopes to play in the NBA after college. He is currently a sports management major.

Progress Toward Goals So Far; Reasons for Progress or Lack Thereof in:

Areas of occupation: Jake usually wears sweats but does wear jeans and shirts with buttons which he can don and doff independently. He is currently using a button hook and loop zipper pulls but wants to dress without these adaptations. His meals are prepared for him and he eats in the dorm cafeteria. He performs grooming and hygiene tasks with his injured hand, but reports it takes longer to do than before his injury. He is keyboarding with both hands, although he is very slow. Using a joystick for video games with his injured thumb is painful. Jake texts using his index finger which has slowed him down. He reports being bored, having low energy and not eating or sleeping well.

Performance skills: Jake's posture is hunched forward and contributes to his neck and back pain. Fine motor coordination is improved but not restored to prior level of function.

Performance patterns: Jake is currently following his class schedule, except when team travel demands interfere. He is not practicing with the team, but he attends all games, home and away. He stays in bed until 15 minutes before his first scheduled class, skipping breakfast on the days he goes to class. He is going to bed around midnight most nights. He plays video games for 2–3 hours per day, but wants to play more. He spends 1 hour a day on the stationary bike while watching TV, another hour running on the track, and an hour in the weight room to keep his legs in shape for basketball.

Client factors: Jake reports pain throughout his R hand and arm, limiting his use of that limb. He is wearing a thumb support splint, limiting movement of his R thumb. The pain in his right thumb had reduced from a 9 (on a 10-point scale) to a 5 at rest and a 7 after 15 min. of activity. Pinch strength is below age norms on his injured hand. ROM measurements as noted below. Energy and drive are currently below what they were before the injury.

ROM	DIP Flexion	DIP Extension	PIP Flexion	MCP Flexion	MCP Extension	Abduction
R thumb	45	0		45	0	35
L thumb	90	10		60	10	70
R index	40	10	90	70	25	10
L index	70	10	100	90	30	20
R middle	40	0	90	80	25	10
L middle	70	0	100	90	30	20

FIGURE 16.1   Jacob Olson's Intervention Plan.

ROM	DIP Flexion	DIP Extension	PIP Flexion	MCP Flexion	MCP Extension	Abduction
R ring	40	0	90	75	20	15
L ring	70	0	90	90	25	20
R little	45	0	90	80	25	15
L little	70	0	100	90	30	20

Contexts: Initially, the desk and chair were not fitted to proper working heights for a person as tall as Jake (6'11"), but that has been corrected. Laptop computer screen was too low but has been elevated to reduce strain on his neck. Jake spends most of his time in class, the gym or his room.

Equipment/orthotics issued: Thumb support splint

Home programs/training: Gentle R hand exercises. Decreased time playing videogames and texting.

INTERPRETATION

Analysis of occupational performance: Jake met his short term goals to engage in 3 hours per day of physical activity, identifying occupations during which his posture is poor, and making three adaptations to his environment to support good posture. He raised his desk, adjusted his desk chair to accommodate his height and reach, and elevated his laptop while using a wireless keyboard. Jake is resistant to attempts to limit his time spent on video games and texting.

PLAN

Long-Term Goals	Short-Term Goals	Methods/Approaches
Jake will return to the basketball team in 6 weeks.	Jake will dribble a basketball for 5 min. with his R hand without pain by March 1, 2014.	Practice dribbling with regulation size basketball Coordinate with team trainer
	Jake will catch and quickly throw a basketball at a target 25 consecutive times using both hands without pain by March 1, 2014.	Practice catch and throw Coordinate with team trainer
Jake will make needed adaptations to his physical environment to support his successful occupational participation by Feb 28, 2014.	Jake will self-correct when he is hunched over during tasks within 3 min. of getting into the poor posture at least 50% of the time by Feb 28, 2014.	Education on body alignment and posture Self-awareness activities
	By Feb 28, 2014 Jake will make adaptations as needed during 3 occupations.	Education on ergonomic principles and types of adaptations that are possible

Expected frequency, duration, and intensity: 3×/wk for 2 wks, 45-min sessions

Location of intervention: OT clinic

Anticipated discontinuation environment: Dorm, gym, and basketball court

Service providers: Ina Second MS, OTR/L and Justa Minute, COTA/L

Ina Second, MS, OTR/L	*2-15-14*
Signature	Date

FIGURE 16.1 (Continued)

OT INTERVENTION PLAN
FUNCTIONAL REHAB, INC

Name: Jamie Shooter   **DOB:** May 18, 1960   **Date of report:** Nov. 3, 2014

Precautions/contraindications: Non-weight bearing for 6 weeks

Reason for referral: Increase mobility for independence in self-care

Occupational profile: Jamie was working as a human cannonball for the circus when he was seriously injured in a freak accident 3 days ago. He has multiple fractures of his lower extremities, a dislocated R shoulder, and numerous contusions, cuts, and scrapes all over his body. He had a severe concussion with loss of consciousness for 10 minutes following the incident. Prior to the injury he was healthy and physically fit.

Analysis of occupational performance: Client is in a great deal of pain and resists moving quickly or through his entire range. He is totally dependent in transfers and dressing. He requires moderate assist for grooming and hygiene and minimal assist for feeding. Jamie expressed frustration with his condition, saying he is not used to lying around and has always been active. He thinks boredom will be one of his biggest challenges because he knows he can recover from the physical injuries, but the recovery will not come as quickly as he would like. He loves his job and hopes to return to circus work, although he thinks the doctor is unlikely to recommend a return to being shot out of a cannon. He says he loves the rush he feels flying through the air, so if he can't do that, then maybe he will consider the trapeze.

Problems prioritized: #1 Needs to increase mobility for self-care skills

#2 Needs to decrease dependence on others for self-care skills

#3 Needs to stay occupied

Long-term goal:

Client will transfer independently from bed to wheelchair by Dec. 15, 2014.

Short-Term Goals for Problem #1	Intervention Approaches/Methods for #1
By Nov 20, client will transfer from the mat table to the wheelchair with moderate assist on three consecutive tries.	Strengthening activities Instruction in safe techniques practice pushing up on arms to bear weight on his arms without moving to another surface
By Dec 1, client will transfer from the mat table to the wheelchair with stand-by assist and verbal cues as needed on three consecutive tries.	Strengthening activities involving weight bearing on arms

Frequency of OT sessions: 2×/day

Duration of OT sessions: 30 min

Expected length of OT services: 6 weeks

Bob Bababaran   *11-3-14*
Signature   Date

FIGURE 16.2   Additional Sample Intervention Plans.

OT INTERVENTION PLAN
FUNCTIONAL REHAB, INC

Name: Loretta Mojo   **DOB:** 4-28-09   **Date of report:** Nov. 3, 2014

Precautions/contraindications: Strong aversion to any touch

Reason for referral: Aversion to touch is interfering with everyday life

Occupational profile: Loretta is a 4-year-old girl with autism. She developed normally until she was 18 months old when she seemed to regress to earlier developmental stages. She has strong aversive responses to any form of touch. General health has been good, with only a few ear infections.

Analysis of occupational performance: According to Loretta's mom, Loretta has become increasingly aversive to almost any touch. She is removing her clothes because they appear to irritate her, making it difficult for Loretta to go out in public. She screams when anyone touches her. She fights her bath, especially getting her hair washed. She walks on tiptoes so that her whole feet do not have to touch the floor. Loretta's mom reports that Loretta is a very picky eater and will not let them hug her. This last point seemed to be of the greatest concern to her mom as evidenced by her tears at this point in the interview. Results of sensory integration testing confirm aversion to touch, and deficits in processing both tactile and proprioceptive input.

Problems prioritized: #1 Needs to tolerate touch so that she can be hugged and give hugs

#2 Needs to tolerate touch so that she can wear clothes of varying textures and get her hair washed calmly

#3 Needs to increase the variety of foods she will eat

Long-term goal:

Loretta will share hugs with parents and loved ones within 1 year.

Short-Term Goals for Problem #1	Intervention Approaches/Methods for #1
Loretta will receive one hug without withdrawal during three consecutive OT sessions within 3 months.	Sensory integrative techniques for tactile processing that will gradually increase in duration and intensity. Begin with her applying the stimuli and moving toward the OT applying them.
Loretta will initiate a hug with a parent following OT sessions on four out of five opportunities within 5 months.	Progressive touching activities such as handshaking, putting her arm around an object or person, and then to a hug.

Frequency of OT sessions: 2×/week

Duration of OT sessions: 45 min

Expected length of OT services: 1 year

Bob Bababaran   _11-3-14_
Signature   Date

FIGURE 16.2   (Continued)

OT INTERVENTION PLAN
FUNCTIONAL REHAB, INC

Name: Yolanda Odor   **DOB:** Jan. 18, 1963   **Date of report:** Nov. 3, 2014

Precautions/Contraindications: None

Reason for referral: Needs to improve personal hygiene

Occupational Profile: Yolanda is a 46-year-old woman with schizophrenia. She has been living in community housing; however, recent complaints of poor hygiene resulting in strong body odor has resulted in increasingly angry exchanges with housemates. According to Yolanda, she would bathe if she needed to, but she sees no need to. She also does not think that her bathing habits are anyone's business but her own. She also says she had been faithful in taking her medications, but has stopped taking them because she feels she no longer needs them.

Analysis of Occupational Performance: Client has a very strong body odor; stringy, greasy hair, and has not shaved her legs or armpits in quite some time (judging by the length of the hair). During observation, she did not wash her hands no matter how soiled they became. She did not wash her hands after going to the bathroom. Client reports not using toothpaste, soap, or deodorant in weeks. She also says she does not notice any particular odor about her. Her clothes had multiple spots where food had landed on them.

Problems prioritized: #1 Needs to improve personal hygiene skills

                                               #2 Needs to improve personal grooming skills

Long-term goal:

Within 1 month, Yolanda will independently complete all personal hygiene tasks.

Short-Term Goals for Problem #1	Intervention Approaches/Methods for #1
Within 1 week, Yolanda will wash her hands with soap and water after each time she uses the toilet.	Visual reminders in the bathroom Coaching and verbal reminders
Within 3 weeks, Yolanda will independently initiate showering at least 4 days per week.	Adaptive equipment and instruction in the safe use of this equipment as needed calendar to keep track of showers coaching and feedback

Frequency of OT sessions: 3x/week

Duration of OT sessions: 60 min

Expected length of OT services: 6 weeks

Bob Bababaran   *11-3-14*
Signature   Date

FIGURE 16.2   (Continued)

or more goals that the practitioner expects client to accomplish in a month or two. While the client may have lots of areas that need work, it would be better to focus on a few and do well with them than try to work on too many goals and not do as well.

▼ REVISING INTERVENTION PLANS ▼

The longer you work with a particular client, the more likely it is that you will need to revise your intervention plan. This is not necessarily a sign that your plan is not working, but it just means that it takes time to effect significant changes in a person. Intervention plans are usually revised on a regular schedule, such as every 30 or 90 days, often depending on the requirements of the third-party payer and/or the condition of the client.

Revising the intervention plan allows you to step back from day-to-day intervention and really evaluate whether the plan is working or not. If it is working, then maybe the time is right to take things to the next level. If it is not working, then this is a good time to figure out what you could do differently. Maybe you were too ambitious in your goal setting and need to set

Exercise 16.3

This exercise is called "Create-a-Client." In this exercise, you will create an imaginary client and develop a mini-intervention plan for this client. I suggest that you create a memorable client, someone you think would be fun to work with. You can create a serious case that is simple or complex, or you can create a bizarre and unique client. Use the following format to write about your client.

First, establish background information on your client. Create a memorable name for your client. Determine the client's age, diagnoses, and occupational profile. Then summarize the occupational needs of the client. Determine what performance skills, performance patterns, contexts, activity demands, or client factors contribute to the problems. Next, prioritize occupational needs and establish goals for this client. Finally, suggest intervention strategies.

Create-a-Client

I. Background information
Name: _____
Age: _____
Diagnoses: _____

II. Findings:
Occupational profile:

Summary of progress (since last intervention plan):

III. Interpretation:
Strengths and need areas:

Prioritize occupational needs:
1.
2.
3.

IV. Plan:
One long-term and two short-term goals for top priority:
LTG:

STG:

STG:

Possible interventions:

Frequency, intensity, duration:

_____
Signature   Date

Exercise 16.4

Write an intervention plan based on the following cases:

1. Butch is a 46-year-old man with autism, seizures, and sensory processing disorder. He lives in a shared apartment and works at a sheltered workshop 5 days a week. At the sheltered workshop, he packages craft kits that will be sold at a chain of craft stores nationally. Butch shares his apartment with two other men; all are autistic, and there is a staff person available from 4 p.m. to 9 a.m., Monday to Friday, and 24 hours a day on weekends. With setup by staff, Butch dresses himself, and he assists with cooking and cleaning. For leisure activities, Butch does jigsaw puzzles, rides the exercise bike, goes for walks, and watches TV. Over the last 2 months, the staff at the workshop and at his home have noticed an increase in Butch's self-stimulatory and noncompliant behaviors. He has increased the frequency and intensity of his rocking and mumbling to himself, and hand-flapping. He is saying "no" when he is asked or told to do something, refusing to comply with instructions about 50% of the time. In the last week, he has started to refuse to shower and has gotten pickier about his food. He has not had any medication changes. At the workshop, about 2 months ago, he was moved into a different room, but the task remained the same. He is now in a room with higher functioning clients. At home, last month, the carpeting was replaced with a laminate floor in the living room, and the walls were painted blue. One of his roommates has been having more visitors lately. The staff at the apartment called for an occupational therapy consultation to evaluate and plan a new sensory diet and environmental adaptations as necessary in an effort to restore Butch to his prior level of function.

2. Marcus is a 3-year-old born with Fragile X syndrome. He is nonverbal. His mother completed a Sensory Profile on him, and he appears to have oversensitivity to noise, but undersensitivity to touch. He bites his wrists. He walks independently, but has problems with balance and motor planning. He is a very picky eater, he drinks out of a sippy cup, and does not chew his food well. Sometimes the food falls out of his mouth. Marcus does not dress himself and he is not potty trained. Bathing him and washing his hair are extremely challenging as he is very resistive; he screams and hits, trying to stop the process. His mom reports that it takes two people to give him a bath or wash his hair, and he is inconsolable when it is over. His pediatrician referred him to a pediatric clinic that specializes in sensory integrative evaluation and interventions.

3. Mariah is an 87-year-old woman with mild congestive heart failure, who fell while walking her dog and broke her right hip. She is cognitively very sharp. She was a college professor (English) who kept teaching into her early seventies. Prior to her fall, she lived independently with her husband (age 89), and wire-haired fox terrier, Scarlett. They live in a small house in the city. They both gave up driving 2 years ago. Mariah had surgery to repair her hip 3 days ago and was transferred from the hospital to a subacute unit in the long-term care facility near her home. She has two daughters and six grandchildren who live within 10 miles of this facility. She hopes to return home in 2 weeks. While in the subacute unit, she will receive both occupational and physical therapy twice a day.

smaller goals. Maybe you were not ambitious enough and you need to set higher goals. Maybe you need to consider taking the interventions in a whole new direction. It is up to the occupational therapist to evaluate the effectiveness of the intervention plan. Any changes in the plan should be made in consultation with the client and/or client's caregiver (AOTA, 2010a).

SUMMARY

In this chapter, you have learned about writing intervention plans. The intervention plan is a vital document that is used by payers to determine whether continued intervention is needed, by coworkers to communicate the client's current status and progress, and by the occupational therapy personnel to evaluate the effectiveness of intervention programs.

Generally speaking, a client receiving ongoing intervention from occupational therapy will have an intervention plan developed immediately after the evaluation, and then periodically until services are discontinued. Except when the client is working on maintenance goals, each successive intervention plan should show progress in the client's areas of occupation. If progress is not made, an explanation for the lack of progress must be given.

The occupational therapist is responsible for writing, revising, and communicating the intervention plan. An occupational therapy assistant contributes to the intervention planning process. It is a client-centered process.

In addition to necessary client identification information, intervention plans usually contain a brief summary of progress, revised goals, and intervention strategies. Intervention strategies include frequency and duration of services, manner of service delivery, place of service delivery, types of adaptive equipment/environmental adaptations, task modifications, home programs, and training for the client and the client's caregivers. While intervention plans are written in ink, they are not engraved in stone. They are expected to change as the client's circumstances and condition changes.

REFERENCES

American Occupational Therapy Association. (2008). Medicare Basics. Retrieved August 8, 2008, from http://www.aota.org/Practitioners/Reimb/Pay/Medicare/FactSheets/37788.aspx

American Occupational Therapy Association [AOTA]. (2009). *Guidelines for supervision, roles, and responsibilities in the delivery of occupational therapy services.* Retrieved from http://www.aota.org/-/media/Corporate/Files/Secure/Practice/OfficialDocs /Guidelines/Guidelines%20for%20Supervision%20Roles%20and%20Responsibilities.pdf

American Occupational Therapy Association. (2010a). Standards of practice for occupational therapy [Supplemental material].*American Journal of Occupational Therapy, 64,* S106–S111. doi:10.5014/ajot.2010.64S106

American Occupation Therapy Association. (2010b). Occupational therapy code of ethics—2010 [Supplemental material]. *American Journal of Occupational Therapy, 54,* S17–S26. doi:10.5014/ajot.2010.64S17

American Occupational Therapy Association. (2013). Guidelines for documentation of occupational therapy. Retrieved from http://www.aota.org/-/media/corporate/files/ secure/practice/officialdocs/guidelines/guidelines%20for%20documentation.pdf

American Occupational Therapy Association. (2014). Occupational therapy practice framework: Domain and process (3rd ed). *American Journal of Occupational Therapy, 68*(Suppl. 1), S1-S48. http://dx.doi.org/10.5014/ajot.2014.682006

Brennan, C., & Robinson, M. (2006). Documentation: Getting it right to avoid Medicare denials. *OT Practice, 11*(14), 10–16.

Centers for Medicare and Medicaid Services [CMS]. (2008). *Pub100-02 Medicare benefit policy: Transmittal 88.* Retrieved from http://www.cms.hhs.gov/transmittals/downloads/R88BP.pdf

Centers for Medicare and Medicaid Services [CMS]. (2012). Physical, occupational, and speech therapy services. Retrieved from http://www.cms.gov/Outreach-and-Education/ Outreach/OpenDoorForums/Downloads/090512TherapyClaimsSlides.pdf

McQuire, M. J. (1997). Excellence and efficiency in documentation. *OT Practice, 2*(12), 36–41.

Moyers, P. A., & Dale, L. M. (2007). *The guide to occupational therapy practice* (2nd ed.). Bethesda, MD: American Occupational Therapy Association.

World Health Organization. (2002). *International classification of function.* Geneva, Switzerland: Author. Retrieved May 22, 2002, from http://www3.who.int/icf

Yamkovenko, S. (2012). *Medicare too strict: Two courts rule "improvement standard" too strict in SNF, HH.* Retrieved from http://www.aota.org/en/Advocacy-Policy/Federal-Reg-Affairs/News/2012/medicare-too-strict.aspx

CHAPTER 17

SOAP and Other Methods of Documenting Ongoing Intervention

INTRODUCTION

Written documentation of ongoing intervention comes in different sizes and formats, but all are intended to provide a record of intervention sessions. In most cases, they are written following each intervention session; however, in some cases, they may be written weekly or at other time intervals. These notes may be called progress notes, progress reports, encounter notes, daily notes, or by similar names, but will be called progress notes in this text. Typically, a progress note covers a longer time interval than a daily, contact, or encounter note (Brennan & Robinson, 2006).

Progress notes should be more than simply a listing of the types of activities in which a client has engaged. They are called progress notes because they are supposed to show progress. Therefore, the notes need to include information about the client's response to interventions and how current performance is different from previous performance (American Occupational Therapy Association [AOTA], 2014; Brennan & Robinson, 2006). Any unusual or significant event, assistive or adaptive equipment issued or tried, and any client/caregiver instruction also need to be documented (AOTA, 2014). Ultimately, a progress note or progress report has to show that the skills of an occupational therapy practitioner contributed to the progress a client has made toward the goals established in the intervention plan; how the client is different as a result of occupational therapy interventions (Brennan & Robinson, 2006).

Contact notes, are intended to be shorter, and reflect the client's response to intervention during that day or that intervention session (Brennan & Robinson, 2006). A contact note may be in any of the formats described in the following sections, or in the form of a log or flow sheet. Since this note reflects one session or one day's sessions, the emphasis is not on progress, but on what services were provided and how the client responded to that intervention, including adaptive equipment issued, and any client or caregiver education provided (Brennan & Robinson, 2006).

There are three main kinds of progress notes: narrative, SOAP, and DAP (FIP). Narrative notes are notes that are written in paragraph form. SOAP and DAP (FIP) notes have specific labeled sections. All three types of notes are discussed in this chapter. In addition, ways to document progress in checklist or graphic forms, such as progress flow sheets and attendance logs, are discussed.

▼ ROLE DELINEATION FOR PROGRESS REPORTING ▼

The occupational therapist, with contributions from the occupational therapy assistant, performs reevaluation during the ongoing intervention process (AOTA, 2010). He or she documents changes in the client's occupational performance, short-term goals, and anticipated discharge environment (AOTA, 2010). The occupational therapy practitioner modifies the interventions as the client's contexts, wants, needs, and responses to interventions change

(AOTA, 2009, 2010). Contact notes may be written by either the occupational therapist or occupational therapy assistant. Progress notes are usually written by the occupational therapist with contributions from the occupational therapy assistant. Notes written by an occupational therapy assistant are usually reviewed and cosigned by the occupational therapist when required by statute, regulation, accrediting agency, payer, or facility/agency policy (AOTA, 2010, 2013).

Documentation of intervention requires that the occupational therapist and occupational therapy assistant work closely together. As mentioned in Chapter 16, in some settings, the occupational therapy assistant works without daily on-site supervision by an occupational therapist. Depending on state licensure or registration laws, the stability of the clients, and the service competency of the occupational therapy assistant, an occupational therapist may provide on-site supervision a couple days a week, once a week, or once every couple weeks. When the occupational therapist does not see the client on a daily basis, he or she relies heavily on the occupational therapy assistant to report changes in the client's condition and client's performance in areas of occupation in the form of contact notes. The occupational therapist uses this information along with his or her observations, interviews, and data gathering to recommend any modifications to the ongoing implementation of intervention. These modifications are documented in progress notes and revised intervention plans.

▼ SOAP NOTES ▼

SOAP notes are another of medicine's acronyms. SOAP stands for **S**ubjective, **O**bjective, **A**ssessment, **P**lan, which are the component parts of this type of progress note. One of the advantages of this type of note is that it is quite common and the reader knows just what kind of information to find in what part of the note. Professionals from all health care disciplines write them. The SOAP format can also be adapted for use as an evaluation report or discontinuation summary (Gateley & Borcherding, 2012; Kettenbach, 2009).

Let's revisit Jacob Olson from Chapters 14 and 16. Jacob was a basketball player who injured his thumb playing video games so many hours a day. Figure 17.1 shows two types of notes written in SOAP format. The first is a contact note written to describe one session of occupational therapy, while the second is a progress note written to summarize a week's worth of service.

Dr. Lawrence Weed is credited with developing SOAP notes in the 1960s as part of his efforts to make client charting more client-centered (Gateley & Borcherding, 2012; Kettenbach, 2009). He reorganized a client's medical record so that there would be a master list of the client's problems from the perspective of all the disciplines working with the client, and then a section for progress notes that all disciplines could write in (as opposed to separate sections of the chart for each discipline). Weed named this system the Problem Oriented Medical Record (POMR). The SOAP note format has become so popular that today, even if facilities do not use POMR, the SOAP note is still the preferred format for note writing (Gateley & Borcherding, 2012). Figure 17.2 shows some additional sample progress notes written in SOAP format.

Subjective

The subjective part of the SOAP note usually refers to the client's subjective comments about problems, complaints, life circumstances, goals, current performance, limitations, or other comments that are relevant to the services you are providing (Gateley & Borcherding, 2012; Kettenbach, 2009; Quinn & Gordon, 2003). You may directly quote the client or paraphrase, but direct quotes must be marked as such with quotation marks. A direct quote can be very effective at illustrating the client's attitude, use of language, denial, or loss of memory. However, simply writing "I feel icky" does not really tell the reader much (Gateley & Borcherding, 2012; Tips on Medical Progress Notes, 2002). If a client says that, ask him or her for clarification, then write down the client's description of his or her aches, pains and

CONTACT NOTE:

S: "I've always had to sit with my knees near my chest. Chairs are just too short for me."

O: Jake sat in an office chair that was adjusted for an "average" person. The occupational therapist instructed Jake on how to adjust the chair for a person his size, and provided a written handout that showed proper body alignment. After the instruction, Jake demonstrated adjusting the chair without any cues from the occupational therapist. Next, Jake demonstrated how he sits on the couch to play his video games. He sat with his hips flexed to 40°, his knees flexed to 50°, he was leaning forward so that his head was almost touching his knees. He held the game controller between his knees. His shoulders were rounded and his head flexed. Discussed ways to change his sitting position or to sit in the properly adjusted desk chair during game playing.

A: Jake's poor posture contributes to his neck and back pain. Jake understands how to adjust a chair to fit his body, and to shift positions while game playing.

P: OT 3×/wk. to decrease pain and improve function of his R thumb. Reinforce ergonomic principles.

PROGRESS NOTE:

S: "I sat in my desk chair while playing last night. It felt weird! I played for four hours. I'm not any more sore than I was before."

O: Jake received three lessons in ergonomic positioning this week. He demonstrated proper adjustment of a desk chair twice without cuing. We discussed strategies for raising seats, shifting positions, and increasing support for his shoulders with pillows. He received ultrasound and gentle stretching on his R thumb. Home program for gentle ROM for R hand and thumb provided.

A: Jake has made progress in his understanding of ergonomic principles and strategies for adjusting furniture to fit his needs.

P: OT 3×/wk. to decrease pain and improve function of his R thumb. Reinforce ergonomic principles.

FIGURE 17.1   Sample SOAP Format Notes for Jacob Olson.

feelings. "I feel tired and my chest and shoulder hurt" conveys more specific information. A relative or caretaker may also say something that is significant, and these comments can also be recorded in the subjective section of the SOAP note. Sometimes a client is nonverbal. If that is the case, you can document nonverbal communication such as smiles, nods, and gestures as appropriate.

Exercise 17.1

Which of these statements belong in the subjective section of the SOAP note?

1. _____ Ndebe appeared tired and listless.
2. _____ Client said she is hearing voices telling her to cut her hair.
3. _____ Raësa got dressed by herself today.
4. _____ Cyndee's mother said that Cyndee has not been sleeping well the past 3 nights.
5. _____ "I am fat and ugly."
6. _____ Client is resistant to all suggestions.
7. _____ "Where am I?"
8. _____ Client made several lewd comments throughout the session, accompanied by sexually suggestive hand gestures.
9. _____ Saji's shirt was misbuttoned, untucked, and stained.
10. _____ Tamara came to the clinic with brown smudges around her mouth and on her hands. She said, "I ate cake for breakfast."

CASE 1: HELEN, ALZHEIMER'S CLIENT IN DAY CARE SETTING

S: "Where do I go? What do I do?"

O: Upon entering the building, Helen waited for her daughter to tell her which way to turn. Once in the room, she helped herself to a cup of coffee. Then she sat down and sipped her coffee until she received further instructions. She imitated the exercises that the group leader demonstrated. Halfway through the exercise group, she stood up, put her coffee cup in the garbage, and thanked everyone for a pleasant experience. She started to leave the room. She blushed and hid her face when told that the group was not over yet.

A: Helen appears to be dependent on the verbal cues of others in her environment to direct her behavior. In the absence of verbal cues, she gets confused.

P: Pair verbal and visual cues for Helen, or use verbal cues alone. Continue to encourage participation in small-group activities. Provide a structured environment with a consistent, posted schedule. Continue monthly occupational therapy consultation.

Bobbi Babinski, OTR/L 11-1-14

CASE 2: 27 Y.O. WITH LCVA (BOB)

S: "I used to be able to do this without thinking about it. Now I have to concentrate so hard on it I wonder if it's worth it."

O: Client participated in a 30-minute occupational therapy session to work on functional activities with his unaffected (nondominant) hand. Bob attempted to use a computer mouse with his left hand by playing a game of solitaire. He moved quickly to the general area that he wants the mouse to be. He moved slowly and hesitantly to the precise spot he needed; however, he often overshot the mark. Bob clicked the mouse with his index finger easily; however, he had minimal success holding the mouse button down while dragging the mouse. It took 20 minutes to complete one game of solitaire.

A: Bob has not yet achieved adequate coordination with either hand to allow him to perform mouse activities to his satisfaction.

P: Try a touchpad mouse. Encourage moving slowly and carefully. Practice using left hand for other activities during the day. Continue twice-daily occupational therapy as per plan of care.

Carrie Ingwater, COTA/L 3-2-14
Bobbi Babinski, OTR/L 3-2-14

FIGURE 17.2 Sample Progress Notes in SOAP Format.

Some people advocate using statements like "Client denies feeling suicidal" (Sample Medical SOAP Note, 2002). I think the word "denies" sounds like you do not believe the client; it sounds judgmental. I prefer wording such as "Client reports she is not having suicidal thoughts."

Pick your "S" carefully. Make sure it is relevant to the intervention addressed in your note. For example, if you are writing a SOAP note about the client's functional skills in meal preparation, an "S" about what the client watched on TV last night is not relevant. If there is nothing relevant to report in the "S" section, you can draw a circle with a line through it (Ø) to indicate that you thought about it but there was nothing relevant to write about. Leaving it blank might look like you forgot to write something there.

Objective

The objective section is the place for recording observations, data collected, and other facts (Gateley & Borcherding, 2012; Kettenbach, 2009; Quinn & Gordon, 2003). The emphasis of this section should be on the client's performance, not simply a listing of activities the client engaged in. The information you record in this section should be the indisputable truth. It is harder than it looks to keep your interpretations out of this section. Remember the Description, Interpretation, Evaluation (DIE) discussion in Chapter 14? This would be a good time to review that material.

The "O" section should contain only descriptive statements. If the client made an attempt to open a carton of milk, but gave up before getting it open, would you say "The client was unsuccessful at opening a milk carton" or "The client is dependent in opening milk cartons"? Both sentences are probably true and accurate statements. The first sentence is descriptive of a particular event. The second is a generalization; it makes the claim that the client would be unlikely to open any milk carton. This makes the second sentence an interpretive statement that belongs in the "A" section rather than the "O" section.

Another consideration when writing the "O" section is that in some settings, the preference is to document only what the client can do, not what the client cannot do. In other settings, it is expected that both strengths and limitations will be documented. However, the "O" section should not read like a list of the client's failings.

The actual intervention is not as important as how the client responded to the intervention (Gateley & Borcherding, 2012). Your powers of observation are essential in writing good progress notes. Record the client's reaction to the intervention. Here are some possible "O" statements:

- Client pulled away from contact with the shaving cream.
- Client was dressed in plaid pants and a striped shirt.
- Jalele made fleeting eye contact with other members of the group.
- Client stacked the plates eight high on the bottom shelf of the overhead cabinet.
- Client was instructed in use of stocking aid; she demonstrated proper use of it.
- Client dressed herself independently, except for minimal assist for shoes and socks.
- Selena entered the room and went straight to the coffee pot.
- Client spontaneously used his right hand to pick up his coffee cup.

Exercise 17.2

Which of the following statements belong in the "O" section of the SOAP note?

1. _____ The client's eyes were red and watery.
2. _____ Bob seemed to be frustrated.
3. _____ He pushed away from the table and left the room.
4. _____ She spit out the strawberries.
5. _____ Pevitra wants to be recognized for good behavior.
6. _____ Esai ate all of one food before eating the next food on his plate.
7. _____ The client appears bewildered when others get annoyed with him for invading their personal space.
8. _____ The client has a habit of twisting her ring around her finger during personal conversations.

Gateley and Borcherding (2012) suggest that the "O" section begin with a statement of where and why the client was seen. Some settings and payers also expect the note to contain the amount of time the client was in occupational therapy since the last progress note. For example, the section might start with this sentence: "Demitri participated in two 45-minute occupational therapy clinic sessions this week to develop age-appropriate social skills." Or "Etta received occupational therapy today for 60 minutes in her home to work on meal preparation and housekeeping skills."

The "O" section can be organized chronologically, that is, describing events in the order in which they happened (Gateley & Borcherding, 2012; Kettenbach, 2009). This gives the reader a good idea of exactly what transpired during occupational therapy intervention sessions. If you are working with a client such as a child with sensory integration dysfunction where the sequence of interventions is important, then this is the best format.

Alternatively, some authors suggest that objective data can be categorized to make the note appear more organized (Gateley & Borcherding, 2012; Kettenbach, 2009). Headings can be used to clearly identify separate topics such as test results, functional activities, or body parts. When reporting range of motion or strength data for multiple joints, a chart can be used to display the information. A chart is easier to read and refer back to than a long sentence with multiple measurements.

Exercise 17.3

Practice organizing the "O" section for the following case.

You are working with a client who has severe rheumatoid arthritis, resulting in joint deformities of the fingers of both hands. He wants to be able to keyboard so he can e-mail his son. On his right hand, the thumb IP joint can flex to 40°. Thumb abduction is 55°. The MCP joint can flex to 30°. The index finger has DIP, PIP, and MCP flexion of 45°, 85°, and 50°, respectively, with 35° of hyperextension at the DIP and 35° of MCP extension. There is ulnar drift of index, middle, ring, and little fingers of 30°, 30°, 35°, and 40°, respectively. Both the middle and ring fingers have 50° of DIP flexion. The little finger has no movement at the DIP joint. The PIP joint of the middle, ring, and little fingers are 50°, 40°, and 30°, respectively. There is 30° of flexion and extension for the MCP joints. On his left hand, the thumb IP joint can flex to 40°. Thumb abduction is 55°. The MCP joint can flex to 70°. The index finger has DIP, PIP, and MCP flexion of 50°, 60°, and 50°, respectively. The index finger has 40° of hyperextension at the DIP joint and 40° of MCP extension. There is ulnar drift of index, middle, ring, and little fingers of 20°, 30°, 30°, and 40°. Both the middle and ring fingers have 30° of DIP flexion. The little finger has no movement at the DIP joint. The PIP joints of the middle, ring, and little fingers flex to 60°, 50°, and 45°, respectively. There is 35° of flexion and 40° of extension for the MCP joints.

Fill in each of the following tables using the data in the previous paragraph.

L	Thumb	R
_____	IP flexion	_____
_____	MCP flexion	_____
_____	Abduction	_____
	Index finger	
_____	DIP flexion	_____
_____	DIP extension	_____
_____	PIP flexion	_____
_____	MCP flexion	_____
_____	MCP extension	_____
	Middle finger	
_____	DIP flexion	_____
_____	PIP flexion	_____
_____	MCP flexion	_____
_____	MCP extension	_____

Ring finger

_____	DIP flexion	_____
_____	PIP flexion	_____
_____	MCP flexion	_____
_____	MCP extension	

Little finger

_____	DIP flexion	_____
_____	PIP flexion	_____
_____	MCP flexion	_____
_____	MCP extension	_____

Ulnar Drift

_____	Index	_____
_____	Middle	_____
_____	Ring	_____
_____	Little	_____

Finger	DIP flexion	DIP extension	PIP flexion	MCP flexion	MCP extension	Abduction	Ulnar drift
R thumb							
L thumb							
R index							
L index							
R middle							
L middle							
R ring							
L ring							
R little							
L little							

Next, answer the following questions:

1. Of the three methods of presenting information (narrative, list, and table), which do you think is the easiest to read and understand?
2. Can you think of another way to organize this information?

Assessment

The assessment or "A" portion of the SOAP note is where you explain what all this data (the subjective and objective) means (Gateley & Borcherding, 2012; Kettenbach, 2009; Quinn & Morgan, 2003). This is where your professional judgment and skills come into play. A good "A" section will provide justification for the continued provision of skilled occupational therapy services.

The assessment section is where data recorded in the "S" and "O" sections is analyzed, summarized, and prioritized. No new information should be added in the "A" section that is not supported by information recorded in the "S" and "O" sections. In some facilities, the "A" section begins with a problem list (Gateley & Borcherding, 2012). By listing the problems in order of importance to the client you let the readers, which often includes payers, know why occupational therapy is involved in this case. There is no need to use complete sentences in the problem list. Examples of problems could be:

- Impaired self-care skills
- Decreased hand function
- Decreased job skills
- Low self-esteem
- Limited access to services in his community
- Difficulty feeding herself
- Limited attention to tasks

The problem list is followed by a summary that explains to readers the correlations between the "S," "O," and "P" sections, justifies your recommendations, clarifies progress made, explains any difficulties in obtaining information, and makes suggestions for further testing.

Here is an "A" section using this type of format:

A: Problem list: Limited ROM in R shoulder, impaired dressing, grooming, and hygiene skills.
Summary: Pt. is using trunk rotation to substitute for R shoulder flexion. He has improved since last visit in that he now is using his R arm for some tasks. Pt. would benefit from continued occupational therapy.

In other facilities, the "A" will be presented in a more narrative way without listing problems. In this method, the "A" would consist of wording similar to what one would write in the summary sections of the "A" part of the preceding note.

Examples of "A" statements would be:

- Client is independent in dressing including shoes and socks.
- Laleh needs verbal cues to stay on task.
- She is ready to go on a home visit.
- He has difficulty with impulse control.
- Client is dependent in toilet transfers.
- Client is able to manage her own medication routine.
- The client has demonstrated gains in using fasteners since last report. She now can button and unbutton buttons 1/2 inch in diameter without assistance.

Gateley and Borcherding (2012) suggest that one way to distinguish an "O" statement from an "A" statement is by structuring the "A" statement to emphasize the factors contributing to the problem identified. The "A" statement would include, in this order, the contributing factor, and then its impact on occupational performance (Gateley & Borcherding, 2012). Examples of "A" statements written in this format include:

- Deficits in shoulder ROM no longer limit U/E dressing
- Inability to tune out distractions around her limit Laleh's ability to stay on task.
- Progress on self-care and socialization skills indicates she is ready to go on a home visit.
- Impulsivity interferes with his ability to plan and execute tasks to completion.
- Poor balance, strength, and coordination result in the client's dependence in toilet transfers.

- Improved organizational skills have enabled this client to manage her own medication routine.
- Improved fine motor skills have resulted in gains in using fasteners since last report. She now can button and unbutton buttons 1/2 inch in diameter without assistance.

It might seem unnecessary to remind you that what you write in the "A" section must directly relate to what you write in the "S" and "O" sections, but this has consistently been one of the hardest things for students to learn to do. Often what happens is that students write great "A" statements, but when you look at the "O" section, there is nothing supporting the conclusions drawn in the "A" section. For example:

S: Client reported pain in his shoulder every time he moves in any direction
O: Client twisted his trunk and extended his R elbow to reach objects in front of him rather than flexing his shoulder. Once positioned, he grasped various objects including a cup, a glass, a fork, a scissors, and a pen.
A: He writes legibly with his R hand.
P: Continue OT sessions 3×/wk to improve functional use of RUE.

While the "O" does mention that he grasped a pen, there are no observations related to actually using the pen. The "A" is a big leap of thinking and it is unsupported by anything in the "O" or "S" sections. A better "A" for this note would be, "He is protecting his shoulder by substituting trunk and elbow movement for shoulder movement. However, this is an improvement over last session when he refused to use the hand/arm at all." The "A" section is not the place to bring in new information (Gateley & Borcherding, 2012). Everything you write in "A" has to be supported with evidence in the "S" and "O" sections.

One technique that can be helpful in writing "A" sections that connect to "S" and "O" sections is asking yourself what it is about what the client said or did that is important enough to write down. What does it tell you about the client's performance in areas of occupation? What does it tell you about performance skills, patterns, or client factors? You may find a difference between what the client said and what the client did. You may notice whether or not there has been an improvement in function. The keys are to not restate the "O" in "A," and be sure that every statement in "A" is supported by evidence in "O."

Exercise 17.4

Which of these make good "A" statements on SOAP notes?

1. _____ She has to be told to come out of her room.
2. _____ Client tried to use the TV remote control to call home.
3. _____ Client completed 75% of the task without assistance.
4. _____ Usha does not interact with peers.
5. _____ He used public transportation independently.
6. _____ Ashton can tolerate a moderately noisy environment for up to 10 minutes.
7. _____ Client's statements are inappropriate to the situation.
8. _____ Benjamin refused to taste the meal.
9. _____ Willow is making good progress.
10. _____ Paula cooked the entire meal one handed.

In addition to the interpretation of data, justification of the goals, inconsistencies, progress, difficulty in obtaining information, and suggestions for further intervention you can also include a statement justifying continuing occupational therapy services (Gateley & Borcherding, 2012). For example, ending with a sentence that starts with "Client would benefit from . . ." (Gateley & Borcherding, 2012). This would show why continuing services are necessary.

Plan

The plan section is where you very clearly spell out what your plan is for helping the client achieve his or her goals. It often states the frequency, duration, and intensity of occupational therapy and suggestions for intervention. It can also include the location of the intervention sessions (i.e., bedside, clinic, or home) and equipment issued to the client (Kettenbach, 2009). The "P" section should be written with sufficient clarity that if you get sick and cannot come to work the next time the client is supposed to be seen, a substitute occupational therapy practitioner could step in and do what you would have done.

Examples of the "P" statements include:

- Continue OT 3×/wk for self-care skills development. Try adaptive feeding equipment such as a plate guard and large-handled utensils.
- Continue OT bid, 5×/wk for brain injury retraining program. See in room in a.m. for dressing, grooming, and hygiene, and in clinic in the afternoon for meal prep, safety, and problem solving.
- As per plan of care, client will be seen 5×/wk for 30-minute sessions for the next 2 weeks. Will work on toilet transfers and manipulation of clothes necessary for toileting next visit. Caregiver instruction will be included.
- Client will participate in activity group and assertiveness group daily.

It is not uncommon to see the "P" section written with differing levels of specificity depending on the writer. Generally, the more specific the better.

Which of these make good "P" statements?

1. _____ Practice writing his name three times per day.
2. _____ Engage client in conversations about child care.
3. _____ She should be more careful in the kitchen.
4. _____ Increase repetitions as tolerated.
5. _____ Instruct in splint care and maintenance.
6. _____ Client needs to spend more time on leisure occupations.
7. _____ Client will work on chewing food at least 10 times before swallowing.
8. _____ Client should do this more often.
9. _____ Continue OT 2×/wk.
10. _____ Talk with caregivers about follow-through on the unit.

Figures 17.3 and 17.4 show some sample progress notes. Read through them and see what you think about the quality of the notes. Consider how useful and informative the information is. Review the criteria for Documenting with CARE (Chapter 6). All the SOAP notes in Figure 17.3 technically have subjective information in the subjective space,

---

The client, Susie, is a 4-year-old girl with cerebral palsy, who is seen in an outpatient rehabilitation center. Although only a few notes are shown here, assume that the notes follow a similar pattern twice a week for several months.

Jan. 4, 2014

    S: No new complaints today.
    O: Today we worked on fine motor skills using blocks and pegs.
    A: Susie tolerated everything fairly well today.
    P: Continue OT 2×/wk per plan of care.

Jan. 6, 2014

    S: No new complaints today.
    O: Today we worked on functional activities for fine motor development including large and small pegs, using hand over hand assistance as needed.
    A: Susie tolerated everything fairly well today.
    P: Continue OT 2×/wk per plan of care.

Feb. 11, 2014

    S: No new complaints today.
    O: Today we worked on:
        1. Grasp and release using small pegs and a pegboard
        2. Gross motor coordination using adaptive scissors
        3. Spatial relationships by stacking measuring cups
        4. Writing
    A: Susie tolerated everything fairly well today.
    P: Continue per POC 2×/wk.

March 17, 2014

    S: No new complaints today.
    O: Today we worked on PNF diagonal patterns by reaching for things while sitting on a large ball, weight-bearing by rocking back and forth while on all fours, throwing beanbags to work on grasp/release, and turning pages of a book.
    A: Susie tolerated everything fairly well today.
    P: Continue OT 2×/wk per plan of care.

FIGURE 17.3 Poorly Written SOAP Notes.

objective information in the objective space, and so on; however, the notes lack any really useful information. Figure 17.4 shows two SOAP notes where the objective and assessment sections contain information that belongs in the other section or have assessment statements that are not supported by objective information.

The client, Susie, is a 4-year-old girl with cerebral palsy, who is seen in an outpatient rehabilitation center. Although only a few notes are shown here, assume that the notes follow a similar pattern twice a week for several months.

Jan. 4, 2014

S: "No"
O: Today we worked on fine motor skills using blocks and pegs. She cannot seem to get a stack of more than 3 1" cubes without knocking it down in the process of adding the fourth block. She lacks coordination to stack them higher. Using a whole hand grip on large pegs, she placed six in a row before she refused to do anymore.
A: Susie did fairly well today. She was less resistive to fine motor tasks.
P: Continue OT 2x/wk per plan of care.

Jan. 6, 2014

S: "No"
O: Today we worked on functional activities for fine motor development including large and small pegs. She needed hand-over-hand assistance with the small pegs. She could pick them up between her thumb and index finger, but could not get them to stand up in the holes.
A: Susie needs to continue to work on fine motor tasks. She was unable to stack four or more 1" blocks.
P: Continue OT 2x/wk per plan of care.

Feb. 11, 2014

S: Ø
O: Today we worked on:
1. Grasp and release using small pegs and a pegboard to make a big square shape. She didn't seem to understand the concept of alternating colors to make a pattern.
2. Fine motor coordination using adaptive scissors. She made a few snips on a piece of paper, but threw the scissors down when the OT tried to guide her to cut along a line.
3. Spatial relationships by nesting measuring cups. She nested 3 cups (1/4 c., 1/2 c., 1 c.). She liked this activity, nesting and unnesting them repeatedly.
4. Writing. She scribbled with a large crayon. She refused to make an S.
A: Susie did fairly well today. She seems to be getting used to working with the occupational therapist.
P: Continue per POC 2x/wk.

March 17, 2014

S: "OK"
O: Today we worked on PNF diagonal patterns by reaching for things while sitting on a large ball. She pulled plastic figures off a shelf and dropped them in a bucket. We worked on weight-bearing by rocking back and forth while on all fours. Once she got started rocking she didn't want to stop; she appeared overstimulated and excited. We worked on throwing bean-bags to work on grasp/release, as well as turning the pages of a book. She is doing better at quickly releasing objects.
A: Susie had a great day! She was happy throughout the session.
P: Continue OT 2x/wk per plan of care.

FIGURE 17.4   SOAP Notes with Misplaced Information.

Exercise 17.7

Write the P section for each of the three cases in Exercise 17.5.

Case 1: Client with severe arthritis

P:

Case 2: Client with sensory defensiveness

P:

Case 3: Client with left-side neglect

P:

Exercise 17.8

Label the following statements according to where they would best belong in a SOAP note. Use "S" for subjective, "O" for objective, "A" for assessment, and "P" for plan. Then use these statements to write one coherent SOAP note. You may add transitional phrases to make the note flow better.

1. _____ The client sat on the side of the bed waiting for dressing direction.
2. _____ The client is unable to initiate dressing.
3. _____ She walks to the kitchen when dressed carrying her purse, ready to go to day care.
4. _____ When told what clothes to put on she gets dressed.
5. _____ What am I supposed to wear?
6. _____ The buttons on her blouse are not lined up.
7. _____ While sitting there, she removes her nightclothes.
8. _____ Clothing will be carefully placed in proper sequence and laid out the night before, so the client can see the clothes on the chair when she gets up.
9. _____ When given cues, can dress herself with minor errors.
10. _____ She puts her anklets on under her TED stockings.

S:

O:

A:

P:

Exercise 17.9

Analyze the following SOAP notes. Tell what is good about them and what needs improvement.

Case 1: Client is a 78-year-old woman who had a stroke affecting her left side 3 months ago. Her left arm has been in a sling with only a little active range of motion in her elbow and shoulder. Then 3 days ago, she fell outside on the sidewalk, breaking her right arm. It is now in a cast. She is now attending an intensive program to facilitate movement in her left arm (constraint induced movement therapy [CIMT]).

S: "I felt so helpless with two useless arms. I can't believe I was able to feed myself with my left arm."

O: Client participated in 6 hours of outpatient occupational therapy today. Fitted with a universal cuff, she was able to feed herself using a spoon, with minimal spillage. It required her to use both elbow flexion and trunk movements to get the applesauce scooped up and into her mouth. It was the first time she had fed herself since breaking her arm.

A: Client is making progress in the functional use of her left arm. She was not able to get the spoon to her mouth yesterday.

P: Continue participation in CIMT program 6 days per week as established in plan of care. Provide adaptive equipment as needed.

Case 2: Client is a 19-year-old man who lost his left arm in a farm accident (he is right-handed) 3 weeks ago.

S: "I still can't believe my arm is gone. It's unreal. There are times I swear I can still feel it, like a fly crawling on it, but when I look there's nothing there. Nothing."

O: Withdraws from light touch within 1.5 inches of wound. He demonstrated proper stump wrapping technique. Instructed on how to massage area in preparation for artificial arm.

A: Stump is healing well, and he is on track for getting an artificial arm. He is ready to be fitted with a temporary arm.

P: OT bid, 6 days per week, to reduce sensitivity of stump, prepare stump for artificial arm, and begin training in the use of an artificial arm.

▼ DAP NOTES ▼

DAP notes are very similar to SOAP notes in that each letter stands for one section of the note: **D**escription, **A**ssessment, and **P**lan. This format is less common than either the narrative or SOAP note. They could also be called FIP notes, as in **F**indings, **I**nterpretation, and **P**lan.

The description (findings) section is much like a combination of the "S" and "O" section of a SOAP note. In this section, you describe what you see and hear during the occupational therapy session. It can include quotes, paraphrases, observations, measurements, and test results. This is where you provide evidence that you are making progress. Be sure that everything in this section is fact based, and not a conclusion or inference on your part.

The "A" and "P" ("I" and "P" for FIP notes) sections are exactly like those in SOAP. Figures 17.5 and 17.6 show examples of DAP and FIP notes.

Note 1: Helen, Alzheimer's client in day care setting

D: Upon entering the building, Helen waited for her daughter to tell her which way to turn. "Where do I go? What do I do?" Once in the room, she helped herself to a cup of coffee. Then she sat down and sipped her coffee until she received further instructions. She imitated the exercises that the group leader demonstrated. Halfway through the exercise group, she stood up, put her coffee cup in the garbage, and thanked everyone for a pleasant experience. She started to leave the room. She blushed and hid her face when told that the group was not over yet.

A: Helen appears to be dependent on the verbal cues of others in her environment to direct her behavior. In the absence of verbal cues, she gets confused.

P: Pair verbal and visual cues for Helen, or use verbal cues alone. Continue to encourage participation in small-group activities. Provide a structured environment with a consistent, posted schedule.

Bobbi Babinski, OTR/L 11/2/2014

FIGURE 17.5   DAP Note Example.

Note 2: 27 y.o. with LCVA (Bob)

F: "I used to be able to do this without thinking about it. Now I have to concentrate so hard on it I wonder if it's worth it." Client participated in a 30-minute occupational therapy session to work on functional activities with his unaffected (nondominant) hand. Bob attempted to use a computer mouse with his left hand by playing a game of solitaire. He moved quickly to the general area that he wants the mouse to be. He moved slowly and hesitantly to the precise spot he needed; however, he often overshot the mark. Bob clicked the mouse with his index finger easily, however, he had minimal success holding the mouse button down while dragging the mouse. It took 20 minutes to complete one game of solitaire.

I: Bob has not yet achieved adequate coordination with either hand to allow him to perform mouse activities to his satisfaction.

P: Try a touchpad mouse. Encourage moving slowly and carefully. Practice using left hand for other activities during the day. Continue twice daily occupational therapy as per plan of care.

Carrie Ingwater, COTA/L 3/2/14

Bobbi Babinski, OTR/L 3/2/2014

FIGURE 17.6   FIP Note Example.

Exercise 17.10

Write concise SOAP notes and DAP (FIP) notes for the following cases.

Case 1: Toddler boy with seizure disorder and sensory processing disorder (sensory hypersensitivity)

Tommy was brought to the therapy clinic today by his father. Although Tommy has been here twice a week for the last 3 months, and has always seen the same occupational therapist, he was resistant to separating from his father and coming with the OT. He held on to his father and refused to let go. His father described breakfast this morning as very difficult. Tommy threw his sippy cup, refusing to drink from it. He spit out his oatmeal and pushed the spoon away. He asked for his bottle, and after a while dad gave up and gave Tommy his bottle. Tommy refused to sit in a chair in the clinic, so Tommy's dad held him in his lap at the table. Cheerios® and Cheetos® were placed on the table. Tommy picked up a piece of the cereal and put it in his mouth. He held it in his mouth while putting two more pieces in. He gagged on them. Next he tried Cheetos®. He smiled when he tasted it, but spit it out rather than swallow it once it softened in his mouth. He saw the orange residue on his hand and started flapping his hand and screaming. He allowed his father to wipe it off with a damp cloth. He took three sips of milk from a covered cup. He withdrew when his father tried to wipe his chin with the same cloth. His father then sat Tommy on the floor (carpeted), but Tommy immediately stood up and started bouncing up and down. The OT tried to engage Tommy in playing with toy cars made of smooth plastic. He held on to one for 5 seconds, another for 3 seconds. He watched the whole minute the OT played with the cars, but did not make any attempt to reach out and grab any cars. When presented with a toy tree that was bristly, Tommy refused to touch it. He kept two fingers (usually his left hand, but occasionally his right) in his mouth throughout most of the session. He cried and tried to jump off a low platform swing. Next Tommy was brought by his dad over to the water table. Tommy watched for a minute or two, but refused to put his own hands in, no matter how the OT or his dad begged him to try it. Tommy rolled a ball between himself, the OT, and his dad for a couple minutes. Although the OT and his dad sat on the floor, Tommy remained standing. He did allow his dad to put him on the floor with his legs spread like the OT and dad, but he only stayed like that for about 10 seconds. This is longer than he has ever stayed on the floor before in the clinic. About halfway through the session, he left dad and held the OT's hand as they walked over to the easel. Dad stayed by the door. After about 2 minutes, Tommy stopped scribbling and began to look for dad, dropped everything, and ran to hug dad around the knees. They sat back down at the table again and tried the Cheetos® again. This time the OT held one while Tommy licked the orange coating. He said it tasted good. The OT asked Tommy to copy her while she demonstrated chewing without food in her mouth. Tommy moved his lower jaw up and down. Then she demonstrated taking a small bite of Cheetos®, chewing and swallowing it. Tommy imitated her, and swallowed a small piece. He did this three times before starting to gag. OT discussed with dad the possibility of trying the copying game at home at mealtime. Also discussed trying to engage Tommy in games where he sits on the floor. First try it with long pants on, then in shorts. Since some progress was observed today, I recommend continuing services twice a week.

S:

O:

A:

P:

D:

A:

P:

Case 2: 82-year-old woman who fractured the head of her left femur and then had a heart attack trying to crawl to a phone in her bedroom. She has been in the hospital for 10 days and is transferring to a transitional care facility in 2 days.

Mrs. Anderssen was seen today in her room for work on toilet transfers and dressing. She transfers from bed to wheelchair with minimal assist using a transfer belt and a pivot transfer. This is an improvement, since she was requiring moderate assist 2 days ago. She propelled herself to the bathroom and washed her face and upper body with a washcloth independently. The toilet seat is raised to same height as wheelchair seat. Toilet also has handrails. Client locked the wheelchair at a right angle to the toilet, put both hands on the arms of her wheelchair, and using both arms and her right leg raised herself to standing. She moved her right hand to the toilet rail, pivoted on her right leg, and sat down on the toilet with stand-by assistance. She independently obtained and used toilet paper. She reached behind her and flushed the toilet while still sitting. Then she again used her arms and right leg to stand and then used a pivot transfer with minimal assist to get back to the wheelchair. She reports that except when OT is in her room, the nurses give her a lot of assist with toilet transfers. She has not yet tried toileting independently while wearing street clothes, which would require her to worry about adjusting her clothing. We will attempt to do it this afternoon.

She propelled herself into her room and in front of her closet. From her closet she used a long-handled reacher to get a hanger down from the hanging rod. She removed a sweat suit and replaced the hanger, again using the reacher. Then she got her bra and panties out of a drawer. She removed her gown and put on her bra (using the hook in front, then twisting it around and pulling up the straps) and sweatshirt without assistance. Next, she used a sock aid to put on anklets. It took three tries and some verbal cues, but she did do it without physical assist. Then she used the dressing stick to put her panties and pants on and pull them just over her knees. This was a slow process and she expressed some frustration at how tired and slow she felt. Until she fell, she was a very active woman and participated in a local mall-walking club. It is probably because she was in good condition for her age that she has made the progress that she has. She slid her feet into Velcro sneakers with a long shoehorn. She pushed herself up to standing, pausing for a couple seconds to make sure her balance was good. She steadied herself with her left hand on the bed. Finally, she pulled her panties and pants the rest of the way up and then sat back down in her chair. The entire process of washing, toileting, and dressing took 35 minutes. She reports that it used to take her 10 minutes to do all that, although she didn't have to use all that extra equipment. She is progressing as planned. OTR left instructions for undressing with both Mrs. Anderssen and the nursing staff.

S:

O:

A:

P:

D:

A:

P:

▼ NARRATIVE NOTES ▼

If the narrative progress note is written directly in the client's medical record, it is usually done in a section of the medical record set aside for that purpose. Notes are entered as close to the time of intervention as possible since the notes are expected to be in chronological order. Therefore, narrative notes written directly in the medical record need to be dated, and often the time the note was written is also recorded (Fremgen, 2011; Ranke, 1998). Since the pages of the progress note section of a client's medical record already contain the client's identifying information, there is no need to repeat it in the note. The length of time of the intervention session is usually recorded.

How do you show that your client is making progress? The easy way would be to write "The client is making progress." However, this would be woefully inadequate. Why should anyone reading the record take your word for it? You have to show that the client is doing something now that he or she could not do before; you have to show a change in the client's occupational performance. Figure 17.7 shows three examples of narrative notes.

Narrative format is often used to write a contact note. This is a note written to document contact with a client, usually, but not necessarily, during a therapy session. For example, a contact note may be written when you instruct a caregiver in proper transfer techniques or splint care. A contact note could be written to document the reason for a missed intervention session. A contact note might also be used to document that you met the client and scheduled the client to come to the occupational therapy room to begin the evaluation (or for you to come to the client's room and begin the evaluation there if that is the plan). In a case like this, the contact note might look like this:

Note 1: Helen is an 84 y.o. female with Alzheimer's disease. She receives OT on a monthly consultative basis.

Helen attended her day program for people with Alzheimer's 5 days a week for the past month. She received social and recreational programming, one congregate meal, a short rest period each day, and occupational therapy consultation. In addition to Alzheimer's, the client has high blood pressure and circulatory problems in her left leg. She wears a TED stocking. Her medications are stable. She is a widow of 2 years.

Helen helped herself to coffee without asking for permission or directions. She stayed with the morning exercise group for about 20 minutes (it is a 45-minute group) each day. At about that time, she typically got up to throw her coffee cup away, and tried to continue on out of the room. Helen allowed the group leader to redirect her back to the group, and then she continued to participate in the exercises until she was told that the group is over. Then she asked what was next. When asked the name of the program, she said she was not sure she ever knew the name of it.

Helen has been consistent in her behavior for the last month. According to staff, she is less agitated since moving into small-group activities instead of the large group she was in 2 months ago. She is dependent on verbal cues for the completion of most activities. She expresses her confusion with frequent questions.

Helen will continue to attend the 5×/wk Alzheimer's program. Staff will provide her with a highly structured, small-group experience. The client will continue to ask many questions, and these will be responded to in short, simple sentences. Staff will post a daily schedule near the clock.

Bobbi Babinski, OTR/L Nov. 1, 2014

Note 2: 27 y.o. with LCVA (Bob)

Bob participated in a 30-minute session to work on functional activities with his unaffected (non-dominant) hand. Bob attempted to use a computer mouse with his left hand by playing a game of solitaire. He moved quickly to the general area that he wants the mouse to be. He moved slowly and hesitantly to the precise spot he needed; however, he often overshot the mark. Bob clicked the mouse with his index finger easily; however, he had minimal success holding the mouse button down while dragging the mouse, such as when he wanted to move a card to a different pile. He expressed concern about how much more he had to concentrate on the movements than he had to when he used his right hand. It took 20 minutes to complete one game of solitaire.

Carrie Ingwater, COTA/L 3/2/14

Bobbi Babinski, OTR/L 3/2/2014

FIGURE 17.7 Narrative Note Examples.

Rina was seen today for a 30-minute session. She did not make eye contact with the occupational therapist, but she did respond to sound and to touch. She did not try to locate a toy by sight, but when a rattle was touched to her fingertips or the back of her hand, she turned her hand to grasp the rattle and shake it. From a prone position, she rolled to the right and to the left in response to noise. She rolled in a straight line to her right but was slower and less direct rolling to her left. Mild ATNR present, stronger when her head is turned to the left. Rina supported her weight on her right arm when prone on elbows with a toy in her left hand. After three attempts, she was not able to support her weight on her left arm when prone on elbows with a toy in her right hand. While she is able to use both arms to reach and grasp for toys, she is showing greater strength and endurance on her right side. Her vision continues to appear impaired. The plan is to continue to see Rina twice a day for the duration of her hospitalization to work on movement and play skills and to monitor for any sign of returning vision.

Stephanie Smith, OTR/L 7/02/14

Saw Mrs. Smith in her room today. Explained what occupational therapy is and that she was referred to occupational therapy to work on her self-care skills. She said she understood her doctor's concern, but that she was sure that her left side was not affected by the stroke and that she really did not want to waste my time when I could be helping someone who really needs my help. She agreed to humor me and come to the occupational therapy clinic this afternoon at 1:30. I told her I would send an aide to come and bring her to the clinic. Britta Farver, OTR/L, 9-23-09

Went to client's room to bring her to the clinic. She said she felt really nauseous today, and a bit light-headed and would prefer to skip this afternoon's session. Checked with the nurse who was aware of the situation and concurred that she should not participate in occupational therapy this afternoon. Mika Vica, OTR/L, 9-23-14

FIGURE 17.7   (Continued)

Exercise 17.11

Write a narrative progress note based on the following cases:

Case 1: Kiki is a 6-year-old receiving occupational therapy following a car accident. She had a severe head injury. Last week she visually tracked a toy while supine over a 60° horizontal arc. She did not reach for the toy. During passive ROM to her upper extremities, she cried out with each movement. She was dependent in all her ADLs. This week, she tracked the toy while sitting over a 90° arc horizontally and 40° vertically. She cried out during shoulder passive ROM, but not during elbow, wrist, or hand PROM. Showing about 10° active ROM in R elbow spontaneously, but not on command. She remains dependent in all her ADLs. She received occupational therapy twice a day, 5 days this week, and once on Saturday.

Case 2: 88-year-old woman with osteoarthritis in her knees, COPD, and diabetic neuropathy, who received home-based occupational therapy following hospitalization for pneumonia, resulting in diminished strength and endurance. She received occupational therapy twice a week, and you write a note after each visit. Her goals are to prepare light meals for breakfast and dinner (Meals on Wheels for lunch), dress and undress herself without fatigue, and safe showers. In addition, the client wants to be able to take care of her houseplants and play solitaire, even though holding things in her hands is difficult. During this 45-minute visit, occupational therapy worked on using a kitchen stool to sit on while preparing a meal, shower transfers using the bath bench you brought for her to try, and trying adaptive equipment for dressing and card playing. (*Write the narrative note, using an educated guess on how much progress she has made since you saw her 3 days ago.*)

▼ PROGRESS FLOW SHEETS ▼

Flow sheets can show the progress a client is making on specific activities in a very concise way. Flow sheets are typically tables or graphs where measurements can be recorded at regular intervals, generally after each intervention session. It makes it easy for the reader to see at a glance whether progress is being made in a particular area of need for a client. For example, you could chart the length of time it takes for your client to complete a meal, the number of dishes the client unloaded from a dishwasher and put away in a cabinet, or the degrees of active range of motion of a client's wrist. When progress flow sheets are used, then the narrative, SOAP, or DAP note may be written weekly or biweekly rather than after every intervention session.

There are several advantages of using flow sheets to track progress. One is that they are easier to read than multiple contact notes. The data recorded is kept to a minimum, and is organized in an easy-to-follow format. Second, instead of relying on someone saying a client has made progress, you have solid, objective data that shows the progress. Another advantage is that a flow sheet contains a lot of data but uses minimal space, so it conserves paper. Using a flow chart keeps the clinician focused on interventions that are specific to the client's goals, and less chance to go off on tangents. It makes it easy for a substitute clinician to know what to expect a client to do in the next occupational therapy session. Finally, flow charts provide reliable data that can be used to write progress summaries. In those settings where progress notes are written weekly or biweekly, a clinician who can reflect that data off the flow sheet will have written a more reliable note than one who writes from memory alone. This is particularly helpful if the client's medical record is ever called into court.

There are also disadvantages to using flow sheets. Often, there is space enough to record a number or other objective measurement, but not room for descriptions of performance. There is no place to record the client's reaction to the intervention. There may be a place to record new interventions, but there may not be, depending on the form used.

Figure 17.8 is a sample progress flow sheet for an adult with mental retardation being seen in a sheltered workshop. In this case, only brief objective data is recorded. Figure 17.9 is a sample of a progress flow sheet for a woman in a nursing home. The therapist records objective data in the appropriate box. It does allow for observations to be recorded as well as number of cues, number of repetitions, time to complete task, or whatever measure is included in the goal. Some forms use short-term goals rather than a problem statement.

Intervention \ Date	6-4-14	6-6-14	6-8-14	6-11-14	6-13-14	6-15-14	6-18-14	6-20-14	6-22-14	6-24-14	6-26-14
Number of correct packets assembled independently	6	6	7	6	7	7	7	8	7	8	
Number of times in a 30-min period client needed redirection	8	9	8	8	7	6	8	6	6	5	
Degree of assist needed in lunch line (dep = 5, max = 4, mod = 3, min = 2, indep = 1, P = physical, V = verbal	3P 4V	3P 4V	3P 3V	3P 3V	2P 3V	3P 3V	3P 4V	2P 3V	2P 3V	2P 3V	

FIGURE 17.8 Sample Progress Flow Sheet in Sheltered Workshop.

Number of times during lunch client engages in self-stimulatory behavior	6	7	6	6	6	6	5	6	5	5	
Initials	KC TC	KC	KC	KC	KC	KC	KC TC	KC	KC	KC	

Signatures:		
Initials:	Name:	Credentials
KC	Katie Clapsaddle	OTS
TC	Thomas Carter	OTD

FIGURE 17.8 (Continued)

In some settings, there may be a separate flow sheet for each goal area. If this is the case, you can graph progress. For example, if you were working on having a client with schizophrenia and attention deficit disorder (ADD) increase attention to task, you could graph the amount of time the client worked on a task before his first redirection, or the number of redirections in a 1-hour session. The graphs might look like Figure 17.10. You can see

Goal area	Date: 7-20-09	Date: 7-22-09	Date: 7-24-09	Date
Dresses self in 15 min or less with no more than 2 cues	21 min 2 v cues 1 phys prompt	21 min 1 v cue 1 phys prompt	19 min 1 v cue 1 phys prompt	
Feed self meal w/o spilling	Breakfast: used fork; no spilling when stabbing meat, but did spill 3× when scooping eggs	Breakfast: used fork for eggs, fingers for meat; eggs fell off 2×	Breakfast: used spoon for oatmeal; no spilling	
Actively participate in one group activity per day	Attended bingo game when aide escorted her, but did not play	Attended current events group, make 1 comment in 30-min session	Attended current events group, made 2 comments in 30-min session	
Develop a repertoire of individual activities (6) in which to engage	Discussed former hobbies; used to enjoy crocheting, knitting, reading magazines and novels, cooking, walking, and dog grooming.	Showed her where magazines are kept for resident use and provided library cart schedule. Provided a large crochet hook and her choice of yarns.	Resident has 6 inches of a scarf crocheted. Reports that her hands hurt after a while. Told her about a program to crochet afghans for kids at homeless shelter.	
Provider name	Mo Chu Yan, COTA/L	Mo Chu Yan, COTA/L	Mo Chu Yan, COTA/L	

FIGURE 17.9 Progress Flow Sheet Long-Term Care.

Maximum Uninterrupted Time Attending to Task:										
15 min										
14 min										
13 min										
12 min										
11 min										
10 min										
9 min										
8 min										▓
7 min										
6 min									▓	▓
5 min				▓	▓	▓	▓	▓		
4 min		▓								
3 min	▓		▓							
2 min										
1 min										
Task	1	1	1	2	2	2	3	3	3	3
Date 2014	9–8	9–9	9–10	9–11	9–14	9–15	9–16	9–17	9–18	9–21
Initials	KS	KS	KS	KS	CJ	KS	KS	KS	KS	KS

Tasks: 1 = wipe tables 2 = put chairs on tables 3 = vacuum
Signatures: _____
Initials: Name:
KS   Katrina Sanchez, MA, OTR/L
CJ   Cecilia Jorgenson, COTA/L

FIGURE 17.10   Progress Flow Sheet Example.

at a glance that progress is being made, even before you read the data. Figure 17.11 shows a type of bar graph, but you could use a line graph where you connect the dots plotted like this as well.

Flow sheets must be signed at the bottom of the page, but each entry is usually simply initialed. There can be a key at the bottom that looks like the one on the bottom of Figure 17.10. This lets readers know who worked with the client on what day.

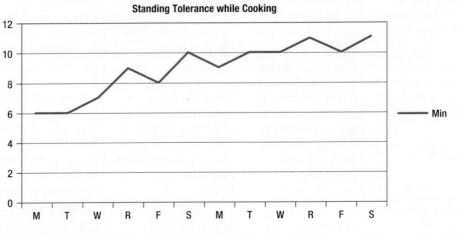

FIGURE 17.11   Line Graph Flow Sheet.
Dates: August 17-29, 2014.

Progress flow sheets cannot entirely replace progress notes. They may decrease the frequency with which progress notes are written from daily to weekly or biweekly in some settings. Not every setting uses progress flow sheets.

Attendance Logs

Attendance logs, at minimum, identify when the client had therapy. Many also identify which occupational therapy personnel worked with the client that day, and how long the therapy session was. Some also identify which type of intervention happened during which intervention session. An attendance log can be used for billing therapy services if it is designed to be compatible with the billing system used at that facility.

Attendance logs may be kept on a clipboard in the department with a separate page for each client. When the client is discontinued, the attendance log may go in the client's permanent record, the department file, or the billing office, depending on facility policy. They may also be built into an electronic health record system.

Attendance logs can be set up much like the first example of a flow chart, with dates across the top and interventions listed along one side. If the attendance log is used for billing, then the interventions are labeled so that they coincide with billing codes. In the box that correlates to the date and intervention, the clinician records the number of billable units of that intervention, or the number of minutes of that intervention. The biggest difference between the attendance log and the flow sheet is the attendance log does not include any data on the client's performance, only that a particular intervention was worked on.

▼ PHOTOGRAPHIC AND VIDEO DOCUMENTATION ▼

It is often said that a picture is worth a thousand words. If that is the case, then it would seem logical that visual evidence of a client's performance would strengthen the documentation. With the availability of digital cameras, visual documentation is getting easier and less cumbersome.

There are several ways in which visual evidence can be used. Still pictures of proper positioning of a client can be used both as an educational aid for clients and/or caregivers and as evidence of the caregiver/client education in the medical record. Before-and-after intervention pictures of resting hand position, posture, range of motion, sensory tolerance, or other intervention provide eloquent evidence of the effect of intervention.

Video can be used to show how a client functions in a particular environment to aid in the evaluation process (Kashman, Mora, & Glaser, 2000). A video camera can be less intrusive than adding a person into an environment for the purpose of observing behavior. The video can capture antecedents to behavior, such as with a child with autism. By using video, an occupational therapist can replay the event to look for details in both the environment and client to help in understanding behavior (Kashman et al., 2000). A video can also be used to document the client carrying out an activity, as proof that the client understood the instructions.

Using video or photographic documentation raises issues of privacy and confidentiality. Many facilities have policies and procedures to govern the use of video or photographic documentation which must be followed very carefully. Some require a separate release form before photos or video can be taken, and some include it in the general release form signed by the client or responsible party upon admission. Always check to see what the facility policy and procedure are before taking any pictures.

▼ MEDICARE COMPLIANCE ▼

Medicare requires a progress report (progress note) at least every 10 treatment days or once every 30 calendar days, whichever is less (Centers for Medicare and Medicaid Services [CMS], 2008, 2012). The progress report must be signed by the occupational therapist providing the interventions or supervising the occupational therapy assistant who is providing the interventions. The progress report should contain a description of progress; plans for continuation or discontinuation of treatment; plans to change long-or short-term goals; and statements of the client's rehabilitation potential—that "maximum improvement is yet to be attained" (CMS, 2008, p. 35) and that the expected improvement is likely to occur in a "reasonable and generally predictable period of time" (CMS, 2008, p. 36). If you are using a SOAP format for your progress note, these items belong in the "A" section, and clear, objective data to support the "A" belong in the "O" section.

Medicare also requires documentation of "all treatments and skilled interventions" (CMS, 2008, p. 36) in a treatment note, also called an encounter note or contact note. The treatment note is written for every treatment session, and will be used to compare to billing statements as verification that the services billed for were delivered (CMS, 2008, 2012). If your treatment note contains the information required in a progress report, you do not need to write additional progress reports. Each treatment note should contain the date of service, the specific interventions provided and billed, the total time the client received treatment during that session, the total of the "timed code treatment minutes" (CMS, 2008 p. 37), and the signature of the occupational therapy practitioner who provided the service. Medicare says that optional information that can be included in the treatment note includes patient self-report (the "S" of your note), any adverse reactions to an intervention, any "significant, unusual or unexpected changes in clinical status" (CMS, 2008, p. 38), equipment provided to the client, communication you have with another provider of services about your client, and anything else you think is important to document (CMS, 2008, 2012).

As with other Medicare compliant documentation, progress reports must demonstrate that the skills of an occupational therapist are required, and that the services are reasonable and necessary (CMS, 2012). Medicare requires that the plan of care demonstrate that the "expertise, knowledge, clinical judgment, decision making and abilities of a therapist" are required (CMS, 2012, p. 23). To demonstrate that the skills of an occupational therapist are required, it is not sufficient for the occupational therapist to simply co-sign the note. The occupational therapist must actively participate in the provision of services to the client at least once during each progress reporting period (CMS, 2012). Medicare considers the following to be skilled services:

- Evaluation and reevaluation
- Establishing treatment goals
- Designing a plan of care
- Ongoing assessment and analysis
- Instruction leading to development of compensatory skills
- Selection of devices to replace or augment a function
- Patient and caregiver training (CMS, 2012, p. 26)

In addition, occupational therapy services must be reasonable and necessary. This means that the occupational therapy services are intended for the recovery or improvement of function, and if possible, to restore prior level of function (CMS, 2012). Ongoing occupational therapy services must meet standards of medical practice, be specific and effective in treating the condition, be of a level of complexity or sophistication, or the care can only be provided by a skilled occupational therapist or occupational therapy assistant under the supervision of an occupational therapist, or the client's condition requires the skills of an occupational therapist. The amount, frequency and duration of intervention must be considered reasonable under accepted professional standards of practice (CMS, 2012). There should be significant potential for rehabilitation in relation to the extent and duration of the occupational therapy service, in other words, an expectation of significant improvement in a reasonable period of time. This is demonstrated by objective measurements over time.

Maintenance services are considered reasonable and necessary if they require the skills of an occupational therapist to carry them out due to the patient's special medical complications or the services are so complex that only an occupational therapist could perform them (CMS, 2012). This may be changing in light of the recent court decisions discussed in Chapter 16.

SUMMARY

In this chapter, we explored documentation of intervention, including three types of progress notes. The narrative note is written in paragraph form, and often reads as if one is telling a story, which is in fact what one is doing. SOAP (subjective, objective, assessment, plan) and DAP (description, assessment, plan) or FIP (findings, interpretation, plan) perform the same function as narrative notes, but do it in a prescribed fashion. Progress notes do not simply list activities, but describe what progress has been made, how the client reacted to the interventions, and what functional skills the client has demonstrated.

SOAP notes are used by many health care disciplines in many settings. The "S" part of the note is where subjective information, such as the client's perspective on the problem, is recorded. The "O" is for objective data, the information about what the client did without judgment or interpretation. In the "A" section, you make sense out of the information in the "S" and "O" sections by interpreting it and assessing it. Finally, in the "P" section, you state what you plan to do with the client so that the client can achieve his or her goals.

DAP notes are also sometimes called FIP (findings, interpretation, plan) notes. They are very similar to SOAP notes. In the "D" section, you combine the subjective and objective information that would normally be recorded in separate sections in a SOAP note. In the "A" section, you assess the meaning of the information in the "D" section, and in the "P" section you record the plan.

Narrative notes contain the same information as SOAP and DAP but the information is not labeled as such; rather, it is written in paragraph format. Narrative notes may be written in great detail, or may only hit the high points. A specific kind of narrative note, a contact note, may be written to document contact with a client or client's caregiver (as part of an occupational therapy session or outside of regular sessions) or to document the reason for a missed intervention session.

Progress flow sheets and attendance logs were also discussed in this chapter. These documents provide information on when a client received intervention and, to a limited extent, what was worked on. These documents can supplement, but not replace, writing progress summaries.

The occupational therapist is responsible for ensuring that progress reports get written in accordance with standards and regulations for timeliness and content and are communicated to the client or other involved party (in accordance with privacy regulations). Occupational therapy assistants, under the supervision of an occupational therapist, contribute to the process. Either the occupational therapist or the occupational therapy assistant may write the progress report. In most situations, as part of routine supervision, the occupational therapist will cosign notes written by the occupational therapy assistant.

REFERENCES

American Occupational Therapy Association. (2010). Standards of practice for occupational therapy [Supplemental material]. *American Journal of Occupational Therapy, 64,* S106–S111. doi:10.5014/ajot.2010.64S106

American Occupational Therapy Association. (2013). Guidelines for documentation of occupational therapy. Retrieved from http://www.aota.org/-/media/corporate/files/secure/practice/officialdocs/guidelines/guidelines%20for%20documentation.pdf

American Occupational Therapy Association. (2014). Occupational therapy practice framework: Domain and process (3rd ed). *American Journal of Occupational Therapy, 68*(Suppl. 1), S1–S48. http://dx.doi.org/10.5014/ajot.2014.682006

Brennan, C, & Robinson, M. (2006). Documentation: Getting it right to avoid Medicare denials. *OT Practice, 11*(14), 10–15.

Centers for Medicare and Medicaid Services. (2008). *Pub100-02 Medicare benefit policy: Transmittal 88.* Retrieved May 8, 2008, from http://www.cms.hhs.gov/transmittals/downloads/R88BP.pdf

Centers for Medicare and Medicaid Services [CMS]. (2012). Physical, occupational, and speech therapy services. Retrieved from http://www.cms.gov/Outreach-and-Education/Outreach/OpenDoorForums/Downloads/090512TherapyClaimsSlides.pdf

Fremgen, B. F. (2011). *Medical law and ethics* (4th ed.). Upper Saddle River, NJ: Prentice Hall.

Gateley, C.A. & Borcherding, S. (2012). *Documentation manual for occupational therapy: Writing SOAP notes* (3rd ed.). Thorofare, NJ: Slack.

Kashman, N., Mora, J., & Glaser, T. (July 3, 2000). Using video tapes to evaluate children with autism. *Occupational Therapy Practice, 5*(14), 12–15.

Kettenbach, G. (2009). *Writing SOAP notes* (4th ed.). Philadelphia, PA: F. A. Davis.

Quinn, L. & Gordon, J. (2003). *Functional outcomes: Documentation for rehabilitation.* St. Louis, MO: Saunders.

Ranke, B. A. E. (1998). Documentation in the age of litigation. *OT Practice, 3*(3), 20–24.

Sample Medical SOAP Note. (2002). Retrieved September 5, 2002, from http://cpmcnet. Columbia.edu/dept/ps/2002/SOAPmed.html

Tips on Medical Progress Notes. (2002). Retrieved September 5, 2002, from http://cpmcnet. Columbia.edu/dept/ps/2002/SOAPmed.html

Visit **www.pearsonhighered.com/healthprofessionsresources** to access the student resources that accompany this book. Simply select Occupational Therapy from the choice of disciplines. Find this book and you will find the complimentary study tools created for this specific title.

CHAPTER 18

Discharge Summaries

INTRODUCTION

When the client achieves all of his or her goals, moves out of the facility, refuses to continue in the program, or achieves maximum benefit from occupational therapy, a discharge summary must be written (American Occupational Therapy Association [AOTA], 2010). This summary, also called a discharge report, needs to show the client's progress from the beginning of occupational therapy services to the end. It is the final justification of your services.

▼ ROLE DELINEATION IN DISCONTINUATION OF SERVICE ▼

The occupational therapist determines when a client is ready to discontinue services (AOTA, 2010). This occurs as part of the ongoing process of intervention review (AOTA, 2014). The occupational therapy assistant may recommend discontinuing services to a client. The occupational therapist prepares, implements, and documents the discontinuation plan, including appropriate follow-up resources and reevaluation needs. The occupational therapy assistant contributes to the process of implementing the discontinuation plan and in documenting the changes in the client's engagement in occupations (AOTA, 2010, 2013).

▼ COMPONENTS OF A DISCHARGE SUMMARY ▼

In some facilities, the discharge summary is an interdisciplinary effort. There is one document and members of the treatment team all contribute to the one discharge document. At other facilities, there may be a paper or electronic form or format that is followed by each profession for discharge summaries. Generally, no matter whether you dictate, fill out a form, or write the report electronically, the same basic information is provided. First, there is, as always, identifying information. Next is a summary of the occupational therapy services provided and the client's response to the intervention (AOTA, 2013). The *Guidelines for Documentation of Occupational Therapy* lists the following items that should be found in this part of the document (AOTA, 2013):

- Client information
- Summary of intervention
- Recommendations

In addition to these elements, a good discharge summary will also include the reason for discontinuation. It may be that the client is being discharged from the facility, is refusing further therapy, or that the client has achieved the outcomes expected. These are good reasons to discontinue services. It may be that the client has reached the maximum insurance coverage, for example, the client may have hit the cap on Medicare outpatient therapy. This is not a good reason to discontinue services because it is not related to the client's outcomes or wishes. If a client chooses to discontinue services for financial reasons, that may be a satisfactory rationale for discharge. The difference between these is that in the case of the payment limit, the decision to discontinue is being made by someone other than the client and occupational therapist. A client can choose to discontinue occupational therapy at any time and for any reason, but the documentation should reflect that it was the client's choice, not a decision made for the client by the occupational therapist or the occupational therapist's employer.

It is important to be comprehensive, yet concise when reporting on progress toward goals and occupational therapy outcomes. If a client has been receiving occupational therapy intervention for several months or more, you may want to focus more on the long-term goals than on each and every adjustment to short-term goals. However, if a client was seen for a few days to a few weeks, you may address each short-term goal.

When addressing the initial and ending status of the client in relation to engagement in occupations, the emphasis will clearly be on occupations rather than on changes in client factors, activity demands, or even contexts. However, contexts, especially those related to the client's discharge disposition, are very important. The client's discharge disposition is the place the client is being discharged to; it could be to the client's home, extended care facility, assisted living facility, home care, outpatient program, or other community-based service (Moyers, 1999). Your evaluation of the client's ending status is dependent on the discharge disposition.

In order to make appropriate recommendations for follow-up or referrals in the discontinuation summary, the discharge disposition is also essential (Moyers, 1999). If a client is being discharged to another facility, you need to know what services are available at that facility in order to make an appropriate referral. If the client will be receiving occupational therapy intervention at the new facility, it is helpful if the occupational therapists can talk with each other. However, in order to do that, permission to discuss the client's status must be obtained from the client or client's legal guardian in order to comply with confidentiality regulations (i.e., HIPAA; see Chapter 6). If a client is being discharged to his or her home, community-based services can be recommended, but the occupational therapist has to know what kinds of services are available in the area. This is where working as a team with a social worker can be a real help. For example, you might recommend that a client participate in a community-based 12-step program (i.e., Alcoholics, Anonymous), join a health club or community-based exercise program, or seek further help from a vocational rehabilitation program (Moyers & Dale, 2007).

You may recommend that the client come back in a few months for a recheck, for example, if you expect the client will progress or regress on his or her own and may need more occupational therapy at a later time or the client may have some medical procedures planned that will result in a change of functional status. Orthotic devices or adaptive equipment may need to be checked periodically for wear and fit. For any of these reasons or others, recommending the client come back in three months for a recheck may be a good idea. However, if you make such a recommendation, be sure it is documented in the discharge summary. Figure 18.1 shows a sample completed discharge summary.

▼ SOAP FORMAT ▼

Some facilities use the SOAP format for their discharge summaries (Gateley & Borcherding, 2012; Kettenbach, 2009). In a discharge note, the "S" would describe something the client said about her progress, or the client's subjective description of current function.

OCCUPATIONAL THERAPY DISCHARGE SUMMARY

BACKGROUND INFORMATION

Date of report: 2-28-14

Date of birth &/or age: 6-25-93

Primary intervention diagnosis/concern: Tendonitis of R thumb; neck, back, and & R arm pain

Secondary diagnosis/concern: Depression

Precautions/contraindications: Thumb immobilized until 1-28-14

Reason for referral to OT: Immobilization of thumb interferes with daily life tasks

Reason for discharge from OT: Goals were met

Therapist: Ina Second, MS, OTR/L

Client's name: Jacob Olsen

Date of referral: 1-14-14

Description of OT intervention: Jake was seen for OT 3×/wk for 6 weeks. R thumb was treated with ultrasound, massage, and gentle stretching. Jake also participated in education on ergonomic principles including adjusting work and play spaces and an exploration of alternative leisure activities. Jake's goals were to return to playing basketball and to learn to make environmental adaptation to support a pain-free lifestyle.

Brief summary of intervention process: For the first 2 weeks of occupational therapy, Jake's thumb was immobilized. Services focused on ergonomic education and exploration of alternative leisure activities. Jake learned to adjust his desk chair, modify the height of work and seating surfaces. He received a set of table leg lengtheners and instructions for ordering a seat cushion. He is aware of the need to pay attention to his posture and avoid positions in which his shoulders are hunched forward. Exploration of alternative leisure activities occurred, but Jake was not open to many of the alternatives. His R thumb has full ROM and pinch strength is 80% of expected. He reports a change in pain in his neck and back from a 7 initially to a 3 at discharge. Pain in his R thumb decreased from an 8 initially to a 2 at rest and 4 after use.

Discharge recommendations: Limit video game playing to 1–2 hours per day. Adjust seating and work surfaces as instructed. Follow up with team trainer for thumb pain. Resume basketball practice.

Ina Second, OTR/L   _2-28-14_

Signature   Date

Justa Minute, COTA/L contributed to this report.

OCCUPATIONAL THERAPY DISCHARGE REPORT

Date of report: Sept. 30, 2014

Date of birth/age: March 26, 1985

Primary intervention diagnosis/concern: Depression with suicide attempt

Secondary intervention diagnoses/concerns: History of cutting

Precautions/contraindications: Do not allow to use sharp instruments without close supervision. Count sharps at end of session.

Reason for referral to OT: Evaluate and treat for depression. Increase self-esteem.

Reason for discontinuation of OT: Completed 7-day inpatient program.

Therapist: Carla McShane, OTR/L

Client's name: Sadie Clapsaddle

Date of initial referral: Sept. 23, 2014   M   F

Description of OT intervention: Sadie was seen in the occupational therapy clinic twice a day for 6 of the 7 days she was here. Provided with unconditional support and encouragement. Participated in self-esteem and assertiveness group as well as task group.

Brief summary of intervention process: Sadie's initial goal for herself was to begin to get involved in activities that interested her in the past. She used to paint, but stopped painting when her children were little. Her children are now teenagers. She also wanted to learn to say "no" to members of her family who demanded that she do things for them, without feeling guilty and changing her mind because of it. She met both goals. Both goals were achieved.

FIGURE 18.1 Sample Discharge Summary Reports, Bifip Format.

Sadie initially sat with her head down; she did not initiate conversation or activities. She was compliant with all therapist requests. She said nothing interested her anymore. Sadie did not initiate any interactions with peers or staff. She did not comb her hair unless she was told to do it.

During her week here, she rehearsed saying "no" during role-playing exercises with the therapist. By the end of the week, when the therapist would ask Sadie for favors like "Could you clean up the sink?" Sadie said "no" and stuck with that answer. If the therapist asked for volunteers to do something, Sadie literally sat on her hands to keep from volunteering. With the help of the occupational therapist, Sadie signed up for a painting class through Sadie's local community education program. Sadie reports that she is excited about taking a painting class. She said she liked the paintings she made in occupational therapy. She met with her husband and children and told them that they had to start doing some things for themselves when she came home. They agreed to take on some of the work she usually does. Sadie said she was amazed that her family was so unaware of her feelings. She made a commitment to express her feelings on a more regular basis, and they agreed not to "blow her off." Sadie is returning to her home with twice-a-week outpatient visits with a counselor. Home has been a stressful place for Sadie, but she and her family say they are committed to making things less stressful by sharing Sadie's load.

Discharge recommendations: Sadie will participate in counseling sessions twice a week. She will attend a painting class through community education.

Carla McShane, OTR/L   _Sept 30, 2014_
Signature   Date

FIGURE 18.1 (Continued)

The "O" would report objective data regarding performance in areas of occupation. This can include both initial and ending data. The "A" would articulate your assessment or interpretation of the data in "O." You would summarize those areas where significant progress occurred and identify areas where progress was not made. The "P" would be where you indicate home program instructions, follow-up recommendations, and referrals to other professionals. Figure 18.2 shows a SOAP-based discharge summary for the same client as in Figure 18.1.

OCCUPATIONAL THERAPY DISCHARGE SUMMARY

BACKGROUND INFORMATION
Date of report: 2-28-14   **Client's name:** Jacob Olsen
Date of birth &/or age: 6-25-93   **Date of referral:** 1-14-14
Primary intervention diagnosis/concern: Tendonitis of R thumb; neck, back, and & R arm pain
Secondary diagnosis/concern: Depression
Precautions/contraindications: Thumb immobilized until 1-28-14
Reason for referral to OT: Immobilization of thumb interferes with daily life tasks
Reason for discharge from OT: Goals were met
Therapist: Ina Second, MS, OTR/L

S: "I understand now how to adjust the height of things to fit me better."
O: Jake was seen for OT 3x/wk for 6 weeks. R thumb was treated with ultrasound, massage, and gentle stretching. Jake also participated in education on ergonomic principles including adjusting work and play spaces and an exploration of alternative leisure activities. Jake's goals were to return to playing basketball and to learn to make environmental adaptation to support a pain-free lifestyle. For the first 2 weeks of occupational

FIGURE 18.2 Sample Discharge Summaries, SOAP Format.

therapy, Jake's thumb was immobilized. Services focused on ergonomic education and exploration of alternative leisure activities. Jake adjusted his desk chair and modified the height of work and seating surfaces. He received a set of table leg lengtheners and instructions for ordering a seat cushion. The therapist explored alternative leisure activities with Jake, but he refused to try 90% of them. The two he tried (hacky sack and fly tying), he did not like and reported that he would not be likely to do them in his leisure time. His R thumb has full ROM and pinch strength is 80% of expected. He reports a change in pain in his neck and back from a 7 initially to a 3 at discharge. Pain in his R thumb decreased from an 8 initially to a 2 at rest and 4 after use.

A: Both goals were met. Jake is aware of the need to pay attention to his posture and avoid positions in which his shoulders are hunched forward. He demonstrated making adjustments to his seating and work surfaces. He is returning to practicing and paying with the team.

P: Limit video game playing to 1–2 hours per day. Adjust seating and work surfaces as instructed. Follow up with team trainer for thumb pain. Resume basketball practice pending physician approval.

Ina Second, OTR/L   _2-28-14_
Signature   Date

Justa Minute, COTA/L contributed to this report.

OCCUPATIONAL THERAPY DISCHARGE SUMMARY

Date of report: Sept. 30, 2014   **Client's name:** Sadie Clapsaddle
Date of birth/age: March 26, 1985   **Date of initial referral:** Sept. 23, 2014   M   (F)
Primary intervention diagnosis/concern: Depression with suicide attempt
Secondary intervention diagnoses/concerns: History of cutting
Precautions/contraindications: Do not allow to use sharp instruments without close supervision. Count sharps at end of session.
Reason for referral to OT: Evaluate and treat for depression. Increase self-esteem.
Reason for discontinuation of OT: Completed 7-day inpatient program.
Therapist: Carla McShane, OTR/L

S: "I am looking forward to the painting class. It will be like taking a 'mini-vacation' twice a week."
O: Sadie was seen in the occupational therapy clinic twice a day for 6 of the 7 days she was here. Provided with unconditional support and encouragement. Participated in self-esteem and assertiveness group as well as task group.

Long-Term Goals	Initial Performance	Ending Performance
Sadie will say "no" and stick to that answer.	Client complied with all requests of the occupational therapist.	Client said "no" to three requests on last 2 days of OT, did not change her answer.
Look people in the eye, maintain eye contact for 10 s.	Client looked down, did not make eye contact.	Maintained eye contact with therapist and peer for 10 s on six occasions in last 2 days of OT.
Engage in painting with watercolors.	Started painting after several prompts.	Independently initiated painting upon entering OT clinic. Signed up to take painting class through community education.

A: Client made good progress. She achieved all of her goals. She is taking steps to take charge of her life, such as taking a painting class, talking with her family and negotiating shared workloads, and not backing down once she says "no"?
P: Sadie will participate in counseling sessions twice a week. She will attend a painting class through community education.

Carla McShane, OTR/L   _Sept 30, 2014_
Signature   Date

FIGURE 18.2 (Continued)

Exercise 18.1

In a narrative format, summarize the progress for each client, given starting and ending data.

Case 1: Woman recovering from a complete mastectomy of her right breast. Received outpatient OT three times a week for 3 weeks, then twice a week for 3 weeks.

Initial data: Shoulder flexion and abduction severely limited. Dependent in grooming and hygiene, moderate assist in feeding and dressing, she is able to use her left arm for some tasks. Client rates pain during movement of right arm as 9 on a 1–10 scale with 10 being excruciating.

Ending data: Nearly full range of motion in right shoulder, it is sufficient to complete most ADLs. Independent in grooming, hygiene, feeding, dressing, and meal preparation. Client rates pain during movement of right arm as 4 on a 1–10 scale with 10 being excruciating.

Summary:

Case 2: Man with low back injury at work (he worked as a carpenter). He has been attending a work-hardening program 5 days per week, 4 hours per day for 4 weeks.

Initial data: Client rates pain as 5 on a 1–10 scale at rest (10 is excruciating), 8 on the same scale when bending. When asked to demonstrate how he lifts a 2 × 4, he bent from the waist, grabbed his back, and dropped the wood. Following instruction in proper body mechanics, he demonstrated lifting the 2 × 4 by bending his knees and keeping his back straight. He lifted one 2 × 4 and carried it 10 feet. He said it hurt too much to do more.

Ending data: Client is lifting and carrying using proper body mechanics without cuing. He lifted and carried twenty 2 × 4s 10 feet without complaining of pain. He assembled and disassembled a wall frame in the clinic using proper body mechanics and without complaints of pain. He rates his pain as 1 at rest and 3 at the end of an OT session. He demonstrates independence in back strengthening exercises and reports that he does the exercise routine twice a day. He was instructed to do it three times a day, but he says he looks like a "doofus" if he does them during the workday in front of his coworkers.

Summary:

Exercise 18.2

Create a complete discontinuation report for each client in Exercise 18.1.

▼ MEDICARE COMPLIANCE ▼

Medicare Part B (outpatient) requires a discharge summary at the end of each episode of care (Centers for Medicare and Medicaid Services [CMS], 2008). If a comprehensive discharge summary is written by the physician, Medicare does not require the occupational therapist to write a separate discharge summary. When the occupational therapist writes the discharge summary, it covers the time period since the last progress report, ending on the day of discharge. If the discharge was "unanticipated in the plan or previous Progress Report, the clinician may base any judgments required to write the report on the Treatment Notes and verbal reports of the assistant or qualified personnel" (CMS, 2008, p. 33). Under Medicare Part A (inpatient) follow the facility's policies for documenting discontinuation.

SUMMARY

The discontinuation of services brings closure to a case. It provides the final justification for the services that were provided. In this document, you provide an overview of the client's progress and plans for the future. Because it is a summary, it does not need to be a session-by-session recap of what happened. Rather, it hits the highlights and reflects progress toward occupational therapy outcomes.

A discharge summary may be written in narrative or SOAP format. Either way, the discharge summary must contain specific information about the client's change in status and recommendations for follow-up and referral to other services. Knowing the client's discharge disposition is essential for making accurate statements about the client's status at discharge and what services can be recommended after discontinuation of occupational therapy services.

REFERENCES

American Occupational Therapy Association. (2010). Standards of practice for occupational therapy [Supplemental material]. *American Journal of Occupational Therapy, 64,* S106–S111. doi:10.5014/ajot.2010.64S106

American Occupational Therapy Association. (2013). *Guidelines for documentation of occupational therapy.* Retrieved from http://www.aota.org/-/media/corporate/files/secure/practice/officialdocs/guidelines/guidelines%20for%20documentation.pdf

American Occupational Therapy Association. (2014). Occupational therapy practice framework: Domain and process (3rd ed). *American Journal of Occupational Therapy, 68*(Suppl. 1), S1-S48. http://dx.doi.org/10.5014/ajot.2014.682006

Centers for Medicare and Medicaid Services. (2008). *Pub100-02 Medicare benefit policy: Transmittal 88.* Retrieved May 8, 2008, from http://www.cms.hhs.gov/transmittals/downloads/R88BP.pdf

Gateley, C.A., & Borcherding, S. (2012). *Documentation manual for occupational therapy: Writing SOAP notes.* Thorofare, NJ: Slack.

Kettenbach, G. (2009). *Writing patient/client notes: Ensuring accuracy in documentation* (4th ed.). Philadelphia, PA: F. A. Davis.

Moyers, P. (1999). The guide to occupational therapy practice. *American Journal of Occupational Therapy, 53,* 247–322.

Moyers, P. A., & Dale, L. M. (2007). *The guide to occupational therapy practice* (2nd ed.). Bethesda, MD: American Occupational Therapy Association.

SECTION IV

School System Documentation

CHAPTER 19

Overview of School System Documentation

INTRODUCTION

In school systems, the requirements for documentation are different than for occupational therapy services provided in clinical settings. There are clear federal guidelines about what to document and when. In this section of the book, we look at the documentation requirements for services provided to children through the school system. Minimal information about the actual delivery of services is covered.

▼ OVERVIEW OF SCHOOL SYSTEM DOCUMENTATION ▼

The Individuals with Disabilities Education Act (IDEA) dictates how educational services are provided to children with disabilities from birth to age 21 (United States Department of Education [USDE], 2006). IDEA also provides guidelines about how to document those services. Under IDEA, there are three types of documents: notice and consent forms, the Individualized Family Service Plan (IFSP), and the Individualized Education Program (IEP). IDEA allows each state to develop guidelines for service delivery to children that further refine the federal law. In most states, services to these children are provided by local school districts. For children birth to age 2, some states provide services to children with special needs through the school district (coordinated by the state Department of Education), but in others, the primary provider of these services could be a home health agency or welfare agency (coordinated by the state Department of Health or Department of Human Services).

Throughout this section of the book, federal laws and regulations will be cited. However, examples of how these federal laws and regulations are implemented will come from individual states. This is because IDEA requires states to offer certain services, document them, and inform families, but allows the states to determine the exact method of implementation and documentation of these services. States used as examples in this section of the book represent those in which information is more readily available on the Internet. It is not meant to imply that the states whose forms or regulations are cited have better systems than those that are not cited. I have tried to present information from different states representing a geographic cross section of this country.

One of the biggest differences between school system documentation and clinical documentation is that school system documentation is intended to be shared with the child's family or guardian. When you document in a school system, you know that the parent or guardian will receive a copy of the document, and will read what you write. In a clinical setting, you know the physician and other team members will read the document, but only if a family asks for access to the documents will they be allowed to read what you wrote.

School systems may bill third-party payers (insurance companies, managed care organizations, or Medicaid), but not every state, or every school district within a state has elected to do so, yet. Billing third-party payers may, but does not always, impact the type and frequency of documentation completed by occupational therapy personnel.

▼ ROLE DELINEATION IN SCHOOL SYSTEM DOCUMENTATION ▼

In school systems, most of the documentation is written through a team effort. The team may include teachers, special education teachers, school nurses, speech clinicians, school psychologists, and administrators, along with occupational and physical therapists. As a member of the team, the occupational therapist may write or verbally contribute to sections of the notice and consent forms, IFSP, or IEP. Occupational therapy assistants may also contribute to development of the IEP and IFSP. If the occupational therapist is serving as the service coordinator for an infant or toddler, he or she will be responsible for ensuring that all required documentation is completed within established timelines. As described in the *Guidelines for Documentation of Occupational Therapy* (AOTA, 2013), the occupational therapist is responsible for completing the evaluation; an occupational therapy assistant may participate in the process. Specific rules for documentation written by the occupational therapist or occupational therapy assistant in school systems may vary from state to state. You can find these rules by checking with your state education agency (i.e., Department of Education). As always, the AOTA *Standards of Practice for Occupational Therapy* (2010) and *Guidelines for Supervision, Roles, and Responsibilities During the Delivery of Occupational Therapy Services* (2009) for role delineation in documentation apply.

▼ OTHER LAWS IMPACTING OCCUPATIONAL THERAPY DOCUMENTATION IN SCHOOLS ▼

No Child Left Behind

Occupational therapy services in schools fall under the No Child Left Behind Act (NCLB, pronounced Nickel-Bee). This law describes how students of all abilities will succeed in school, and how schools will be held accountable for the achievements of all students (United States Department of Education, n.d.). In recent years, the law has been revised to allow more flexibility by states while still requiring state accountability, teacher excellence, and evidence-based practice (United States Department of Education, n.d.). Under NCLB, any modifications required for a student to participate in achievement testing need to be documented in the child's Individual Education Program (United States Department of Education, 2013). An occupational therapy practitioner, as a member of the team working with a child with a disability, will contribute to documenting the student's exemption from or modification of standardized achievement testing.

Section 504 of the Rehabilitation Act of 1973

Section 504 of the Rehabilitation Act of 1973, as amended (29 U.S.C. § 794 [Section 504]), is intended to protect the rights of people with disabilities, including children in school (United States Department of Education, Office for Civil Rights, 2010). According to the United States Department of Education, Office for Civil Rights (2010):

> The Section 504 regulations require a school district to provide a "free appropriate public education" (FAPE) to each qualified student with a disability who is in the school district's jurisdiction, regardless of the nature or severity of the disability. Under Section 504, FAPE consists of the provision of regular or special education and related aids and services designed to meet the student's individual educational needs as adequately as the needs of nondisabled students are met (para 4, Introduction).

A student who does not meet the qualifications for special education services may still be eligible for services under Section 504. For example, a first grader with ampliopia (lazy eye) who wears a patch over her "good eye" but has no other physical, intellectual, or emotional disability might benefit from occupational therapy services to help adapt the student's environment to better support her participation in classroom activities but would not qualify for special education services. These adaptations might include adjusting where the student sits in relation to the smartboard, adjusting font sizes on the computer, providing adapted writing paper, and other modifications. To qualify for a 504 plan, the student's disability cannot be transient. In other words, the disability must be expected to last for at least 6 months (United States Department of Education, Office for Civil Rights, 2010).

A student receiving services under Section 504 will have the services documented on a 504 plan. The 504 plan cannot be written until an evaluation has been documented (United States Department of Education, Office for Civil Rights, 2010). Students receiving services under Section 504 have rights and schools must provide the families of these children with notice and consent forms, similar to those provided to parents of students receiving special education services. The Los Angeles Unified School District (LAUSD) has a document that explains the process and has examples of notice and consent forms and the 504 plan at http://www.lausd.k12.ca.us/lausd/offices/eec/pdfs/BUL_4045.pdf (LAUSD, 2008). Additional sample forms can be found at http://doe.sd.gov/oess/documents/sped_section504_Guidelines.pdf

Response to Intervention

Response to intervention is part of IDEA, but it happens before students qualify for special education. Response to intervention (RtI) is an early intervening service, meaning it occurs before a student is evaluated for special education (AOTA, 2008). There are three levels of service under RtI. The first level involves the overall curriculum, looking at overall supports for all children. The next level is for those students who do not appear to be benefiting from the broader intervention. The third level is intensive interventions for individual students. Occupational therapy practitioners may be involved at any or all of these levels as part of the problem-solving team. Each intervention on every level is documented. Each intervention also must be based on evidence (AOTA, 2008). AOTA offers members several resources to help occupational therapy practitioners understand their role in RtI.

▼ STRUCTURE OF THIS SECTION OF THE BOOK ▼

Under IDEA, the contents of educational documentation, including notice and consent forms, the IFSP, and the IEP, are specified; however, the specific forms may be developed by the state education agency or the school district/local agency. Just as with documents in medical model settings, these are legal documents and can be called into court when there are lawsuits. It seems lately that there are more and more lawsuits involving the provision of special education and related services, especially issues around who will be responsible for paying for what services.

Notice and consent forms are designed to guarantee that the rights of the child and his or her family are respected. Some of these forms provide information or notice to the family; others seek parental consent to evaluate, provide, or change services (USDE, 2006). These are discussed in Chapter 20.

Documentation for children birth through age 2 is covered in Chapter 21. Each infant or toddler who qualifies for services under IDEA must have a written plan, called an IFSP, for the services he or she will receive. This chapter discusses the IFSP.

The last chapter of this section, Chapter 22, discusses the IEP. This is generally written for children with special needs ages 3–21. For these children, occupational therapy is a related service rather than a special education service (USDE, 2006).

REFERENCES

American Occupational Therapy Association. (2008). *FAQ on response to intervention for school-based occupational therapists and occupational therapy assistants.* Retrieved from http://www.aota.org/-/media/corporate/files/secure/practice/children/rtifinalrevise12-21-08.pdf

American Occupational Therapy Association. (2009). *Guidelines for supervision, roles, and responsibilities during the delivery of occupational therapy services.* Retrieved from http://www.aota.org/-/media/corporate/files/secure/practice/officialdocs/guidelines/guidelines%20for%20supervision%20roles%20and%20responsibilities.pdf

American Occupational Therapy Association. (2010). Standards of practice for occupational therapy [Supplemental material]. *American Journal of Occupational Therapy, 64,* S106–S111. doi:10.5014/ajot.2010.64S106

American Occupational Therapy Association. (2013). *Guidelines for documentation of occupational therapy.* Retrieved from http://www.aota.org/-/media/corporate/files/secure/practice/officialdocs/guidelines/guidelines%20for%20documentation.pdf

Los Angeles Unified School District. (2008). *Section 504 and students with disabilities.* Retrieved from http://www.lausd.k12.ca.us/lausd/offices/eec/pdfs/BUL_4045.pdf

United States Department of Education. (2006). *Building the legacy of IDEA, 2004.* Retrieved from http://idea.ed.gov/explore/home

United States Department of Education. (2013). *Modified academic achievement standards: Non-regulatory guidance.* Retrieved from http://www2.ed.gov/admins/lead/account/saa.html#regulations

United States Department of Education. (n.d.). *No child left behind: Elementary and secondary education act (ESEA).* Retrieved from http://www2.ed.gov/nclb/landing.jhtml

United States Department of Education, Office for Civil Rights. (2010). *Guidelines for educators and administrators for implementing Section 504 of the Rehabilitation Act of 1973, Subpart D.* Retrieved from http://doe.sd.gov/oess/documents/sped_section504_Guidelines.pdf

---

Visit **www.pearsonhighered.com/healthprofessionsresources** to access the student resources that accompany this book. Simply select Occupational Therapy from the choice of disciplines. Find this book and you will find the complimentary study tools created for this specific title.

CHAPTER 20

Procedural Safeguards: Notice and Consent Forms

INTRODUCTION

Whenever you work with children, you are working with a vulnerable population. As such, the federal government has developed regulations that protect the rights and interests of the child and his or her family. The term *procedural safeguards* refers to both the process and the forms used to protect those rights. The forms that are used to protect the rights of recipients, inform families, and obtain consent are called notice and consent forms. Generally, the school system or agency will have these forms available for obtaining parent consent and providing legally required notices.

Some states mandate that school districts use a prescribed set of forms; others allow each school district to develop its own set of forms. Box 20.1 shows the language of the federal law (20 U.S.C. 1400 et seq.) relating to Procedural Safeguards, including the types of notices and consent forms and their contents (United States Department of Education [USDE], 2006). No matter what type of form parents are asked to read or sign, they must be provided in the families' native language, including Braille or orally (Pacer Center, 2006; 34 C.F.R. § 300.503[c]; 34 C.F.R. § 303.403[c]).

BOX 20.1 Procedural Safeguards. (20 U.S.C. 1400.615)

SEC. 615. PROCEDURAL SAFEGUARDS

(a) ESTABLISHMENT OF PROCEDURES. Any State educational agency, State agency, or local educational agency that receives assistance under this part shall establish and maintain procedures in accordance with this section to ensure that children with disabilities and their parents are guaranteed procedural safeguards with respect to the provision of a free appropriate public education by such agencies.

(b) TYPES OF PROCEDURES. The procedures required by this section shall include the following:

(1) An opportunity for the parents of a child with a disability to examine all records relating to such child and to participate in meetings with respect to the identification, evaluation, and educational placement of the child, and the provision of a free appropriate public education to such child, and to obtain an independent educational evaluation of the child.

(2) A Procedures to protect the rights of the child whenever the parents of the child are not known, the agency cannot, after reasonable efforts, locate the parents, or the child is a ward of the State, including the assignment of an individual to act as a surrogate for the parents, which surrogate shall not be an employee of the State educational agency, the local educational agency, or any other agency that is involved in the education or care of the child. In the case of—

(i) a child who is a ward of the State, such surrogate may alternatively be appointed by the judge overseeing the child's care provided that the surrogate meets the requirements of this paragraph; and

(ii) an unaccompanied homeless youth as defined in section 725(6) of the McKinney-Vento Homeless Assistance Act (42 U.S.C. 11434a(6)), the local educational agency shall appoint a surrogate in accordance with this paragraph.

(B) The State shall make reasonable efforts to ensure the assignment of a surrogate not more than 30 days after there is a determination by the agency that the child needs a surrogate.

(3) Written prior notice to the parents of the child, in accordance with subsection (c)(1), whenever the local educational agency—

(A) proposes to initiate or change; or

(B) refuses to initiate or change, the identification, evaluation, or educational placement of the child, or the provision of a free appropriate public education to the child.

(4) Procedures designed to ensure that the notice required by paragraph (3) is in the native language of the parents, unless it clearly is not feasible to do so.

(5) An opportunity for mediation, in accordance with subsection (e).

(6) An opportunity for any party to present a complaint—

(A) with respect to any matter relating to the identification, evaluation, or educational placement of the child, or the provision of a free appropriate public education to such child; and

(B) which sets forth an alleged violation that occurred not more than 2 years before the date the parent or public agency knew or should have known about the alleged action that forms the basis of the complaint, or, if the State has an explicit time limitation for presenting such a complaint under this part, in such time as the State law allows, except that the exceptions to the timeline described in subsection (f)(3)(D) shall apply to the timeline described in this subparagraph.

(7) (A) Procedures that require either party, or the attorney representing a party, to provide due process complaint notice in accordance with subsection (c)(2) (which shall remain confidential)—

(i) to the other party, in the complaint filed under paragraph (6), and forward a copy of such notice to the State educational agency; and

(ii) that shall include—

(I) the name of the child, the address of the residence of the child (or available contact information in the case of a homeless child), and the name of the school the child is attending;

(II) in the case of a homeless child or youth (within the meaning of section 725(2) of the McKinney-Vento Homeless Assistance Act (42 U.S.C. 11434a(2)), available contact information for the child and the name of the school the child is attending;

(III) a description of the nature of the problem of the child relating to such proposed initiation or change, including facts relating to such problem; and

(IV) a proposed resolution of the problem to the extent known and available to the party at the time.

(B) A requirement that a party may not have a due process hearing until the party, or the attorney representing the party, files a notice that meets the requirements of subparagraph (A)(ii).

(8) Procedures that require the State educational agency to develop a model form to assist parents in filing a complaint and due process complaint notice in accordance with paragraphs (6) and (7), respectively.

(c) NOTIFICATION REQUIREMENTS.

(1) Content of prior written notice. The notice required by subsection (b)(3) shall include—

(A) a description of the action proposed or refused by the agency;

(B) an explanation of why the agency proposes or refuses to take the action and a description of each evaluation procedure, assessment, record, or report the agency used as a basis for the proposed or refused action;

(C) a statement that the parents of a child with a disability have protection under the procedural safeguards of this part and, if this notice is not an initial referral for evaluation, the means by which a copy of a description of the procedural safeguards can be obtained;

(D) sources for parents to contact to obtain assistance in understanding the provisions of this part;

(E) a description of other options considered by the IEP Team and the reason why those options were rejected; and

(F) a description of the factors that are relevant to the agency's proposal or refusal.

(Continued)

BOX 20.1   Continued

(2) Due process complaint notice.

(A) Complaint. The due process complaint notice required under subsection (b)(7)(A) shall be deemed to be sufficient unless the party receiving the notice notifies the hearing officer and the other party in writing that the receiving party believes the notice has not met the requirements of subsection (b)(7)(A).

(B) Response to complaint.

(i) Local educational agency response.

(I) In general. If the local educational agency has not sent a prior written notice to the parent regarding the subject matter contained in the parent's due process complaint notice, such local educational agency shall, within 10 days of receiving the complaint, send to the parent a response that shall include—

(aa) an explanation of why the agency proposed or refused to take the action raised in the complaint;

(bb) a description of other options that the IEP Team considered and the reasons why those options were rejected;

(cc) a description of each evaluation procedure, assessment, record, or report the agency used as the basis for the proposed or refused action; and

(dd) a description of the factors that are relevant to the agency's proposal or refusal.

(II) Sufficiency. A response filed by a local educational agency pursuant to subclause (I) shall not be construed to preclude such local educational agency from asserting that the parent's due process complaint notice was insufficient where appropriate.

(ii) Other party response. Except as provided in clause (i), the non-complaining party shall, within 10 days of receiving the complaint, send to the complaint a response that specifically addresses the issues raised in the complaint.

(C) Timing. The party providing a hearing officer notification under subparagraph (A) shall provide the notification within 15 days of receiving the complaint.

(D) Determination.—Within 5 days of receipt of the notification provided under subparagraph (C), the hearing officer shall make a determination on the face of the notice of whether the notification meets the requirements of subsection (b)(7)(A), and shall immediately notify the parties in writing of such determination.

(E) Amended complaint notice.

(i) In general. A party may amend its due process complaint notice only if—

(I) the other party consents in writing to such amendment and is given the opportunity to resolve the complaint through a meeting held pursuant to subsection (f)(1)(B); or

(II) the hearing officer grants permission, except that the hearing officer may only grant such permission at any time not later than 5 days before a due process hearing occurs.

(ii) Applicable timeline. The applicable timeline for a due process hearing under this part shall recommence at the time the party files an amended notice, including the timeline under subsection (f)(1)(B).

(d) PROCEDURAL SAFEGUARDS NOTICE.

(1) In general.

(A) Copy to parents. A copy of the procedural safeguards available to the parents of a child with a disability shall be given to the parents only 1 time a year, except that a copy also shall be given to the parents—

(i) upon initial referral or parental request for evaluation;

(ii) upon the first occurrence of the filing of a complaint under subsection (b)(6); and

(iii) upon request by a parent.

(B) Internet website. A local educational agency may place a current copy of the procedural safeguards notice on its Internet website if such website exists.

(1) Contents. —The procedural safeguards notice shall include a full explanation of the procedural safeguards, written in the native language of the parents (unless it clearly is not feasible to do so) and

written in an easily understandable manner, available under this section and under regulations promulgated by the Secretary relating to—

(A) independent educational evaluation;

(B) prior written notice;

(C) parental consent;

(D) access to educational records;

(E) the opportunity to present and resolve complaints, including—

    (i) the time period in which to make a complaint;

    (ii) the opportunity for the agency to resolve the complaint; and

    (iii) the availability of mediation;

(F) the child's placement during pendency of due process proceedings;

(G) procedures for students who are subject to placement in an interim alternative educational setting;

(H) requirements for unilateral placement by parents of children in private schools at public expense;

(I) due process hearings, including requirements for disclosure of evaluation results and recommendations;

(J) State-level appeals (if applicable in that State);

(K) civil actions, including the time period in which to file such actions; and

(L) attorneys' fees.

▼ TYPES OF NOTICE AND CONSENT FORMS ▼

The Individuals with Disabilities Education Act (IDEA) requires that notice be given to parents (or designated surrogates) whenever there is a proposal to initiate or change services, or when the agency refuses to initiate or change services (USDE, 2006; 20 U.S.C. 1400.615[b]). The law requires that notices must be provided in the family's native language (USDE; 34 C.F.R. § 300.503[c]; 34 C.F.R. § 303.403[c]) in writing or by other approved method such as e-mail (USDE, 2006). Providing notice means that the agency has notified the parent or guardian; it does not mean that the parent has agreed to anything. Whether you are the service coordinator or not, it is important to know the different types of forms a family might be asked to sign, so that if a family member asks you about a form, you will know how to respond.

Evaluation (and Reevaluation) Notice and Consent

Parental consent is needed before an evaluation or reevaluation can be conducted (USDE, 2006; 34 C.F.R. § 300.505[a][1]; 34 C.F.R. § 300.505[a][1]; 34 C.F.R. § 300.503[b]; 34 C.F.R. § 303.404). The notice has to include what action is being proposed, a rationale for that action, what procedural safeguards are available, and procedures for filing a complaint in that state (34 C.F.R. § 303.403[b]). This document may be called a Prior Written Notice (California Department of Education [CDE], 2009) or a Notice of Recommendation (New York State Education Department [NYSED], 2012).

    The service coordinator completes the form including details about what areas are to be evaluated. Areas to be evaluated may vary from state to state in terms of wording, but usually include academic achievement, functional performance, cognitive functioning, communication status, health, hearing/vision, motor abilities, and social/emotional status (Illinois State Board of Education [ISBE], 2008). For each area to be assessed, the members of the team who will be involved in conducting the evaluation are listed. Finally, a reason for evaluating that area and a plan for doing so are documented. A copy of the form is presented to the child's family, and sometimes to the referral source. An example of a consent form can be found in Appendix C (see website) and at http://idea.ed.gov/static/modelForms.

Since the family or guardian will be reading this document, it is imperative that the writer use clear language, avoid abbreviations and jargon, and be especially careful to keep evaluative language out of any written document. The hardest part of the form to word appropriately is the explanation of the reason for assessing a particular area. You do not need to be very specific. You could say that you want to do a motor assessment to "determine student's ability to participate in movement related preschool learning activities" or "determine the child's ability to move about and interact with environment in preparation for learning." For an older child, it might say that you want to do an assessment of motor function to "determine the student's ability to participate in instructional activities/programs and complete class work requirements" or an assessment of transition skills to "determine vocational skills for possible employment after graduation."

Exercise 20.1

Write a reason for doing the following assessments:

1. Peabody Developmental Motor Scales for a 5-year-old who has difficulty with both gross and fine motor skills, which cause her to stand out as "different" in her kindergarten class.

2. Test of Visual Perceptual Skills on a 6-year-old with attention deficits and mental retardation.

3. Clinical observations of neuromotor skills for a 7-year-old with cerebral palsy.

4. Erhardt Developmental Prehension Assessment for a 2-year-old with Down syndrome.

Meeting Notice

Since parents and guardians are so involved in this process, they need to be notified and invited to participate in all team meetings, especially meetings for developing the Individualized Education Program (IEP) or Individualized Family Service Plan (IFSP). Parents/guardians are vital to the success of school-based programs. The service coordinator must be sure that proper forms for notifying parents/guardians of team meetings are completed and delivered to the parents/guardians. At minimum, the notice of a team meeting must include the purpose, time, and place of the meeting, as well as identifying who will be at the meeting in addition to the parents (34 C.F.R. § 300.345[b][1]; CDE, 2009; NYSED, 2012).

Other Notices

In addition to notifying parents when an evaluation is being conducted or a team meeting is being held, notices are required whenever services are initiated, changed, discontinued, or refused, for example, if a school district proposes to make significant changes to the IEP or refuses to make changes requested by the family, or proposes to change a student's placement or refuses to change a placement (34 C.F.R. § 300.503; CDE, 2009; NYSED, 2012), notice is required.

Here is a sample list of notice and consent forms used by school districts or state agencies (Minnesota Department of Education [MDOE], 2008):

- Referral for an initial evaluation
- Procedural safeguards notice
- Parental permission for initial evaluation/reevaluation

- Report of IEP/IFSP meeting
- Manifestation determination form
- Notice of a team meeting
- Consent to release private data
- Documentation of significant changes to IEP plan
- Permission to start the program

Not every state agency or school district will require all of these forms. Complete information on which forms are required in your state, visit your state's education department and enter the search term *procedural safeguards*.

▼ SERVICE COORDINATION ▼

Providing educational services to children is a team effort. It includes professionals from several disciplines as well as the parents and, when possible, the child. Because of the many people who could be involved in the team, there needs to be one person who takes responsibility for ensuring that everything that needs to be done gets done in a timely fashion. This person is referred to as the service coordinator (team leader). An occupational therapist can serve as the service coordinator for a child from birth through age 2 if designated as such by IFSP team (34 C.F.R. § 303.6). However, because occupational therapy is a related service (rather than a special education service) for children ages 3–21, an occupational therapist is usually not the service coordinator for preschool through school-age children. However, if designated by the IEP team, the occupational therapist can be the case manager (National Early Childhood Technical Assistance Center [NECTAC], 2008).

The service coordinator prepares the documents for parent notification and consent (NECTAC, 2008). The service coordinator must provide parents with written information about procedural safeguards upon initial referral or evaluation, each notification of IFSP or IEP meetings, every reevaluation, and when the parents request it (34 C.F.R. § 300.504[a]). This information accompanies notice and consent forms presented to families to ensure that families are fully informed about their rights.

Exercise 20.2

Go to the website for the Department of Education for your state. See if you can locate information about the notice and consent forms or procedural safeguards that are used in your state. You are looking for state regulations about special education services. Once you find where the regulations are posted, locate and read the requirements for parental notifications and consents. Some state websites are more difficult to navigate than others, but do not get discouraged. Keep digging until you find what you are looking for.

SUMMARY

In school systems, there are several forms that are used to ensure that a child and his or her family's rights to notice and consent are protected. For children under age 3, an occupational therapist may be the service coordinator, thereby being the person responsible for the completion of notice and consent paperwork. For children over the age of 3, an occupational therapist may contribute to the notice and consent documents, but would not usually be the service coordinator (case manager). As with all school system documentation, the writer needs to be sure that they are written so that parents of all educational levels can read them.

REFERENCES

California Department of Education. (2009). *Notice of procedural safeguards.* Retrieved from http://www.cde.ca.gov/sp/se/qa/documents/pseng.pdf

Illinois State Board of Education. (2008). *Parent/guardian consent for evaluation.* Retreived from http://www.isbe.net/spec-ed/pdfs/nc_id_34-57bc.pdf

Minnesota Department of Education. (2008). *Recommended due process forms.* Retrieved October 24, 2008, from http://education.state.mn.us/MDE/SchSup/ComplAssist/Forms/

National Early Childhood Technical Assistance Center. (2008). *Service coordination under IDEA 2004.* Retrieved from http://www.nectac.org/topics/scoord/scoord.asp

New York State Department of Education. 2012. *Procedural safeguards notice.* Retrieved from http://www.p12.nysed.gov/specialed/publications/psgn1211.htm#pwn

Pacer Center. (2006). Informed parent consent for pre-school and school-aged children with disabilities. Retrieved from http://www.pacer.org/publications/pdfs/ALL40.pdf

United States Department of Education. (2006). *Building the legacy: IDEA 2004.* Retrieved October 1, 2008, from http://idea.ed.gov/explore/home

Visit **www.pearsonhighered.com/healthprofessionsresources** to access the student resources that accompany this book. Simply select Occupational Therapy from the choice of disciplines. Find this book and you will find the complimentary study tools created for this specific title.

CHAPTER 21

Individualized Family Service Plans

INTRODUCTION

The Individuals with Disabilities Education Act (IDEA), Part C (2004 revision, 20 U.S.C. 1400 et seq.), states that services provided to children with disabilities, birth through age 2, are provided under an Individualized Family Service Plan (IFSP) (Jackson, 2007; Stephens & Tauber, 2005; 20 U.S.C. 1400 Part C Sect. 634). An IFSP is a written document that specifies the unique strengths and needs of a child and his or her family, the steps that will be taken to help the child achieve the outcomes desired by the child's family, and who is responsible for implementing and paying for services needed to meet those outcomes (Stephens & Tauber, 2005; 20 U.S.C. 1400 Part C Sect. 636[d]). AOTA offers a range of documents that support occupational therapy practice in early intervention, including *Occupational Therapy Services in Early Childhood and School Settings* that would be a helpful document to read along with this chapter (AOTA, 2011). This chapter is based on the rules for Part C under IDEA.

▼ IFSP REQUIREMENTS ▼

Specifically, the IFSP must contain the following eight elements:

1. A statement of the infant or toddler's present level of performance of physical development, cognitive development, communication development, social or emotional development, and adaptive development, based on objective criteria;

2. A statement of the family's resources, priorities, and concerns relating to enhancing the development of the family's infant or toddler with a disability;

3. A statement of the major outcomes (measurable results) expected to be achieved for the infant or toddler and the family, and the criteria, procedures, and timelines used to determine the degree to which progress toward achieving the outcomes is being made and whether modifications or revisions of the outcomes or services are necessary;

4. A statement of specific evidence-based early intervention services necessary to meet the unique needs of the infant or toddler and the family, including the frequency, intensity, and method of delivering services;

5. A statement of the natural environments in which early intervention services shall appropriately be provided, including a justification of the extent, if any, to which the services will not be provided in a natural environment;

6. The projected dates for initiation of services and the anticipated frequency and duration of the services;

7. The identification of the service coordinator from the profession most immediately relevant to the infant's or toddler's or family's needs who will be responsible for the implementation of the plan and coordination with other agencies and persons; and

8. A description of how the toddler with a disability will be transitioned to preschool or other appropriate services (20 U.S.C. 1400.636[d][1–8]).

Under certain circumstances, children who are between the ages of 3 and 5, at the request of their family, can have an IFSP written instead of an Individualized Education Program (IEP), which is the document usually written for children ages 3 through 21 (see Chapter 22) (34 CFR § 300.342[c]).

As noted in Chapter 20, for each IFSP written, there must be a person designated as the service coordinator who is responsible for ensuring the implementation of the IFSP and coordination of care with other service providers (Jackson, 2007; 20 U.S.C. 1400.636[d][7]). If the infant's or toddler's needs are best served by intervention from an occupational therapist (e.g., an infant with cerebral palsy or a toddler who had a stroke), then the occupational therapist can serve as the service coordinator. As service coordinator, the occupational therapist would be the person responsible for completing all notice and consent forms as well as the IFSP. The order in which the required information appears on the IFSP document may vary from state to state or agency to agency.

Documentation for services provided under an IFSP minimally consists of the notice and consent forms (see Chapter 20) and the IFSP document. In some states and under some circumstances (such as when a third-party payer is involved) additional documentation may be required. When birth-through-age-2 services are provided in a child's home, it is common for the occupational therapist to also write visit or contact notes that describe what occurred during the intervention session and recommendations for follow-through (i.e., home programs). These notes can be written in either a narrative or a SOAP format.

Exercise 21.1

Get on the Internet and look up the rules governing how services are delivered to infants and toddlers with disabilities in your state. The rules may be posted by your state's Department of Education, Department of Human Services, Department of Health, Department of Public Health, Department of Health and Human Services, Department of Children and Families, Department of Public Instruction, or State Board of Education. Read the section on IFSP services. If you live in a state that mandates or recommends use of a particular form for writing the IFSP, download it to look at as you work your way through the rest of this chapter.

▼ EVALUATION ▼

The evaluation is the first step in preparing the IFSP (after consent to evaluate is obtained). Based on the results of the evaluation, the IFSP is developed and implemented. The occupational therapist and other members of the IFSP team use the evaluation to develop statements of the present level of development in the areas of "physical development (including vision, hearing, and health status), cognitive development, communication development, social or emotional development, and adaptive development" (Clark, Lucas, Jackson, & Nanof, 2008; 34 C.F.R. § 303.344[a]).

If the occupational therapist is the service coordinator for a particular child and family, he or she will be responsible for ensuring the quality of the assessment process (Stephens & Tauber, 2005). This means that the occupational therapist has to ensure that the assessment process meets certain criteria (Clark et al., 2008; Stephens & Tauber, 2005):

- The evaluation is conducted by qualified personnel;
- It is based on the criteria established by the state;
- The child's medical and health histories are included;
- The report includes levels of development, unique needs of the child and family, and services recommended to improve the cognitive, physical, communication, social, adaptive and emotional development of the child;

- The evaluation is conducted in the child's natural environment; and
- Evaluation procedures and materials must be administered in the parent's native language (nondiscrimination).

The service coordinator must also gather data about available family resources, family priorities, and the concerns the family has regarding the child's development (Clark et al., 2008; Stephens & Tauber, 2005; 30 C.F.R. 303.344[b]).

The evaluation process is conducted by members of a multidisciplinary team (Clark et al., 2008; Stephens & Tauber, 2005). The evaluation must be completed within 45 days after the agency receives the referral for services (Clark et al., 2008; Waisman Center, 2008; 30 C.F.R. 303.321[a][2]). If an interim IFSP is developed, the child may begin to receive early intervention services prior to the completion of the evaluation process (Jackson, 2007; 30 C.F.R. 303.345).

▼ PRESENT LEVELS OF DEVELOPMENT ▼

Based on professionally acceptable, objective criteria, the infant or toddler's physical, cognitive, communication, social or emotional, and adaptive (e.g., self-care skills) development are summarized using both descriptive and interpretive statements (34 C.F.R. 303.344[a]). These summaries identify the infant or toddler's present levels of performance and include both strengths and areas in need of improvement. It is important to note that not every child will have needs in every area.

An example of a present level of development in the physical area:

Cole is rolling to the right and left independently. At this time he requires assistance to move from prone to all fours and prone to sit. Once positioned, he can maintain the sitting position for up to a minute. He uses his whole hand to grasp objects and bring them to midline. He does not weight shift to reach objects; rather, he grasps for only those objects within range of an outstretched arm.

▼ FAMILY INFORMATION, RESOURCES, AND CONCERNS ▼

In addition to what professionals identify as the present levels of development, the family's input is recorded on the IFSP. There is space to identify the resources that the family has, the family's priorities, and concerns the family has related to the child's development (Clark et al., 2008; National Dissemination Center for Children with Disabilities [NICHCY], 2012; Waisman Center, 2008; 20 U.S.C. 1400.636[d][2]). Families contribute to identifying the child's strengths as well as desired outcomes of early intervention. Because this document is written for families as well as the providers of early intervention services, it can be helpful to use the parent's words to the extent that you can. Family resources can include people, skills, capacities, and assets (such as private health insurance) that can help the family of an infant or toddler with a disability. You can ask the family to share this information with you, but it would be unethical to pressure the family to divulging more than they want to. Whatever concerns, worries, or distresses the family expresses gets recorded on the IFSP. Other members of the team can identify concerns, but unless the family agrees with them, they are not recorded on the IFSP. The family determines the priorities for their infant or toddler. It is not necessary to prioritize every individual concern; only those that are of the greatest concern to the family right now.

Some IFSPs identify each member of the team working with the client, including school system personnel; physician; private physical, occupational, or speech therapists; county social workers; and others involved in the care of that child (Waisman Center, 2008). This page is a wonderful resource for families because it lists names, addresses, and phone numbers of all these key people all on one page.

Next, the IFSP documents the expected outcomes for the child and his or her family, based on input from both health or education professionals and the family. These outcomes can be for either the child or the family (Clark et al., 2008; NICHCY, 2012; Waisman Center, 2008; U.SC. 1400.636[d][5]). The outcomes should be specific and have criteria, procedures, and a timeline for meeting them. While the outcomes are written annually, they are reviewed at 6-month intervals (USDE, 2006).

An outcome is a statement of change that relates to the infant or toddler's development, which the family can see. This requires using the family's language rather than professional jargon. For example, use the phrase "brothers and sisters" rather than "siblings" or "sit without support" instead of "improve muscle tone." The outcomes are written by the team; they are not intended to be specific to one profession (Shelden & Rush, 2009).

The exact format for wording the outcomes will vary from state to state, and perhaps within a state from agency to agency. Usually, there is an annual outcome that identifies what the child will be doing 1 year from the start date of the IFSP, although some states, such as Nebraska, use a 6-month time frame instead (IFSPWeb, n.d.). An annual outcome is sometimes referred to as the annual goal.

One format for writing the annual goal includes both the starting and ending performance. For example, Ebony will appropriately play with a variety of toys, moving from simple manipulation of toys/objects to consistent intentional use of toys/objects as observed by the occupational therapist. Notice that this goal is worded differently than any of the formats talked about in Chapter 15. It does not include a measure of time. The time frame is implied since a new goal is written every year when the IFSP is rewritten. Figure 21.1 shows the elements of an annual goal (outcome) written in this format. The instructional objectives that lead to meeting

Annual Goal	State	Examples
Direction of Change	• Increase • Improve • Decrease • Maintain	• Calvin will increase the time he stays engaged in play activities while positioned on his stomach from <1 min to 10 min.
Skill or Behavior	• Measurable skill • Observable behavior • Developmental milestone	• Marni will improve her tolerance of getting her hair combed from crying immediately when she sees the comb to letting her mother comb her hair for 1 min without crying.
Present level	From _____	
Expected level of achievement	To _____ (measurement)	

Objectives	State	Examples
Context	• Physical environment • Sociocultural environment • Human assistance • Adaptive equipment or assistive technology	• Given an interesting toy while placed prone on his mother's lap, Calvin will play with the toy for 2 min or more on 3 consecutive days as reported in a log kept by his mother.
Skill or Behavior	• Observable behavior • Measurable skill	• When Marni sees her mother pick up Marni's comb, Marni will cry for less than 10 seconds on 50% of trials as recorded in a daily journal kept by her mother.
Criteria for attainment	• Measurement in terms of a number	
Procedure for attainment	• Tool used to measure • Who will measure	

FIGURE 21.1   IFSP Annual Goals and Objectives, Direction of Change Format.

Family Identified Outcome	Annual Outcome	Objective
Eat finger food	Jacinta will eat finger foods by herself	Jacinta will eat pieces of cereal by using her fingers to put it in her mouth.
Play with sisters	Romeo will play with his sisters	Romeo will play ball games with his sisters when they come home from school.
Sleep through the night	Norichika will sleep through the night	Norichika will sleep through the night in his bed after following the same bedtime routine each night.

FIGURE 21.2 IFSP Annual Goals and Objectives, Participation-Based Format.
Source: Shelden and Rush (2009).

the annual goal simply state the desired behavior, the contexts under which the behavior will be performed, and the criteria and procedures that will be used to measure attainment (Clark et al., 2008; Southwest/West Central Service Cooperatives [SWCSC], 2006).

Some states prefer a participation-based format. Since it is the family that will be measuring the progress, they recommend using a significant family event as the time marker, rather than 6 or 12 months (Shelden & Rush, 2009). Shelden and Rush (2009) recommend that the outcome be something the family can measure. They recommend a "third word" approach to writing the outcome statement. In this approach, the first two words are the *child's name* and *will*. The third word describes the functional outcome rather than a specific skill. It is something that occurs in real time and in the context of the family (Shelden & Rush, 2009). The functional outcome is an active verb (Shelden & Rush, 2009). Figure 21.2 shows examples of this type of outcome statement.

Another format takes a very different approach from the other two. In this format, the team identifies a skill set for each need area that they would like the child to obtain in the next year (SWCSC, 2006). The annual goal then states how much (number or percentage) of that skill set the child will obtain during the year. Shorter term objectives identify the increasing number or percentage of the identified skills the child will obtain (SWCSC, 2006). Figure 21.3 shows an example of this type of outcome setting.

The most important considerations when writing outcomes in an IFSP is that they address both the child's and the family's needs, state why the outcomes are important to the family, and the goals are written so that the family can understand them (Waisman Center, 2008).

Exercise 21.2

Family-Friendly Outcome Statements

For each poorly written outcome statement, translate it into clear, measurable language any parent could understand.

1. Torii will transition from prone to sitting with moderate assistance by the end of the school year.

2. Lynette will don and doff her jacket, including fasteners, in less than 3 minutes by December 1, 2014.

3. Ione will demonstrate improved muscle tone so that she can sit unsupported while engaging in bilateral occupations for 5 minutes or longer by March 1, 2014.

4. Edgar will engage in age-appropriate play activities with a peer on a regular basis within 6 months.

5. Angelina's parents will access available community support services to take the stress off the family for caring for a child with multiple disabilities.

Skill Set	Annual Goal	Objectives
Move around in his environment		
1. Transition between prone on belly and sitting independently 2. Rock while on hands and knees for 30 seconds 3. Crawl forward 10 feet 4. Pull self up to standing independently 5. Walk while holding on to furniture 10 feet in each direction 6. Take 5 steps forward independently	Calvin will improve from performing 0 skills to performing 5 of 6 skills identified.	1. Calvin will perform 2 of the 6 skills identified on 90% of trials as observed and documented by the occupational therapist on an observation checklist. 2. Calvin will perform 4 of the 6 skills identified on 90% of trials as observed and documented by the occupational therapist on an observation checklist.
Play with toys		
1. Hold a toy in one hand for 1 min 2. Hold a toy in each hand for 1 min 3. Remove an object from inside an open container 4 out of 5 times 4. Place an object inside another 4 out of 5 times 5. Push a button to activate a toy 4 out of 5 times 6. Stack 3 objects on 3 out of 5 trials 7. Hand a toy to another person when asked on 90% of trials	Edo will improve play skills by going from performing none of the skills listed to satisfactorily performing 5 of the 7 skills listed.	• When presented with a toy, Edo will successfully complete 3 of 7 skills as observed by the occupational therapist and recorded on a play checklist. • When presented with a toy, Edo will successfully complete 5 of 7 skills as observed by the occupational therapist and recorded on a play checklist.

FIGURE 21.3   IFSP Annual Goals and Objectives, Skill Set Format Examples.

Exercise 21.3

Writing Outcome Statements

For each child and family, write an outcome statement that is clear, measurable, and written in language any parent could understand. Write an outcome statement for the child and another for the family.

1. Soren's father is in the Army reserve and has just been recalled up for active duty, soon to be deployed for a third time to Iraq. His mother works as a manager at a local fast-food restaurant. Soren's grandmother functions as his PCA (personal care attendant). Soren is 2.5 years old; he is nonverbal, and has difficulty attending to any task for more than a few seconds before moving on to something new. The only time he sits still for a few minutes at a time is when grandma puts in a cartoon on TV or DVD. He does not dress himself, but does feed himself finger food. He drinks from a sippy cup. He is a very picky eater and has several food allergies. He walks independently, but cannot jump. Each time his father deploys or comes home, Soren has trouble sleeping, and negative behaviors increase (e.g., throwing things, hitting himself, or biting others).

2. Denay was a normally developing child when her mother's boyfriend got frustrated with her crying while he was babysitting, and he threw her into a wall. She sustained a serious head injury. She is now 18 months old and living with a foster family. The foster family also cares for four other children with special needs. She commando crawls to move around a room, but her right leg is dragged behind her while she uses her arms to pull her body forward. When she stands, she puts most of her weight on her left leg and arm, and her right heel does not touch the floor. She has seizures that are not completely controlled by medication. She grasps objects with either hand, but does not cross midline. She is beginning to learn some signs like "more," "please," and "mother."

▼ SERVICES PROVIDED ▼

The specific services provided under the IFSP must, to the extent possible, be based on peer-reviewed research (USDE, 2007). The frequency, intensity, duration, length, and method of intervention provided by each service provider involved in that child's care must be explicitly stated (Clark et al., 2008; NICHCY, 2012; USDE, 2007; Waisman Center, 2008; 20 U.S.C. 1400.636[d][4]). Frequency refers to how often the child is seen (Waisman Center, 2006). In some states you need to differentiate between direct and indirect minutes. Direct minutes are those in which the service provider spends directly with the child. Indirect minutes are spent on a case but without working directly with the child; it could be time spent in observation and consultation with the child's parents or other caregivers, cooperative planning, or modifying environments (SWCSC, 2006). Intensity is stated in terms of the average number of minutes per session the child will receive services; it is stated specifically rather than a range of minutes (Waisman Center, 2006). Duration means how long the service will be offered from the date of the IFSP meeting or the date of initiation of the service (Waisman Center, 2006). The IFSP must include information about the date the plan will take effect and the anticipated length of time the plan will cover (almost always a year) (Waisman Center, 2006). This task usually falls to the service coordinator.

The IFSP also includes a place to document proposed methods of intervention, the location of the services, and any payment arrangements that may affect or be affected by the services provided (Waisman Center, 2006). The methods of intervention would be written just as the methods of intervention are written in clinical settings (see Chapter 16). Methods of intervention are the things you plan to implement when you are working with the child; they are your best guess as to what will work to move the child toward achievement of the established goals and objectives.

▼ ENVIRONMENTAL STATEMENT ▼

Location of service is exactly what it sounds like. You identify where each service will be provided. Often for young children, services are provided in the most natural environment for an infant or toddler, the child's home. Services may also be provided in a clinic, a preschool, on the playground, in an early childhood classroom, or in a day care facility. IDEA does require that services to these young children be provided in natural environments or justification be provided explaining why the natural environment is not the best place to provide a service (USDE, 2007). A natural environment is a setting that would be considered natural or normal for a child that age without disabilities (Waisman Center, 2006).

TABLE 21.1   Websites with Sample Completed IFSP Forms

Website	Host
http://dese.mo.gov/se/fs/pdfs/IFSPGuidance Exemplars.pdf	Department of Elementary and Secondary Education (Missouri)
http://www.waisman.wisc.edu/birthto3/forms/ documents/EmmasIFSP.pdf	Waisman Center (Wisconsin)
http://nmhealth.org/ddsd/nmfit/Providers/ documents/IFSP_TA_Doc_Nov2011.pdf	New Mexico Department of Health (sample starts on page 47)
http://www2.ku.edu/~kskits/training/webinars/ IFSPalooza/IFSP_GuidanceDocument.pdf	University of Kansas; includes section by section samples of the IFSP
http://www.eipd.vcu.edu/pdf/sample_ifsp_ dashawn.pdf	Virginia Early Intervention Professional Development Center
http://ectacenter.org/topics/families/ stateifsp.asp	National Early Childhood Technical Assistance Center

▼ TRANSITION PLAN ▼

Finally, there must be documentation in the IFSP of steps that will be taken to help the child make the transition from home-based or center-based early intervention services to preschool or other appropriate services, (Waisman Center, 2006). Transition planning can also address other transitions in the child's life, such as moving from hospital to home, biological family to foster care, or vice versa, or a move to a new community (IFSPWeb, n.d.). Planning for any transition should begin as soon as a child is identified for transition; there is no need to wait for an IFSP team meeting. The 2004 revision of IDEA allows for changes to the IFSP to be made without a full team meeting, as long as the frequency and intensity of the new or revised services are unchanged from the original IFSP. The transition plan is intended to help families feel more comfortable throughout the change process, minimize disruptions to the family, and ensure continuity of services (IFSPWeb, n.d.). You can view examples of completed IFSP forms by visiting the Web sites in Table 21.1.

▼ OTHER DOCUMENTATION ▼

Since the natural environment for most infants and toddlers is the home, most IFSP services are provided in the home. Rarely will these services be provided on a daily basis; once or twice a week is usually adequate. However, in providing services only a couple times a week, the occupational therapist may want to see some kind of follow-through on the infant's program by the family or personal care attendant. This is where a visit note (contact note) comes in.

The occupational therapist can use a visit note to communicate with the child's family. The occupational therapist can document what happened during the intervention session, how the child reacted, and what the family can do to supplement or enhance the occupational therapy program. The note can be written in either narrative or SOAP format.

While the law does not require this documentation, it is recommended because it does create a paper trail should there ever be questions about how a family was instructed. If an occupational therapist does write visit notes, it is a good idea to do it on "magic-carbon" (NCR) paper so that both the family and the occupational therapist can retain a copy. Electronic documentation may be an alternative to paper copies.

Preprinted exercise/activity sheets can also be given to families to help them follow through on occupational therapy programs. These may be in addition to or in place of visit notes. Several vendors sell reprintable handouts. Be careful not to copy and distribute pages of books or journal articles that are copyright protected (see Chapter 10).

SUMMARY

The IFSP is written annually to show the child's current level of performance, set goals to move the child's development forward, and determine the frequency and intensity of services. Since an infant or toddler is totally dependent on his or her family, the family plays a big role in the development and implementation of the IFSP. The IFSP must be written in words the family will understand. The goals (outcomes) established in the IFSP can be for the child or the family to achieve. The IFSP contains specific information on what services will be provided, who will provide them, who will pay for them, where they will be provided, and the frequency and duration of those services.

An occupational therapist can be the service coordinator for birth-to-age-2 services. A service coordinator is the person responsible for the development, coordination, and implementation of the plan. Writing the IFSP is a team effort, with the family included as part of the team. While much of the IFSP is similar to an intervention plan in a clinical setting, it differs in that it is written for the family rather than being written for other professionals or third-party payers as the primary audience. While an intervention plan usually represents the services of one provider, an IFSP represents the integrated plan of everyone working with that child.

REFERENCES

American Occupational Therapy Association. (2011). *Occupational therapy services in early childhood and school-based settings.* Retrieved from http://www.aota.org/-/media/Corporate/Files/Secure/Practice/OfficialDocs/Statements/OT-Services-Early-Childhood-and-Schools.PDF

Clark, G. F., Lucas, A., Jackson, L., & Nanof, T. (2008, April). *School system annual program: IDEA part C: Early intervention & occupational therapy.* Paper presented at the meeting of the American Occupational Therapy Association Annual Conference, Long Beach, CA.

IFSPWeb. (n.d.). *Developing a great IFSP.* Retrieved December 1, 2012, from http://www.ifspweb.org/developing.html

Jackson, L. L. (2007). *Legislative context of occupational therapy practice in schools and early childhood settings.* In L. L. Jackson (Ed.), *Occupational therapy services for children and youth under IDEA* (3rd ed., pp. 1–22). Bethesda, MD: American Occupational Therapy Association.

National Dissemination Center for Children with Disabilities. (2012). *Writing the IFSP for your child.* Retrieved from http://nichcy.org/babies/ifsp

Shelden, M. L., & Rush, D. D. (2009). Tips and techniques for developing participation-based IFSP outcome statements. *BriefCASE, 2*(1), 1–6. Retrieved from http://www.fippcase.org/briefcase/briefcase_vol2_no1.pdf

Southwest/West Central Service Cooperatives. (2006, January). *Related services: Decision-making and service provision.* Paper presented at the DAPE and Related Services Network Meeting, Marshall, MN.

Stephens, L. C., & Tauber, S. K. (2005). Early intervention. In J. Case-Smith, (Ed.), *Occupational therapy for children* (5th ed., pp. 771–793). St. Louis, MO: Mosby.

United States Department of Education. (2006). *Building the legacy: IDEA 2004.* Retrieved October 1, 2008, from http://idea.ed.gov/explore/home

United States Department of Education. (2007). *Federal register May 9, 2007(34 CFR Part 303).* Retrieved October 10, 2008, from http://edocket.access.gpo.gov/2007/pdf/07-2140.pdf

Waisman Center. (2006). *Guidelines completing Wisconsin's Individualized Family Service Plan.* Retrieved October 10, 2008, from http://www.waisman.wisc.edu/birthto3/Guidelines.pdf

Waisman Center. (2008). *Welcome to unit 3: The IFSP document.* Retrieved October 10, 2008, from http://www.waisman.wisc.edu/birthto3/WPDP/Unit_Three.html

Visit **www.pearsonhighered.com/healthprofessionsresources** to access the student resources that accompany this book. Simply select Occupational Therapy from the choice of disciplines. Find this book and you will find the complimentary study tools created for this specific title.

CHAPTER 22

Individualized Education Program

INTRODUCTION

The Individualized Education Program (IEP) is the guiding document for special education and related services for children with special needs. It is written for children with special needs ages 3–21 and administered by the school district. The Individuals with Disabilities Education Act (IDEA) (20 U.S.C. 1400 et seq.) allows children between the ages of 3 and 5 to have an Individualized Family Service Plan (IFSP) written instead of an IEP as long as the IFSP contains the same information as would be contained in an IEP (United States Department of Education, 2006; 34 C.F.R. §303.342[c]). Because the IEP is individualized, it takes a great deal of planning and interdisciplinary coordination to produce and implement the document. Specific information on the content of the IEP is found in Part B of IDEA (Polichino, Clark, Swinth, & Muhlenhaupt, 2007). AOTA offers a range of documents that support occupational therapy practice in school-based settings including *Occupational Therapy Services in Early Childhood and School Settings* that would be a helpful document to read along with this chapter (AOTA, 2011).

The IEP has some similarities to the IFSP. Both are written by a team of professionals and include input from the parents of the child involved; both are written annually and both start with an evaluation of the child. Both require parent notification, consent (see Chapter 20), and involvement throughout the process. There are also some differences. While the IFSP is family-centered, the IEP is student-centered. The IFSP looks at the overall development of the child; the IEP looks at levels of educational development, the ways in which a student's disability affects his or her ability to participate in learning (20 U.S.C. 1400.614[b][2][A]; 20 U.S.C. 1400.614[d][1][A][i][I]; 34 C.F.R. §300.347[a][1]).

Occupational therapy is considered a related service under Part B of IDEA (AOTA, 2011; Jackson, 2007; Rebhorn & Küpper, 2007; 20 U.S.C. 1400.602[22]). This means that usually the occupational therapist would not be the service coordinator, but rather would be a contributor to the IEP process. In this instance, the child must first qualify for special education before receiving occupational therapy. An IEP is not a guarantee that the maximum amount of service will be provided; it identifies the necessary services to allow the student to participate in learning. In other words, it provides need-to-have services, not want-to-have services.

Every IEP must include certain information. While IDEA does not mandate the use of one particular form or format, it does mandate the content required in each IEP. Box 22.1 shows the minimum content required by IDEA (34 C.F.R. §300.347). The order in which the information appears in the IEP document is irrelevant. Essentially, the minimum content can be summarized as follows:

- Present level of academic achievement and functional performance
- Annual goals
- Special education and related services
- Participation with nondisabled children
- Participation in state- and district-wide tests
- Starting date and location of services
- Transition services
- Measurement of progress

BOX 22.1   Required Content of the IEP

§300.320 DEFINITION OF INDIVIDUALIZED EDUCATION PROGRAM

(a) *General.* As used in this part, the term individualized education program or IEP means a written statement for each child with a disability that is developed, reviewed, and revised in a meeting in accordance with §§300.320 through 300.324, and that must include—

(1) A statement of the child's present levels of academic achievement and functional performance, including—

(i) How the child's disability affects the child's involvement and progress in the general education curriculum (i.e., the same curriculum as for nondisabled children); or

(ii) For preschool children, as appropriate, how the disability affects the child's participation in appropriate activities;

(2) (i) A statement of measurable annual goals, including academic and functional goals designed to—

(A) Meet the child's needs that result from the child's disability to enable the child to be involved in and make progress in the general education curriculum; and

(B) Meet each of the child's other educational needs that result from the child's disability;

(ii) For children with disabilities who take alternate assessments aligned to alternate achievement standards, a description of benchmarks or short-term objectives;

(3) A description of—

(i) How the child's progress toward meeting the annual goals described in paragraph (2) of this section will be measured; and

(ii) When periodic reports on the progress the child is making toward meeting the annual goals (such as through the use of quarterly or other periodic reports, concurrent with the issuance of report cards) will be provided;

(4) A statement of the special education and related services and supplementary aids and services, based on peer-reviewed research to the extent practicable, to be provided to the child, or on behalf of the child, and a statement of the program modifications or supports for school personnel that will be provided to enable the child—

(i) To advance appropriately toward attaining the annual goals;

(ii) To be involved in and make progress in the general education curriculum in accordance with paragraph (a)(1) of this section, and to participate in extracurricular and other nonacademic activities; and

(iii) To be educated and participate with other children with disabilities and nondisabled children in the activities described in this section;

(5) An explanation of the extent, if any, to which the child will not participate with nondisabled children in the regular class and in the activities described in paragraph (a)(4) of this section;

(6) (i) A statement of any individual appropriate accommodations that are necessary to measure the academic achievement and functional performance of the child on State and districtwide assessments consistent with §612(a)(16) of the Act; and

(ii) If the IEP Team determines that the child must take an alternate assessment instead of a particular regular State or districtwide assessment of student achievement, a statement of why—

(A) The child cannot participate in the regular assessment; and

(B) The particular alternate assessment selected is appropriate for the child; and

(7) The projected date for the beginning of the services and modifications described in paragraph (a)(4) of this section, and the anticipated frequency, location, and duration of those services and modifications.

(b) *Transition Services.* Beginning not later than the first IEP to be in effect when the child turns 16, or younger if determined appropriate by the IEP Team, and updated annually, thereafter, the IEP must include—

(1) Appropriate measurable postsecondary goals based upon age appropriate transition assessments related to training, education, employment, and, where appropriate, independent living skills; and

(2) The transition services (including courses of study) needed to assist the child in reaching those goals.

(Continued)

BOX 22.1 (Continued)

(c) *Transfer of Rights at Age of Majority*. Beginning not later than one year before the child reaches the age of majority under State law, the IEP must include a statement that the child has been informed of the child's rights under Part B of the Act, if any, that will transfer to the child on reaching the age of majority under §300.520.

(d) *Construction*. Nothing in this section shall be construed to require—

(1) That additional information be included in a child's IEP beyond what is explicitly required in section 614 of the Act; or

(2) The IEP Team to include information under one component of a child's IEP that is already contained under another component of the child's IEP.

While IDEA does not require the use of a particular format, the USDE does offer a model form for states or school districts to use (see Appendix C [see website] and http://idea.ed.gov/static/modelForms). Many states have developed their own model forms as well.

Exercise 22.1

Get on the Internet and look up the rules governing how services are delivered to children with disabilities in your state. The rules may be posted by your state's Department of Education, Department of Children and Families, Department of Public Instruction, or State Board of Education. Read the section on IEP services. If you live in a state that mandates or recommends use of a particular form for writing the IEP, download it to look at as you work your way through the rest of this chapter.

▼ EVALUATION PROCESS ▼

The IEP process begins with an evaluation. For a student receiving services under an IEP, a reevaluation is done at least every 3 years (Küpper & Rebhorn, 2007; USDE, 2006; 20 U.S.C. 1400.614[a][2][A]). The initial evaluation is done to determine the child's disability and educational needs (Küpper & Rebhorn, 2007; USDE, 2006 20 U.S.C. 1400.614[a][1][B][i–ii]). Subsequent evaluations identify the child's current level of performance and determine whether the child continues to have a disability, whether the child continues to need special education services, and whether changes or additions to the special education and related services the child receives are needed to enable participation in the general curriculum (Küpper & Rebhorn, 2007; USDE, 2006; 20 U.S.C. 1400.614[c][1][B][i–iv]). The evaluation must be completed within 60 days of the parents' giving their consent for the evaluation (USDE). At minimum, the evaluation must contain information about the child's

- health,
- vision and hearing,
- social and emotional status,
- general intelligence,
- academic performance,
- communicative status, and
- motor abilities (Küpper & Rebhorn, 2007)

IDEA contains legal requirements for conducting an evaluation of a child (20 U.S.C. 1400.614[b][2][A–C]):

A. Use a variety of assessment tools and strategies to gather relevant functional, developmental, and academic information, including information provided by the parent, that may assist in determining—
   i. whether the child is a child with a disability; and
   ii. the content of the child's individualized education program, including information related to enabling the child to be involved in and progress in the general education curriculum, or, for preschool children, to participate in appropriate activities;

B. Not use any single measure or assessment as the sole criterion for determining whether a child is a child with a disability or determining an appropriate educational program for the child; and

C. Use technically sound instruments that may assess the relative contribution of cognitive and behavioral factors, in addition to physical or developmental factors.

In addition, IDEA requires tests and evaluation materials to be nondiscriminatory, or not contain racial or cultural bias, and be administered in the child's native language whenever feasible (Polichino et al., 2007; 20 U.S.C. 1400.614[b][3][A]). Standardized tests have to be valid for the purposes they are being used for, be administered by someone who is knowledgeable and trained in the use of the test, and be administered according to the instructions provided by the test producer (Polichino et al., 2007; 20 U.S.C. 1400.614[b][2][B]). Besides standardized tests, other evaluation methods include information provided by the parents, observation, work samples, interviews, and a review of the student's cumulative educational record (Küpper, Rebhorn, 2007).

If the results of the evaluation show that the child qualifies for special education services, the school then has 30 calendar days in which to meet with the parents to discuss evaluation findings and write the IEP (USDE, 2006; 34 C.F.R. §300.343[b][2]). Often, the sharing of results of the evaluation and writing the IEP occur at the same meeting. If the evaluation results show that the child does not qualify for special education services, but the parents feel the child should have qualified, the parents have the right to ask for an independent education evaluation or appeal the decision using due process as established in IDEA (USDE, 2006).

▼ PRESENT LEVEL OF EDUCATIONAL PERFORMANCE ▼

The results of the evaluation may be incorporated into the IEP, in the section on present level of academic achievement and functional performance. IDEA is quite specific about the kind of information that must be included in the IEP. In the present level of academic achievement and functional performance section, federal law requires the IEP to consider three components (Rebhorn & Küpper, 2007; USDE, 2006; 614 [d][1][A][i][I][aa–cc]):

I. A statement of the child's present levels of academic achievement and functional performance, including—
   (aa) how the child's disability affects the child's involvement and progress in the general education curriculum;
   (bb) for preschool children, as appropriate, how the disability affects the child's participation in appropriate activities; and
   (cc) for children with disabilities who take alternate assessments aligned to alternate achievement standards, a description of benchmarks or short-term objectives.

Present levels of academic achievement and functional performance reflect what the student is able to do now, regardless of what that child was able to do or not do in the past. In this sense, it is very different from a summary of the client's progress or pertinent history in a clinical setting.

Current evaluation results are shared with the IEP team (including parents/guardians). The specific areas that an occupational therapist looks at include activities of daily living (e.g., toileting, eating lunch, putting a coat on and taking it off), instrumental activities of daily living (e.g., safety, using computers and communication devices), education (e.g., ability to access and use learning materials), work (e.g., vocational exploration, work habits), play (e.g., ability to access and use the playground, participation in games), leisure (e.g., ability to participate in extracurricular activities), and social participation (ability to interact with peers, express a need) (Jackson, 2007). The evaluation results need to show any identified deficits that interfere with the education process. If no connection to the educational needs of the child can be drawn, then occupational therapy services may not be necessary in the school setting. This does not mean that occupational therapy services would not in some way benefit the child; it simply means that those services would not be part of the IEP services provided by the school. An example would be that a child has deficits in tying his or her shoe. Tying one's shoes is not essential for participating in school. The child could wear slip-ons or shoes with Velcro® closures. Occupational therapy to work on shoe tying would not be educationally relevant, so it would not be part of the IEP. However, the child could receive occupational therapy services to work on shoe tying from another provider (other than the school district). If the occupational therapist can make a connection between the child's inability to motor plan the act of tying his or her shoes to the inability to motor plan in other situations that are necessary for learning (such as handwriting), then occupational therapy services might be justifiable. It is the responsibility of the occupational therapist to show how the deficits identified in the evaluation process have the potential to interfere with the learning process and that occupational therapy services are necessary to help the child overcome those deficits.

Anyone who has spent any time in a school or preschool classroom will tell you that a student's behavior can interfere not only with that child's learning but the learning of other students in the room as well. In the present level of performance section, a clear and specific description of observed behaviors and how they may interfere with learning must be documented (Polichino et al., 2007). For example, you observe that a child is repeatedly getting up and down off his chair, moving around his chair, and jumping up and down whenever he is asked to stand in line. This is distracting to the other children in the room, and the teacher questions whether the boy is paying attention when he moves around like that. The present level of educational performance would reflect exactly what the behavior looks like. Refer to *Occupational Therapy Services in Early Childhood and School-Based Settings* (AOTA, 2011) for more information on the types of services occupational therapy provides in school settings.

As discussed in Chapter 21, the present level of performance can include both a description of the performance and the occupational therapist's interpretation of that performance. The Massachusetts Department of Education (2001) uses the following examples to show proper wording of a present level of educational performance:

Less than helpful: Joe is not committed to his school program.
More helpful: Joe submits fewer than half of his required homework assignments. He starts most assignments but lacks the organizational skills to complete them by the required due dates (p. 18).

Less than helpful: Jill has a short attention span.
More helpful: Jill typically interrupts the work of others five times per hour. She interrupts when she requires teacher assistance (p. 18).

▼ GOAL WRITING ▼

On the IEP, the team writes annual goals for the child. For children with disabilities who will require alternate assessments (of statewide testing in accordance with the No Child Left Behind Act), short-term objectives or benchmarks are required in addition to the annual goals (Jackson, 2007). These short-term objectives or benchmarks help the IEP team, including the parents, to measure the child's progress throughout the year. Benchmarks describe expected progress at a given point in the year. Unlike the IFSP (Chapter 21), the goals and objectives/benchmarks are written to describe only what the student will do; they cannot be written to address family needs (Jackson, 2007). The annual goals must relate to the child's needs that result from the child's disability (USDE, 2006). They must enable the child to participate in and make progress in the general education curriculum (USDE, 2006; 614 [d] [1] [A] [i][I]).

Goals are not written for each discipline involved in the child's education; rather, they are written to address student's needs and may reflect a multidisciplinary approach to the problem addressed by the goal (Jackson, 2007).

How the goals are worded will vary by state and, to some degree, the school district you work for. You may be the member of the team to draft the wording of the goals, or your services may be provided under a goal written by other members of the team. Either way, the occupational therapist has input into the goal-writing process (Jackson, 2007).

The main components of an IEP annual goal, like the IFSP annual goal, are the behavior or skill to be performed, the direction of the change, and the level of performance expected at the end of the year. The present level of performance may be explicit or implied. For example, if the performance level is explicit, an annual goal might read: Jalena will decrease self-stimulating behavior from ten episodes per day to two episodes per day. If the performance level is implied, the goal could be: Jalena will decrease self-stimulating behavior to two episodes per day. The advantage of making it explicit is that if the goal page gets separated from the rest of the IEP document, you will know where you started from and be better able to identify progress. The advantage of making it implicit is that it takes fewer words to write it.

Once the annual goals have been established, if the child will have alternative testing, the objectives or benchmarks can be developed. While there is no federal legal requirement regarding the number of objectives/benchmarks per goal, two to four for each annual goal seems to be a good range. One objective seems insufficient to allow stepwise progression toward an annual goal, but more than four seems like too many steps to accomplish in 1 year.

Here is an example:

Goal: Anna will consistently maintain her balance while walking on uneven surfaces from walking in a high-guard position and losing her balance five times in 50 feet, to walking in medium-guard without losing her balance at all in 50 feet.

Objective 1: Anna will consistently walk from the playground, up over a curb, to the grassy area around the playground while holding on to an assistant with one hand as observed by teacher or occupational therapist.

Objective 2: Anna will walk from the playground, up over a curb, to the grassy area around the playground without assistance but with arms in high-guard position as observed by the teacher or occupational therapist.

Objective 3: Anna will consistently walk up and down the hill next to the school with arms in high-guard but without assistance as observed by the teacher or occupational therapist.

You may have noticed that the objectives in the above examples contained the phrase "as observed by the teacher or occupational therapist." Not every state or school district requires that the objectives include procedures for evaluation, but some do. Some states use a checkoff system for identifying how the goal will be measured (Virginia Department of Education [VDOE], 2008). Possible ways that progress could be measured include:

- Classroom participation
- Checklist
- Classwork
- Homework
- Observation
- Special Projects
- Test and Quizzes
- Written Reports
- Criterion-referenced test: _____
- Norm-referenced test: _____
- Other: _____ (VDOE, 2008, p. 8)

In general, objectives need to include the conditions under which the behavior or activity occurs, what behavior is to be performed, and the criteria (measurement) for the performance (Case-Smith & Rogers, 2005). The conditions can include the environment(s),

---

Exercise 22.3

For each goal, list two objectives that would help a student with disabilities meet the goal.

Goal 1: Keyshawn will improve his penmanship so that he can write his name legibly on unlined paper, as observed by his regular classroom teacher.

Objective 1a:

Objective 1b:

Goal 2: Miriam will improve her attention to task from going off task eight times during a 15-minute task to going off task once during a half-hour of task participation, as observed by her special education teacher.

Objective 2a:

Objective 2b:

Goal 3: Paul will improve scissors use from hand-over-hand assistance to independently cutting along a curved line, as observed by the occupational therapist.

Objective 3a:

Objective 3b:

INDIVIDUALIZED EDUCATION PROGRAM FOR: <u>Tran Vang</u>
IEP Dates: from <u>Sept. 29, 2014</u> to <u>Sept. 29, 2015</u> DOB: <u>July 17, 2007</u>

CURRENT LEVEL OF PERFORMANCE/MEASURABLE ANNUAL GOALS/BENCHMARKS
Goal # 3

Educational need area: _____ Academic/cognitive _____ Behavior _____ Communication
X Motor _____ Self-help _____ Social _____ Vocational

CURRENT LEVEL OF PERFORMANCE:
Tran uses a rolling walker to move around inside the school building, and a wheelchair for longer distances out of doors. He has very high muscle tone in all four limbs. When he gets excited, he throws his head back, arches his back, and straightens his arms and legs. He uses a whole hand grasp with large-diameter writing utensils. His writing is illegible; the letters are misshapen; letters do not rest on the bottom line; letter size varies.

MEASURABLE ANNUAL GOAL:
Tran will write his name (first and last) legibly on a line 80% of the time, as observed by his classroom teacher.

BENCHMARK/OBJECTIVES:
1. Tran will write his first name legibly on a line 50% of the time, as observed by the occupational therapist.
2. Tran will write his first name legibly on a line 80% of the time, as observed by the occupational therapist.
3. Tran will write his last name legibly on a line 50% of the time, as observed by the occupational therapist.

METHODS OF INTERVENTION:
Tran will practice writing his name on a large scale, such as on the white board, in sand in a sandbox, and other types of materials.
Tran will be instructed in techniques for forming letters.
Tran's sitting posture will be modified to decrease muscle tone in his trunk and arms.
Tran will try different types of writing utensils and papers (with and without raised lines) to see which feels best to him and which yields the best results.

LOCATION OF INTERVENTION:
In his regular education classroom and in the occupational therapy room.

ASSISTIVE TECHNOLOGY NEEDS:
Various writing utensils
Assorted writing papers
Keyboard with key guard for beginning computer use

FIGURE 22.1 Sample IEP Goal Page.

specialized instruction or cuing, specialized materials or equipment, and any assistance needed. The behavior to be performed needs to be observable; it can be qualitative or quantitative. The criteria have to show how the student will demonstrate successful completion of the goal, which means there has to be a measurement, and, in some states, who will evaluate the student's performance and document it (Case-Smith & Rogers, 2005). Figure 22.1 shows a sample goal page from an IEP.

▼ SPECIAL EDUCATION AND RELATED SERVICES IN THE IEP ▼

The IEP must specifically state the type and amount of special education, related services, and supplementary aids and services a child will receive, "based on peer-reviewed evidence to the extent practicable" (USDE, 2006; [34 CFR 300.320(a)]; [20 U.S.C. 1414.614(d)(1)(A)(i)

(IV)]). If an IEP says that a special education or related service is needed, there should be evidence in the scholarly literature that shows that the service is effective for a child with disabilities.

School districts will vary in how they want the frequency stated; most will want the number of minutes per week. Often, the minutes per week or per session will be further specified as either direct or indirect or as individual, group, or consultative.

When appropriate for the unique needs of a child, the IEP includes a statement of whether or not the child will need an extended school year or other calendar modification (USDE, 2006; 34 C.F.R. §300.106). Because of special health needs or other reasons, some students may need shorter school days or a shorter school year. Most school districts will have guidelines that explain under what conditions (how to justify it) this service is offered. Federal regulations require that school districts do not limit this option to any particular category of disability or the type, amount, or duration of those services (USDE, 2006; 34 C.F.R. §300.106).

Sometimes the recording of the details of this section occurs on the same page as the goals; in other cases it may appear on a page that lists services and supports. Since each school district has forms or a format for what information goes where in the IEP, simply follow the form. Follow the school district's lead in terms of how specific or general to be in describing the intervention plans.

▼ PARTICIPATION WITH CHILDREN WITHOUT DISABILITIES ▼

IDEA requires that the IEP contain specific information on the extent to which a child with a disability will participate with children without disabilities in a regular classroom, the general curriculum, and extracurricular/nonacademic activities (Rebhorn & Küpper, 2007; USDE, 2006). The IEP must explain why, if participation in the above-mentioned activities is limited in any way, full participation is not possible. Under IDEA, the preference is that the student spend as much time as possible with peers without disabilities, which means that IEP team members must have good reasons for providing services outside of the regular classroom. The IEP team must determine whether the child could participate in a regular classroom or extracurricular activities with the use of supplementary services and aids. Removing a child from a regular classroom cannot be done only because of needed modifications in the curriculum. The child's transportation needs can be addressed in this section or on a separate page (Rebhorn & Küpper, 2007; USDE, 2006). While the occupational therapist is not usually the person on the team responsible for documenting this, her knowledge and experience in adaptation of tasks and environments make her a great contributor to this process.

▼ PARTICIPATION IN STATE- AND DISTRICT-WIDE TESTS ▼

If the unique needs of that child would make participation in state- or district-wide tests inappropriate, this needs to be documented in the IEP (Rebhorn & Küpper, 2007; USDE, 2006). If the child cannot participate in the state- or district-wide testing, the IEP states the way in which the child will be assessed. Additional rules for which children can be exempt from state- or district-wide tests can be found in the "No Child Left Behind" legislation, President George W. Bush's education reform law.

▼ DATES AND PLACES ▼

The date the IEP takes effect and the location of the services provided are identified in writing. The IEP needs to specify whether the child will receive special education and related services in the regular classroom, special education or other separate room, or a separate setting, such as a hospital, special school, or home (Rebhorn & Küpper, 2007; USDE, 2006). Decisions about the location of services require discussion of the "least restrictive environment" (LRE) (Jackson, 2007; Rebhorn & Küpper, 2007; USDE, 2006). The least restrictive environment refers to the place where a child with a disability has the greatest exposure to children without disabilities yet where the child with a disability can get his or her needs met. For many children, this means they spend some portion of their day in a regular classroom, some in a separate location. The occupational therapist must make a recommendation to the IEP team as to whether occupational therapy intervention will happen in a regular classroom, in a separate room, or both.

▼ TRANSITION ▼

Transition planning and services typically begin when a child is age 16 (Rebhorn & Küpper, 2007;USDE, 2006). These services are designed to help the child move from school to life after school, such as preparing for a job and independent living (Orentlicher, 2007; Rebhorn & Küpper, 2007; USDE, 2006). These services are based on the student's wants, needs, and preferred lifestyle. Again, the expertise of an occupational therapist can be of great help in planning for such a move. While the occupational therapist may not write this part of the IEP, he or she will have good ideas to contribute to the planning process.

▼ MEASURING PROGRESS ▼

If you set goals, it stands to reason that you would want to do some evaluation of the child's progress toward meeting those goals throughout the year. The IEP team must have a method of reviewing progress and communicating that progress to the child's parents and/or guardians (Rebhorn & Küpper, 2007; USDE, 2006). If the child is not making the progress that was expected, the IEP must be revised to address that lack of progress (USDE, 2006; 20 U.S.C. 1400.614[d][4][A]). Both the occupational therapist and occupational therapy assistant participate in this process. Table 22.1 has links to some Websites that have samples of completed IEPs.

TABLE 22.1 Websites with Sample IEPs

Website	Host
http://www.eed.state.ak.us/tls/sped/handbook/FORMS/appg_sec4.pdf	Alaska Department of Education and Early Development
http://dese.mo.gov/se/compliance/IEP/Index.html	Missouri Department of Elementary and Secondary Education
http://sped.sbcsc.k12.in.us/IEPForms.html	South Bend, Indiana school district
http://www.doe.mass.edu/sped/iep/forms/pdf/IEP1-8.pdf	Massachusetts Department of Education
http://www.tea.state.tx.us/index2.aspx?id=2147504486	Texas Education Agency
http://www.k12.wa.us/SpecialEd/Data/ModelStateForms.aspx	Washington Office of Superintendent of Public Instruction
http://www.ritap.org/iep/publications/publication.html	Rhode Island Technical Assistance Project (Rhode Island Department of Education), scroll down for samples

▼ MEDICAID COMPLIANCE ▼

Federal law (PL 100-360, the Medicare Catastrophic Coverage Act) allows school districts to bill Medicaid for certain health-related services, including occupational therapy, provided under an IEP (Prince Georges County Public Schools [PGCPS], 2012).The school district must have an agreement with the state agency that oversees Medicaid in that state (AOTA, 2014).In order to bill Medicaid for school-based occupational therapy services, several criteria must be met:

- The child is eligible for Medicaid,
- The services meet the state's definition of *medically necessary* services,
- The services are provided by a qualified provider under Medicaid,
- The services are documented on the child's IEP, and
- The services are billed according to state guidelines as described in the agreement between the state education agency and the state agency overseeing Medicaid in that state (AOTA, 2014).

Occupational therapy services that are documented in the IEP are educationally related, but they may also meet the criteria for medical necessity under Medicaid, and those are the services that may be billed to Medicaid (AOTA, 2014). Each state has a different definition of medical necessity, so it is important to check with the state Medicaid agency to find that definition.

If the school district is billing Medicaid for occupational therapy services, then there may be additional requirements, such as physician referral, that must be documented.This will depend on both occupational therapy licensure laws and state Medicaid laws. AOTA (2007) recommends that occupational therapy practitioners in school settings keep therapy records to document the specific services provided, including evaluation and re-evaluation reports, intervention plans, contact notes, progress reports, transition plans, and discharge reports. Some states or school districts may require additional documentation. For example, PGCPS (2012) requires that the occupational therapist also include copies of written permission to evaluate (see Chapter 20), and test protocols. The Wisconsin Department of Public Instruction (2011) requires occupational therapy practitioners also document attendance, data collected on the child's response to intervention, and notes documenting contact with the child's parents, physicians, and teachers. AOTA (2007) further recommends, regardless of school district policy, that occupational therapy practitioners maintain therapy records for five years.

SUMMARY

The Individual Education Program (IEP) is the guiding document for services provided by school system personnel, including occupational therapy. Careful wording of goals and objectives or benchmarks is essential. Goals and objectives/benchmarks often follow a specific formula for wording. Goals are the outcomes the child is expected to meet a year from when they are written. Objectives are steps to help the child meet the goals. Occupational therapy practitioners contribute to many parts of the IEP, but are usually not responsible for writing the entire document.

All of this demonstrates just how explicit school system documentation is. Nothing can be assumed. Be clear and direct because not everyone reading the IEP will have the same level of education and understanding of the material as you do.

Because of the amount of specificity in goal setting—specifying minutes per week for every service provider involved with the child in the school, identifying the least restrictive environment, and listing curricular, environmental, and programmatic modifications—the IEP can become a lengthy document. If the school district is billing Medicaid for occupational therapy services, additional documentation may be required.

REFERENCES

American Occupational Therapy Association. (2011). *Occupational therapy services in early childhood and school-based settings.* Retrieved from http://www.aota.org/-/media/Corporate/Files/Secure/Practice/OfficialDocs/Statements/OT-Services-Early-Childhood-and-Schools.PDF

American Occupational Therapy Association [AOTA]. (2014). *Medicaid school-based billing FAQs.* Retrieved from http://www.aota.org/Advocacy-Policy/Federal-Reg-Affairs/Pay/Schools/Medicaid.aspx

Case-Smith, J., & Rogers, J. (2005). School-based occupational therapy. In J. Case-Smith (Ed.), *Occupational therapy for children* (5th ed., pp. 795–824). St. Louis, MO: Mosby.

Jackson, L. L. (2007). Legislative context of occupational therapy practice in schools and early childhood settings. In L. L. Jackson (Ed.), *Occupational therapyservices for children and youth under IDEA* (3rd ed., pp. 1–22). Bethesda, MD: American Occupational Therapy Association.

Küpper, L., & Rebhorn, T. (2007).Initial evaluation and reevaluation (Module 10). *Building the legacy: IDEA 2004 training curriculum.* Washington, DC: National Dissemination Center for Children with Disabilities. Retrieved from http://www.parentcenterhub.org/wp-content/uploads/repo_items/legacy/10-trainerguide.pdf

Massachusetts Department of Education. (2001). *IEP process guide.* Retrieved March 28, 2003, from www.doe.mass.edu/sped/iep/proguide.pdf

Orentlicher, M. L. (2007). Legislative context of occupational therapy practice in schools and early childhood settings. In L. L. Jackson (Ed.), *Occupational therapy services for children and youth under IDEA* (3rd ed., pp. 187–212). Bethesda, MD: American Occupational Therapy Association.

Polichino, J. E., Clark, G. F., Swinth, Y., & Muhlenhaupt, M. (2007). Legislative context of occupational therapy practice in schools and early childhood settings. In L. L. Jackson (Ed.), *Occupational therapyservices for children and youth under IDEA* (3rd ed., pp. 23–58). Bethesda, MD: American Occupational Therapy Association.

Prince Georges County Public Schools [PGCPS]. (2012). *Health related services Medicaid billing handbook 2012-2013.* Retrieved from http://www1.pgcps.org/uploadedFiles/Offices/Business_Management_Services/Medicaid/HEALTH%20RELATED%20HANDBOOK%202011-2012.pdf

Rebhorn, T., & Küpper, L. (2007). Content of the IEP (Module13). *Building the legacy: IDEA 2004 training curriculum.* Washington, DC: National Dissemination Center for Children with Disabilities. Retrieved from http://www.parentcenterhub.org/wp-content/uploads/repo_items/legacy/13-trainerguide.pdf

United States Department of Education. (2006). *Building the legacy of IDEA 2004.* Retrieved October 10, 2008, from http://idea.ed.gov/explore/home

Virginia Department of Education. (2008). *Virginia department of education's sample IEP form.* Retrieved from www.doe.virginia.gov/.../**iep**.../**iep**/.../sample_transition_**iep_**form.doc

Wisconsin Department of Public Instruction [WDPI]. 2011. Occupational therapy and physical therapy: A resource and planning guide. Retrieved from http://sped.dpi.wi.gov/files/sped/pdf/ot-pt-guide-2nd-edition.pdf

Overview of Administration Documentation

INTRODUCTION

In addition to clinical or school-based documentation, there is documentation related to administrative tasks such as getting paid for services; documenting workplace injuries; and writing grants, policies and procedures, and job descriptions. Some of these documents may be written by anyone in the department; they are not necessarily the sole domain of supervisory personnel. They are referred to as administrative documentation because they are not part of a clinical or educational record, but are part of the documentation of the ongoing operations of a department or program.

Administrative documentation varies greatly from facility to facility and setting to setting. The chapters in the section deal with several different types of administrative documentation, but these are by no means the only administrative documentation that gets done. Specifically, documents like productivity reports and staffing reports are so individualized by each facility/setting it would be impossible to do justice to them here; therefore, they are not included in this book. As you read the chapters in this section, realize that the information is intentionally general. You can expect modifications in form and content by the facility/setting.

▼ STRUCTURE OF THIS SECTION OF THE BOOK ▼

Chapter 24 deals with incident reports. Incident reports are written whenever there is an injury, no matter how slight, to a client, visitor, or a staff member. Incident reports are used by the facility to help learn from accidents or errors in an effort to prevent them from happening again.

Chapter 25 discusses ways to word appeal letters. Appeal letters are used when an occupational therapist or client thinks that a third-party payer (like Medicare or an HMO) has denied reimbursement unjustly. These letters explain why occupational therapy services are needed for a particular client.

Chapter 26 presents various ways to take minutes at a meeting. It has been said that if it was not documented, it did not happen. One way to demonstrate that a supervisor provided instruction to staff or that a policy was reviewed is to document it in meeting minutes. The minutes need to be retained in such a fashion that they can be easily retrieved and that everyone in the department has access to them.

Chapter 27 deals with grant writing. Grants are funds made available to an organization for a specific purpose, such as developing a new program or to fund services for clients who do not have the financial resources to pay for services (like scholarships for occupational therapy intervention). Usually, grants are awarded to facilities, departments, or nonprofit organizations. Grant money does not need to be repaid, but there are usually conditions for the award of the money. There is always a process for applying for grant money. This chapter discusses a common process for requesting grant money, but there may be details that are unique to particular funding sources that are not covered here.

Chapter 28 presents a format for writing policies and procedures. Policy and procedure manuals are used to guide employees in their on-the-job performance. They explain what must be done and how it must be done. Following policies and procedures is essential for the orderly conduct of the workplace. When an occupational therapy practitioner fails to follow policies and procedures, he or she weakens his or her defense if a client should decide to sue.

Finally, Chapter 29 discusses job descriptions. Occupational therapy practitioners may not only write job descriptions for occupational therapy positions, but they might be called upon to assist with writing job descriptions for other disciplines or industries. Because of their expertise and skill in breaking down occupations into specific tasks and identifying environmental factors influencing job performance, occupational therapy practitioners are excellent at writing job descriptions.

Visit **www.pearsonhighered.com/healthprofessionsresources** to access the student resources that accompany this book. Simply select Occupational Therapy from the choice of disciplines. Find this book and you will find the complimentary study tools created for this specific title.

CHAPTER 24

Incident Reports

INTRODUCTION

Imagine this scene:

> An occupational therapist is working on toilet transfers with a teenager who recently had a hemispherectomy (to reduce seizures). The client is much taller than the clinician, and when he starts to lose his balance, the occupational therapist tries in vain to lower him gently to the floor. Instead, he falls and hits his head on the sink, causing a gash on his forehead before landing in a heap on the floor with the occupational therapist still holding on to his transfer belt. She immediately summons help.

After attending to the immediate medical needs of the client and the occupational therapist (if he or she is hurt during this event), it will be necessary to document this incident. The person who is most directly involved in the incident is the person who documents it. Generally, the facility will have a form, usually called an incident report, which will have to be completed in addition to documenting the incident in the medical (or school) record. In this case, the occupational therapist would document it. Usually, after the occupational therapy practitioner completes this form, a supervisor will review the form and may complete a section of the form designed for supervisor input. The form is then routed to the person designated by the facility as the risk manager (or someone with a similar title). It will be used to help the facility investigate possible corrective actions to prevent such incidents, sometimes called "adverse events" (Scott, 2013).

The incident report is confidential; it should not be entered into the client's health record (Scott, 2013). The incident is recorded in the record, but there should be no mention of an incident report. Just what should be documented in the clinical record will be discussed later in this chapter. No matter how big or small, all incidents involving clients should be reported including, but not limited to, burns from modalities involving heat or cooking, falls, sores that develop from an ill-fitting orthotic or prosthetic, or allergic reactions to lotions. In addition, any incident resulting in injury involving visitors, staff, vendors, or others who are on the property needs to be reported (Scott, 2013). If this event had happened in a school setting, the procedure is much the same; an incident report would also be required. An incident report is completed if any student, faculty, visitor, or staff member is injured on school property. If the incident took place on school property, the principal usually needs to be notified as soon as possible, in addition to the designated risk manager for the school district. In addition, schools may also require incident reports to be completed for incidents of fighting, bullying, cheating, or weapons violations.

Whenever a client, visitor, or employee is injured, there is the possibility of a lawsuit. The incident report is the primary source of documentation of what happened (Scott, 2013). It may be considered a quality improvement document or simply a record of the incident in case of litigation. Incident reports should be clearly labeled as a " 'confidential quality assurance/improvement report' or a 'document prepared at the direction of the facility attorney in anticipation of or in preparation for litigation.' " (Scott, 2013, p. 186). How the document is labeled will be decided by the facility or agency attorney, administrator, or risk manager. Labeling the document as confidential may not exempt it from discovery by the prosecuting attorney; however, quality assurance documents are more likely to be exempt than a document prepared for litigation (Scott, 2013).

An incident report is completed whenever a client, visitor, or staff member is injured, no matter how big or how small the incident. There may be slightly different forms for when the injured party is a client/visitor or a staff member, but both forms will want similar information. I have always been told that an incident report should be completed for any injury, even a paper cut. One risk manager told me that what looks like a simple paper cut could get infected, and could turn into a big problem, so always fill out the form.

In reality, many staff members fail to complete the report for such a small thing as a paper cut. In cold, dry climates, paper cuts can be a daily occurrence. If a staff member filled out an incident report for each cut, he or she would be doing it several times a week. It seems like a waste of paper and a waste of time. You cannot prevent paper cuts. However, you need to follow the policies and procedures of the facility. If the person in charge of risk management at your facility says it is not necessary to complete an incident report for a paper cut, then that is fine. If the risk manager says that incident reports are necessary regardless of the size of the injury, then you have to do it.

As with all documentation, timeliness is important. Write in the client record and on the incident report as soon as possible after the incident (Grant & Ballard, 2011). Do not wait until the end of the day to document it. Each incident has the potential to end up in court, and as stated earlier in this book, documentation that is written closest to the event is more likely to be viewed as the more accurate documentation.

▼ RECORDING INFORMATION ON AN INCIDENT REPORT FORM AND CLIENT RECORD ▼

Any lawyer I've ever talked to has told me that if I am ever questioned about an event that has occurred, simply answer the questions and do not volunteer *additional* information. It would be wise to view the incident report in the same way. Answer the questions directly, but do not volunteer additional information. The more information you provide, the more likely you are to add embellishments, exaggerations, and extraneous information that could be turned against you by a skilled attorney. As concisely as possible, simply provide the necessary facts on the incident report itself. If you are concerned that the incident could wind up in court, there is nothing that prohibits you from recording a more thorough description of what transpired, including your impressions (as opposed to facts), for your own records, as long as you protect the confidentiality of those involved in the incident.

That said, you still have to provide enough information to adequately describe what happened. You must be objective. Remember the "Descriptive, Interpretive, and Evaluative" discussion from Chapter 14? Keep it descriptive, avoiding interpretive or evaluative statements. Examples of interpretive or evaluative statements would include speculating on the cause, drawing conclusions, or taking or assigning blame (Guido, 2006; Scott, 2013). You can talk to the safety coordinator later about your impressions, but impressions do not belong on the form. Only record what you experienced, not what others tell you that they saw, unless you put the other statements in quote marks and identify the statement as hearsay (Guido, 2006; Scott, 2013). If the incident involves a client or student, and the client or student says something about his or her role in the incident, record it in quote marks and identify the speaker (*Evidence-Based Nursing Guide*, 2009). You will also be asked to specify the time, to the nearest minute, that the incident occurred.

Only record what you actually see, what you witnessed, do not assume anything. For example, if you walk into a room and see a client on the floor, simply describe what you saw, not what you think might have happened, no matter how obvious it seems. Describe the position the person was in when you discovered him or her and the time you found the person. Do not say that you walked into the room and it looked like the person had fallen. You do not know that the person fell; that will be determined when the incident is investigated. Keep it factual (*Evidence-Based Nursing Guide*, 2009; Grant & Ballard, 2011; Guido, 2006; Scott, 2013).

If the incident involves a client, then in the clinical record, documentation would reflect the nature of the injury and any aid provided to the client (Guido, 2006; Scott, 2013). There should be congruence between what is written in the clinical record and in the incident report (*Evidence-Based Nursing Guide*, 2009). Document what the client or client's family says about the incident. Do not offer suggestions for how to prevent this type of event from happening again (*Evidence-Based Nursing Guide*, 2009; Scott, 2013).

Let's look at another case:

> Korpo is an occupational therapy assistant who was born in Somalia and immigrated to this country 10 years ago. She has been assigned to work with a man who recently suffered a head injury, dislocated right shoulder, and two cracked ribs as a result of a motorcycle accident. He is in an agitated state, but needs to relearn grooming, hygiene, and dressing skills. He is a large man with many tattoos and body piercings.
>
> When Korpo enters the room, he immediately begins name-calling and refusing to cooperate. His exact words are "Get out of here, you bitch! I don't do nothin' for n-g---s!" As she brings him a warm, wet washcloth, he hurls it at her, and then shoves the over-bed table into her stomach, knocking her down hard. His face gets red, his eyes are open wide, his teeth are bared, and the veins in his neck are standing out. He picks up the phone on the bedside table and throws it at her, hitting her in the head. She crawls out of the room, a small cut on her forehead.

What would be documented in the medical record, and what would be recorded in the incident report? Here is one possibility.

In the health record, a narrative note might read:

> *2/4/14, 10:03 AM. Patient refused to participate in self-care training at bedside. He shoved the bedside table into her stomach, knocking her down. He swore and threw a washcloth and the telephone at the occupational therapy assistant. OTA will attempt to work with him again bedside tomorrow as per the plan of care. Korpo Bohla, OTA/L*

A SOAP note might look like this:

S: "Get out of here, you b---h! I don't do nothin' for n-----s!
O: Client refused occupational therapy self-care training at bedside. He knocked her down with the bedside table. He swore and threw a washcloth and the telephone at the occupational therapy assistant.
A: Client is agitated and uncooperative.
P: Continue to attempt bedside intervention.

Korpo Bohla, OTA/L 2/4/14.
In the narrative portion of the incident report, you would see:

> When I entered the room, he immediately began name-calling and refusing to cooperate. His exact words were "Get out of here, you b---h! I don't do nothin' for n-g---s!" When I brought him a warm, wet washcloth, he hurled it at me, and then shoved the over-bed table into my stomach, knocking me down hard. His face got red, his eyes were open wide, his teeth were bared, and the veins in his neck were standing out. He picked up the phone on the bedside table and threw it at me, which hit me in the head. I crawled out of the room. There was a small cut on my forehead. The cut was cleaned, antibiotic cream was applied, and the wound was closed with steri-strips.

There are some obvious differences between what gets written in the health record and what is written in the incident report. The contact note is very concise, only the bare minimum of information is written (Distasio, 2000; *Evidence-Based Nursing Guide*, 2009; Scott, 2013). While the contact notes do not convey the entire picture, you do get some sense of the anger expressed by the client. In a client recovering from a brain injury, this is a predictable phase that many clients go through. It is essential that the agitation and anger be documented. Notice that neither progress note mentions the incident report form.

If the incident results in a client needing medical intervention, that intervention must be documented in the client's health record; if that information is not recorded in the client's health record, then the incident report may be called into court (Guido, 2006). If you are working in a setting without a health record, such as at a school, then the incident report may be the only document you write on, depending on the facility's (school's) policy. Of course, in either case, you need to talk to your supervisor as soon as possible after the incident, and in a school, you need to notify the principal as well.

The question that remains is, if a trigger for the explosive behavior can be identified, should it be documented on the incident report? One side of the issue, using this case as an example, is if the trigger is identified, it can be avoided in the future, cutting down on the risk of injury to staff (Distasio, 2000). On the other hand, what if the trigger is identified, but it casts the client or the healthcare provider in a negative light? For example, what if the trigger in this case is that the client is prejudiced against people of color? To decrease agitation, one could make an argument that only white staff should work with the client. But that would be discriminatory, and might cause staff of all colors to have negative feelings toward the client. This is a really delicate issue. Most facilities have policies on discrimination. Whether or not to document the trigger would not be a decision that occupational therapy staff would make alone. Guido (2006) suggests that if there is a space to describe what could be done to prevent such an incident in the future, leave it blank. The rationale for this is that indicating how something could be prevented in the future may imply liability (Guido, 2006).

An incident report is also likely to include some checklists for the employee to mark. There may be a checklist that asks the writer to check off what precautions were taken,

Exercise 24.1

1. Using the case from the beginning of this chapter (post-hemispherectomy client during toilet transfer training), write a narrative progress note and a narrative entry for the incident report.

    Narrative progress note:

    Incident report:

2. Using the following case, write a SOAP note and a narrative entry for the incident report.

    You are working in a community-based program for persons with mental health disorders. The program focuses on development of job skills. The client you are working with on completing job applications begins to get frustrated with the number of errors she is making. On the second application, she begins to scribble across the whole page, saying "Dammit" repeatedly. You calm her down and have her try again. This time, about halfway through, she picks up the application and begins to tear it into pieces while yelling, "I quit. I can't do this. I'm never going to get a job." Before you can stop her, she gets a paper cut. Then she starts cursing, "F---ing S---, A--hole moron, S---" and then more of the same. She starts to hit the wall with her fist. You interrupt her tirade to tell her she has a cut, and when she sees it, she stops and stares at it. You take her to the sink, run it under cold water for a bit, gently dry it off, and then put an adhesive bandage on it. You have her sit calmly for a while before engaging her in another task.

    S:

    O:

    A:

    P:

    Incident report:

3. Write either a SOAP or narrative progress note and a narrative portion of an incident report about the following scene.

> You are an occupational therapist working in a preschool program. You are co-leading a group of 3-year-old. It is snack time. There will be sliced apples and peanut butter. While you are putting peanut butter on the plates, the special education teacher is sitting at the table with the children, showing them what the inside of an apple looks like. She is using a 10-inch cook's knife to cut the apple. Her hands are getting sticky from the apple's juice, so she gets up to get a napkin, setting the knife down on the table. You are at the other end of the table. Just as you are about to remind the teacher to take the knife with her, 3-year-old Tyla picks it up by the blade end, cutting the palm side of three fingers. The special education teacher never saw anything; her back was turned, so she tells you that you have to fill out the paperwork. You take the screaming child to the sink, but realize the child will need medical attention. You wrap up the hand in a clean towel while the special education teacher calls the child's mom and you keep pressure on the wound. Clearly the special education teacher was negligent and bears full responsibility for what happened.

Progress note:

Incident report:

where the incident occurred, what kind of medical attention was required, and what measures could be taken to prevent further incidents. Of course, with any checklist, there is usually a space for "other" with a blank to fill in, where the writer could add to the list something that had not been considered before.

SUMMARY

When the unexpected happens, it needs to be documented in two ways. First, a concise note explaining the event is written in the client's record. The narrative or SOAP/DAP note must contain only objective information that does not lay blame on anyone. Then there is the incident report. You need to provide all the relevant facts on an incident report, but do not volunteer any extra information. Do not lay blame or accept blame anywhere on an incident report. The information you provide may be used by the facility for quality or risk management purposes.

REFERENCES

Distasio, C. A. (2000). Workplace violence: Part II: Documentation and reporting—how to paint the picture. *Maryland-Nurse, 1*(2), 12.

Evidence-based nursing guide to legal and professional issues (2009). Philadelphia, PA: Lippincott Williams & Wilkins.

Grant, P. D., & Ballard, D. C. (2011). *Law for nurse leaders: A complete reference.* New York, NY: Springer Publishing.

Guido, G. W. (2006). *Legal and ethical issues in nursing* (4th ed.). Upper Saddle River, NJ: Pearson Prentice Hall.

Scott, R. (2013). *Legal, ethical and practical aspects of documenting patient care: A guide for rehabilitation professionals* (4th ed.). Sudbury, MA: Jones and Bartlett.

Visit **www.pearsonhighered.com/healthprofessionsresources** to access the student resources that accompany this book. Simply select Occupational Therapy from the choice of disciplines. Find this book and you will find the complimentary study tools created for this specific title.

CHAPTER 25

Appeal Letters

INTRODUCTION

It is not unusual for an occupational therapy practitioner and a third-party payer to disagree about a client's need for services. In some cases, the occupational therapy practitioner may not know until after the service is delivered that the payer does not think that occupational therapy services were medically necessary (or whatever that payer's standard is). Third-party payers may deny payment based on medical necessity, or on a technicality such as not properly completing a required form, not sending in the billing in a timely manner, errors in completing the billing forms, or because the insurer considers the service to be experimental or investigational (Government Accountability Office [GAO], 2011). According to the GAO, insurers reverse their decision upon appeal about half the time (GAO, 2011).

Most occupational therapy services must be paid for in order for the provider to stay in business and continue to serve other clients. If the claim is denied on the basis of a technicality, correcting the error may be all that is required. If the occupational therapy practitioner thinks that a client needs services and that those services reasonably fall within the scope of what the payer customarily pays for, he or she can appeal the decision not to pay for services. In addition to providing additional clinical documentation (if there is any that was not submitted with the initial claim), the occupational therapist writes an appeal letter that explains the rationale for occupational therapy for that particular client, describes the nature of the skilled service needed, and makes an explicit request to overturn the denial (Brennan & Robinson, 2006).

Medical necessity is a concept that has been embraced by government (e.g., Medicare and Medicaid) and nongovernmental agencies (e.g., private health insurance, managed care, or worker's compensation insurance) as the standard for determining whether or not to pay for a service. Every payer uses a slightly different definition of medical necessity, so it is important to find out what the definition is for the specific payer to whom you want to appeal a denial. Medicare defines medically necessary as follows: "Services are medically necessary if the documentation indicates they meet the requirements for medical necessity including that they are skilled, rehabilitative services, provided by clinicians (or qualified professionals when appropriate) with the approval of a physician/NPP, safe, and effective (i.e., progress indicates that the care is effective in rehabilitation of function)" (Centers for Medicare and Medicaid Services [CMS], 2008, p. 23).

▼ APPEAL LETTERS AS OPPORTUNITIES TO EDUCATE ▼

It is critically important that the appeal letter is clear, to the point, and states what you want done about the original denial. In some cases, the person reading the appeal letter may be the same person who wrote the denial in the first place, so you have to be very careful to appear professional and respectful of the initial decision. In other cases, there may be levels of review, and a nurse, an occupational therapist, or a physician may conduct the second or third review.

It is helpful to look at an appeal as a learning process for the reviewer. If the reviewer is not an occupational therapist, as is usually the case, this is an opportunity for you to teach him or her something about it. Not so many years ago, when I called an insurance company to check on coverage for an outpatient, I was told the insurer did not cover occupational therapy services for outpatients (only for inpatients) because "who needs underwater basket weaving anyway?" The person actually said that! After a few calming breaths and a couple more phone calls to the insurer and the client's employer (the insurance was through the client's work), the insurer did pay for occupational therapy, explaining that it had inadvertently left occupational therapy out of the policy. Since it was not listed specifically as an excluded service, they had to cover it.

You have a fighting chance of getting coverage for occupational therapy if the insurance policy is silent on occupational therapy coverage. The insurer can be convinced of the need for occupational therapy and save face by saying the omission of occupational therapy was simply an oversight. If the policy specifically says that occupational therapy services are excluded from coverage, then it is hard to get the insurer to pay for occupational therapy services no matter how strong your arguments are.

As part of the Affordable Care Act, all new and many existing insurance policies are required to have an internal appeals processes, provide enrollees with a description of both the internal and external claims review processes and how enrollees can receive assistance with those processes, allow the enrollee to present evidence and testimony in an appeals process, and allow continued coverage while a claim is being appealed (National Conference of State Legislators [NCSL], 2010). This took effect on October 23, 2010. Insurers are required to make their rulings on appeals within 45 days for regular appeals, and 72 hours for appeals in medically urgent situations (NCSL, 2010). If a denial of coverage occurs following an internal review (within the insurer's organization), the consumer is entitled to request an external review from an independent decision maker (Center for Consumer Information & Insurance Oversight [CCIIO], 2012). These rights belong to the consumer not the provider, but there is no reason why a provider, such as an occupational therapy practitioner, could not assist the consumer if writing the appeal letter.

BOX 25.1 Simple case

You are working with an elderly man in an outpatient clinic. He has coverage through Medicare. The Medicare contractor determines that occupational therapy services are no longer medically necessary and should have been discontinued. You had continued to work with the man until you heard that the last 2 weeks of occupational therapy were not paid for. He is recovering from a hip replacement on his left side (6 weeks ago), complicated by a below-knee amputation of his right leg (5 years ago), diabetic neuropathy (decreased sensation in all remaining limbs), and cataracts in both eyes. Occupational therapy services have been provided twice a week for 6 weeks to improve self-care skills. Physical therapy has also been involved with this client, working on ambulation and transfers. Physical therapy has discharged the client, saying that he has plateaued; he was not making any more progress. You want to continue to see the client to work on more kitchen skills, lower-extremity dressing, and problem solving related to day-to-day challenges he faces. He lives with his wife of 60 years who has been his caretaker but has been showing signs of dementia and has multiple health issues of her own. Their children live 3 hours away and do not visit often. You have seen the client make good progress in all areas. Since it is inappropriate for you to write about another person in your client's documentation, you have not documented his wife's deteriorating health and cognitive state. Your client is cognitively intact. However, you know that the client needs to learn to cook because he has expressed concern about his wife leaving the gas stove on when cooking is done, burning food, and misplacing food items. You decide to appeal this decision.

▼ WRITING AN APPEAL LETTER ▼

In the above case, you are privy to information that the payer does not know. The payer has read all your intervention plans, but is unaware of other contextual factors affecting this case. You have done a good job documenting the client's progress in the stated need areas. The payer has assumed that since the client reached a plateau in physical therapy, a plateau

Part B Reviewer
Best Deal Health Plan
1234 Frugal Street
New Money, NJ 07666-7666

April 15, 2014

Dear Reviewer,

I am the occupational therapist working with Mr. J. Doe, case #246810. I am writing to request that the decision to deny further occupational therapy services be reversed on the basis of the following additional information.

Mr. Doe has been making steady gains in lower-extremity dressing, meal preparation and cleanup, and problem solving. He has progressed from being totally dependent in lower-extremity dressing to needing minimal assist and adaptive equipment. Meal preparation has progressed from needing step-by-step instruction to Mr. Doe initiating meal planning and preparation. He still has difficulty transporting food from the stove to the table or counter and opening some packaging. He provides instruction to his wife in cleaning up after meals. Mr. Doe has expressed concern for allowing his wife to use the stove. She is showing significant episodes of memory loss and confusion about daily chores leading to some dangerous situations in the kitchen. Mr. Doe wants to take over some of her kitchen responsibilities. Teaching Mr. Doe to plan and prepare meals is essential in order for the Does to live in their own home safely.

In addition to the plans of care you have already reviewed, I am enclosing copies of the contact notes for each of the occupational therapy sessions from the last 6 weeks. If I can provide you with any additional information, please let me know.

Sincerely,

Carin Provider, OTR/L
Carin Provider, OTR/L

FIGURE 25.1 Sample Appeals Letter.

in occupational therapy cannot be far behind, and in most cases, 6 weeks of occupational therapy is usually sufficient. In your letter you will outline progress made so far, what additional progress you expect in the next 4 weeks, and justify it by explaining the social environmental factors that affect this case. Your letter will be formal and professional. Figure 25.1 shows an example of what it might look like.

▼ MEDICARE APPEALS ▼

Medicare made significant changes to its appeal processes in 2005 (Brennan & Robinson, 2006). The biggest change is that the process is the same for both Part A and Part B Medicare. Timelines for responding to appeals have been shortened (Brennan & Robinson, 2006). This means that occupational therapy practitioners need to be timely in their responses to denials if they want to get paid for their services. All appeals must be done in writing (CMS, 2011, 2013). Minor errors or omissions that cause an initial denial are handled through a reopening process rather than the appeals process (CMS, 2013).

Medicare sends an initial determination of coverage called a Medicare Summary Notice (MSN) to the beneficiary (CMS, 2013). It is important to have a mechanism for the beneficiary to share this information with you, the provider, since you will not receive this

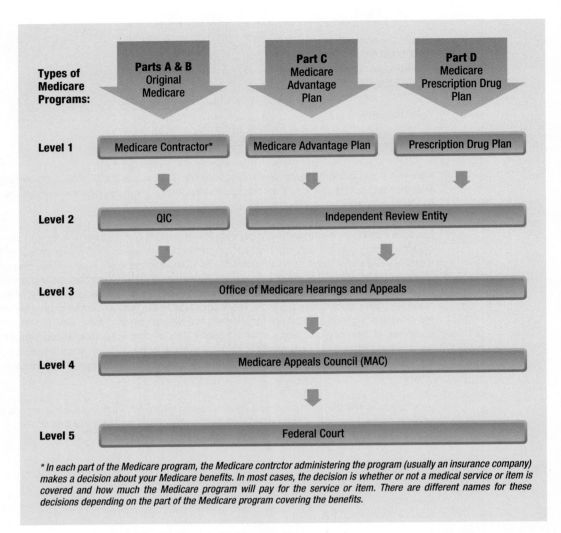

FIGURE 25.2 Levels of Medicare Appeals.

Source: Centers for Medicare and Medicaid Services (n.d.).

notice. A beneficiary can transfer his or her right to appeal to the provider, as long as Form CMS-20031 is completed and signed by the beneficiary and provider (CMS, 2011). A provider receives a remittance advice (RA) that shows what was paid and what was denied. An appeal may be filed based on either an MSN or RA (CMS, 2013). Figure 25.2 shows the levels of appeals for each type of Medicare program.

Under Medicare rules, a provider or client has 120 days to send a request for a redetermination (form CMS 20027) to the office that sent the MSN or RA (CMS, 2011). The person filing the appeal attaches supporting documentation to the form. The redetermination is an examination of the request by the Medicare contractor (formerly called the fiscal intermediary [Part A] or carrier [Part B]) (CMS, 2011). The Medicare contractor who will make the redetermination has 60 days to do so. The notice of redetermination will come in a new MSN or RA (CMS, 2013).

The notice of redetermination must include information on the facts in the case, the laws and policies which apply to the case, and the rights to and process for further appeal (AOTA, 2005). If there is missing documentation, it will be identified in the notice of redetermination. The burden of supplying missing documentation is given to the provider, not the beneficiary. If the provider or beneficiary are not satisfied with the outcome of the redetermination review, they can file form CMS 20033 to request a reconsideration (CMS, 2011).

The reconsideration is conducted by Medicare Qualified Independent Contractors (QICs), independent physician or other health care professional reviewers (CMS, 2011, 2013). The beneficiary, the beneficiary's representative, or the provider has 180 days to request reconsideration of the redetermination from the office that is specified on the notice of redetermination. This is a paper review only, so the documentation has to speak for itself. The request has to explain why the provider or beneficiary disagrees with the redetermination. The QIC has 60 days to make a determination based on any new evidence, as well as the original claim. If the QIC does not rule within the 60-day limit, the beneficiary or provider may request the claim be automatically reviewed at the next higher level (CMS, 2011, 2013).

An administrative law judge (ALJ) conducts the next level of the appeals process (CMS, 2005, 2011). A claim can only get to this level if the amount of the claim is over $140 (CMS, 2013). The request for an ALJ hearing must be filed within 60 days of the QIC's decision. The ALJ usually decides the appeal within 90 days of receiving the appeal, but the timeframe may be extended (CMS, 2011). ALJ hearings are usually conducted by video teleconference or telephone, but if there is a good reason, one may be held in person (CMS, 2011).

There are additional levels of appeal, including going to court, and the reader can learn more by visiting the CMS Web site. Since no new evidence or no new documentation can be submitted at these levels, they are not addressed here.

Always make a copy of all documents associated with the appeal to keep for your records. In wording your reasons for appealing the decision, be clear and direct. Do not imply anything, say it explicitly. If the MSN says that your services are not medically necessary, say that you feel the services are medically necessary and give a clear and concise reason you feel the services are necessary. The reasons you feel your services are medically necessary may include the fact that the services require the skills of an occupational therapist or occupational therapy assistant under the supervision of an occupational therapist (no other professionals or aides could safely and effectively provide the service), that the service is required for the patient's progress, and that the patient's functional goals can be achieved in a reasonable amount of time. Explain how the specific services you are providing have functional outcomes, usually in areas of occupation such as activities of daily living (ADLs) or instrumental activities of daily living (IADLs) and are appropriate to the setting, the client's condition, and the skills of the person providing the services.

Obviously, the Medicare appeals process is complicated and time-consuming. The best option is to document so well that there are no questions of medical necessity or the need for skilled services. Submit your documentation on time and in the right place.

▼ APPEALS TO PRIVATE INSURERS (INCLUDING MANAGED CARE ORGANIZATIONS) ▼

Insurers have appeals processes written into each of their health plans (and worker's compensation plans, auto insurance plans, etc.). If it is at all possible, a good first step is to contact the insurer and find out exactly why the claim was denied (Appeal Solutions, 2002). Find out what the insurer's definition of medical necessity is and build your arguments for covering the service around that definition. For example, some insurers routinely deny coverage for sensory integration intervention. They say it is experimental (often insurers say experimental procedures are not medically necessary); that there is not conclusive evidence that it is an effective, medically acceptable intervention. I know of one insurer who will deny an entire claim if even one unit of sensory integration intervention shows up on a claim, even if there are other procedures used during the same intervention session.

The occupational therapist could do one of two things here. One is that he or she could find as much evidence in the literature supporting the use of sensory integrative techniques and attach those to the letter of appeal. This could be a lengthy process, and you have no guarantee the reviewer will read any of the supporting literature since it may not relate specifically to this case. But it is better than doing nothing. Another would be to make an argument that the other procedures used during that intervention session are reasonable and necessary for the child's condition, and that the insurer has paid for those services in the past. In this case, you might get paid for some part of the session, but probably not the whole session. If I were going to advocate for occupational therapy with an insurer who considers sensory integration to be experimental, I would also enlist the support of the parent and referring physician, asking them to write letters explaining the potential benefits of the denied services.

If you find out that the denial is for all services of a type, such as sensory integration, you can enlist the support of your state occupational therapy association (if you are a member). The association can try to work with the insurer's medical director to change corporate policy. The American Occupational Therapy Association also has resources for members to help in challenging insurance companies.

Insurers deny payment for occupational therapy services for many reasons, not just because they consider an intervention experimental. Other reasons for denial include exceeding coverage limits (e.g., number of allowed visits), failure to complete the required forms in a timely manner, and poor documentation that does not demonstrate medical necessity (Glomstad, 2006). Many insurers post their documentation requirements online, so ignorance of the rules is no excuse. For example, Aetna posts its policy on occupational therapy coverage, including the type and frequency of documentation required at its Web site. (http://www.aetna.com/cpb/medical/data/200_299/0250.html). Be aware that not all private insurance or managed care plans cover the same services. One managed care company in Minnesota will cover occupational therapy services for ADLs, but not for IADLs. This company feels that help is easily available for people with deficits in IADLs, such as grocery shopping. There are home delivery services, so a person would not need to be able to go to the store for food.

Just as with Medicare appeals, a well-written letter of appeal and supporting documentation are needed to try to reverse a denial of coverage. Make sure that your documentation supports your claim of medical necessity and that the skills of an occupational therapist or occupational therapy assistant under the supervision of an occupational therapist are required to address the client's needs. The best defense is a good offense, so take the offensive and use principles of good documentation all the time.

Exercise 25.1

Give reasons to overturn a coverage decision for each of the two cases below.

Case 1: Shevan

Shevan is a 6-year-old child with fetal alcohol syndrome seen for occupational therapy at an after-school program. She has trouble concentrating and is quite active. She is tactilely defensive and fearful of movement through space when both feet are not on the ground (i.e., swings, slides, etc.). She does receive special education services at school, but there are reports that she hits other children and frequently gets off her chair to walk around when she should be sitting and listening. At the after-school program, you have observed her improve at sitting for longer stretches of time, up to 5 minutes sometimes. She has been in the program for 2 months. She is beginning to appear more relaxed on a swing, as long as her feet can touch the ground and she can control the distance the swing goes with her feet. Just yesterday she allowed the swing to go back and forth gently twice before stopping it. She was scribbling on a coloring book page when she first came to the program, but now she attempts to stay roughly within the lines.

    The insurance company said that the services of an occupational therapist are not medically necessary. They say that the services could be provided by lesser-skilled personnel.

Case 2: Seiki

Seiki is an elderly man who had a brain tumor removed from the right side of his brain 2 weeks ago. He is now at a long-term care facility for rehabilitation and then plans to return home to his farm after 4 to 6 weeks of rehab. He has a grandson who is looking after his cows for him. His grandson lives on a neighboring farm. As a result of the surgery, Seiki has some limitation in the movement and coordination of his left arm and side. He also has left-side neglect. He is beginning to accept that he has left-side neglect, but at the time of the last evaluation report/plan of care the neglect was strong, and he denied he had it. His left arm is flaccid, but in the last 2 days you have noticed some spasticity has set in. Seiki is making steady gains in dressing, feeding, grooming, and hygiene. His wife visits every day, but she is a worrier, and says they will have to give up the farm if he does not get better. This agitates Seiki. He is sure that he will recover and be able to go back to farming. In fact, he says that where there is a will, there is a way, and he will rig something up to help him do the work. He has always been a bit of an inventor, and has invented several helpful farm implements in his day. You gave your word to Seiki that you would help him come up with some adaptation that would allow him to do some of the work he used to do in the barn. Then the denial notice came.

The Medicare contractor says that Seiki's potential for recovery is poor at best. The contractor says that Seiki should move to a lower resource utilization group (RUG-III) level with fewer therapy minutes.

SUMMARY

You and your client have the right to appeal any payer's decision to deny coverage for occupational therapy services. Each payer will have a process for appealing such a decision. Writing a letter of appeal requires tact, clarity, and the powers of persuasion. You have to remain respectful regardless of how angry the decision makes you. You have to clearly state your reasons for wanting a coverage determination to be overturned. You have to construct sound arguments for the necessity of occupational therapy interventions in this specific case. Well-written appeal letters are extremely important to getting a denial overturned. You cannot overturn a denial unless you appeal it.

REFERENCES

Appeal Solutions. (2002). Case study: Responding to insurance denials due to lack of medical necessity. *The Appeal Letter.* Retrieved November 21, 2002, from http://appealsolutions .com/tal/medical-necessity-case-study/htm

Brennan, C., & Robinson, M. (2006). Documentation: Getting it right to avoid Medicare denials. *OT Practice, 11*(14), 10–15.

Center for Consumer Information & Insurance Oversight (CCIIO). (2012). *External appeals.* Retrieved from http://cciio.cms.gov/programs/consumer/appeals/index.html

Centers for Medicare and Medicaid Services. (2005). *MLN Matters Number MM4019.* Retrieved June 2, 2007, from http://www.cms.hhs.gov/mlnmattersarticles/downloads/mm4019.pdf

Centers for Medicare and Medicaid Services. (2008). *Pub 100-02 Medicare benefit policy: Transmittal 88.* Retrieved May 9, 2008, from http://www.cms.hhs.gov/transmittals/downloads/R88BP.pdf

Centers for Medicare and Medicaid Services. (2011). *The Medicare appeals process: Five levels to protect providers, physicians, and other suppliers.* Retrieved from http://www. cms.gov/Outreach-and-Education/Medicare-Learning-Network-MLN/MLNProducts/downloads/medicareappealsprocess.pdf

Centers for Medicare and Medicaid Services. (2013). *The Medicare appeals process: Fact sheet.* Retrieved from http://www.cms.gov/Outreach-and-Education/Medicare-Learning-Network-MLN/MLNProducts/downloads/MedicareAppealsprocess.pdf

Centers for Medicare and Medicaid Services. (n.d.). *Appeals process by Medicare type.* Retrieved from http://www.hhs.gov/omha/process/Appeals%20Process%20by%20 Medicare%20Type/appeals_process.html

Government Accountability Office. (2011). *Private health insurance: Data on application and coverage denials.* Retrieved from http://www.gao.gov/new.items/d11268.pdf

Glomstad, S. (2006). Keeping it covered. *Advance for Occupational Therapy Practitioners, 22*(11), 16.

National Conference of State Legislators (NCSL). (2010). Right to health insurance appeals process. Retrieved from http://www.ncsl.org/documents/health/hrhealthinsurapp.pdf

Visit **www.pearsonhighered.com/healthprofessionsresources** to access the student resources that accompany this book. Simply select Occupational Therapy from the choice of disciplines. Find this book and you will find the complimentary study tools created for this specific title.

CHAPTER 26

Meeting Minutes

INTRODUCTION

As has been said many times before, if it isn't documented, it didn't happen. While taking minutes may make some meetings feel more formal than the actual tone of the meeting, it is necessary to keep a record of what was discussed. When surveyors of any type (Joint Commission, CARF, Department of Health, Department of Education, etc.) come to evaluate a facility or department, they usually ask to see copies of meeting minutes. Sometimes they are looking to verify that staff have been instructed in certain policies and procedures; other times they may be looking to see that continuing education has occurred. Meeting minutes also "give all group members the chance to see how issues that were discussed were finally resolved" (Mosvick & Nelson, 1987, p. 169).

▼ OVERVIEW OF MEETING MINUTES ▼

Most facilities, departments, or organizations have an already established system for taking minutes. For the sake of tradition, that system is continued. This is fine most of the time, but occasionally a new note taker will look for a different system. This chapter presents a couple of systems. Which system is used is often a reflection of the management style of that facility, department, or organization.

Meeting minutes can also be used as evidence in legal proceedings. There may be a question of when staff was informed about an administrative decision or policy change. Often, if there is a question about the level of training received by staff, meeting minutes can be used to see how much training (i.e., about a new policy or procedure) was provided and when.

Sometimes, the minutes are documentation of decisions made by a department, facility, or organization. It is not unusual for a topic of discussion that is raised today to have been discussed last year or a couple years ago. By going back over the minutes, time can be saved and the results of the last discussion shared. If there is nothing new to add, the group can move on to the next topic.

▼ COMMONALITIES ▼

All meeting minutes contain certain information, but the format may vary. One very important piece of information on every meeting minute is the date, including the year. Meeting minutes are not much good if you cannot tell when the meeting occurred. Minutes should also reflect who was present at the meeting. If the names of attendees and the date of the meeting are documented, then there is proof that a particular person was informed of whatever the topic was on that date. That person cannot claim ignorance as a means of defending himself or herself.

Topics of discussion are a main component of meeting minutes. Obviously, minutes are more than just a listing of people and dates. They have to contain something of substance. Some minutes try to capture the entire discussion; some summarize the discussion. How much of the discussion is captured in the minutes will vary from place to place.

Finally, the action items are included in the minutes. Action items are the tasks that people must do as a result of the discussion. Examples of action items include the following:

- Ellie will clean the refrigerator and Chris will clean the microwave.
- Jane will meet with the nursing staff to present our program revisions for post-mastectomy patients.
- Arica will represent the department on the interprofessional quality improvement team looking at improving customer service.
- Tanya will contact the vendor for splinting materials about presenting an in-service for the department.

Some organizations follow Roberts Rules of Order, Newly Revised, as a standardized way to run their meetings. Roberts Rules also offers direction for how to take minutes at formal meetings. According to Roberts Rules, minutes are a record of action taken (e.g., motions and amendments to motions, points of order, and the chair's rulings on them) at a meeting, not a record of who said what. In addition to actions taken, the minutes should include the type of meeting, who attended the meeting, when the meeting took place, and when the meeting adjourned (Parlipro.org, 2013; RobertsRules.com, 2011).

▼ TAKING MINUTES ▼

If you are the person taking minutes at a meeting, the recorder, you have some special responsibilities. Because of the amount of concentration that it takes to record the discussion, it is difficult for one person to both lead a discussion and write minutes at the same time. The recorder is responsible for asking for clarification when discussions seem confusing or start going off on tangents (Mosvick & Nelson, 1987). The recorder can ask the group to verify the conclusions or summaries he or she draws at the end of a discussion. At the same time, the recorder needs to be ready to read back portions of the minutes to the group at the request of a group member.

If you are the recorder, be prepared with proper materials and be on time. If the agenda is provided ahead of time, use it to prepare the format or outline for taking minutes (Meetingwizard.org, 2012). Be careful that your opinions on a particular subject do not color the minutes that you are taking. Use as few adjectives and adverbs as possible; it is fine if the minutes are dull to read (Effectivemeetings.com, 2004). Words that signal that your opinions are surfacing include *inspiring, interesting, wonderful, insightful, undoubtedly,* and *antagonistic.*

You may take minutes by writing longhand, using a laptop computer, or by tape-recording the meeting and transcribing it later. If you take minutes with paper and pen, be sure to number your pages. If you have a tendency to abbreviate words or use your own cryptic system, be sure to transcribe the minutes into usable form as soon as possible after the meeting. If you wait too long, you may not be able to make sense of your own minutes (Meetingwizard.org, 2012). If the minutes refer to other documents, be sure to attach these documents to the official set of minutes or state where the documents can be found (Effectivemeetings.com, 2004).

While you may make copies of minutes to distribute to each person who attended or should have attended the meeting, there is usually one set of minutes that is kept as the official record of the meeting. In some places, it may be a three-ring binder kept in the office. In others, it may be a Website or folder on a shared drive on a computer. If a paper copy of the minutes is kept, some organizations require that the official minutes contain the signature of the minute-taker. In some organizations, the minutes do not become official until the Board of Directors or the membership of the committee approves them.

▼ FORMATS ▼

The simplest, but perhaps the wordiest, way to take minutes is to keep a narrative record of the meeting. In this format, after the date and list of attendees, the minute-taker writes down as much of what happened at the meeting as possible. It may include who said what. The paragraphs may be numbered when they represent a new topic.

Figure 26.1 shows an example of narrative minutes of a department meeting.

Date: 11-25-13
Present: E. Bay, J. Kay, G. Whiz, and A. Ging

1. Announcements
   a. Ellie announced that she would be taking Friday off and a sub would be called in.
   b. Jane announced that the United Way fund drive would be starting next week.
   c. Gina reminded staff that rounds this week are changed to Thursday at 9:00 A.M.

2. New patient transportation policy
   Jane presented the proposed new hospital policy on patient transportation. Rehabilitation therapies are to send the next day's schedule to each nursing unit, medical imaging, the lab, and the transportation pool by 3:00 P.M. each day. Unless otherwise noted on the schedule, nursing will have the patients dressed, in a wheelchair, with hearing aids and glasses on as needed by the scheduled pick-up time. Transportation pool personnel will transport those patients who are ready at their appointed time. If a patient is not ready, the transporter may wait for up to 5 minutes. If the patient is still not ready, then nursing will be responsible for finding a volunteer or aide to do the transporting. Patients must be finished with therapy at the time they are scheduled to go back to their rooms (or to other appointments), the transporter can only wait up to 5 minutes if the patient is not ready. After that, therapy is responsible for finding a volunteer or aide to do the transporting. Jane said the new policy was designed to encourage everyone to try to stick to the schedule. The policy is expected to go into effect in 30 days unless there is overwhelming negative feedback. The transportation improvement team is accepting written comments for the next 2 weeks. Gina asked if compliance to the policy would be tracked. Jane said yes, there would be forms that transporters fill out whenever they complete a transportation. Jane asked for a show of hands of people who were supportive of the proposed new policy. The department gave unanimous support to the policy. The policy is attached to these minutes.

3. Infection control
   Jane conducted the annual review of infection control policies and procedures for the department. We reviewed hand washing, and each member was asked to demonstrate proper technique. We discussed cleaning of supplies and equipment, including which cleaning solution is used for which items we clean and which items need to be sent to central sterile supply to be cleaned. We reviewed policies for working with patients in isolation rooms, when to wear protective gear (gloves, masks, and gowns), and proper technique for donning and doffing them. Finally, universal precautions were reviewed in detail. Each member of the department signed an annual review of infection control training confirmation sheet. Jane will forward these to the human resources department for placement in employee files.

4. Parking
   Jane asked for a volunteer to serve on a task force looking into issues regarding employee parking. Parking complaints have risen dramatically in the last year. Everyone in the department agrees that parking has gotten worse lately. Ellie said she tries to get to work 20 minutes early to find a decent spot. Arica said she has noticed that some employees get really competitive about parking spaces and that she has been cut out of a space on several occasions by an aggressive parker who works in the lab. The task force will look at existing parking options and consider alternatives for parking in the future. Arica volunteered to serve on the task force. The first meeting is next Friday at 2:30 P.M.

5. Budget request
   Ellie asked if there was any room in the budget for buying the newest revision of the Peabody Motor Scales. The test has new norms and a few new test items. Our competitors have all switched to the newer version. We use the test about 2–3 times per month, more often in summer. It would be a good investment. Jane said that she would need more information about the cost of the test and ordering information. There is some money in the budget, but there may not be enough for the test kit. We may have to delay or eliminate other expenses if we want it this year. If we cannot fit it in this year's budget, we should make it a priority for next year's budget.

FIGURE 26.1 Sample Narrative Meeting Minutes

Date: 11-25-13
Present: E. Bay, J. Kay, G. Whiz, and A. Ging

1. Announcements
    a. Ellie announced that she would be taking Friday off and a sub would be called in.
    b. Jane announced that the United Way fund drive would be starting next week.
    c. Gina reminded staff that rounds this week is changed to Thursday at 9:00 A.M.

2. New patient transportation policy
   Jane presented the proposed new hospital policy on patient transportation, which was designed to encourage everyone to try to stick to the schedule. The policy is expected to go into effect in 30 days unless there is overwhelming negative feedback. The transportation improvement team is accepting written comments for the next 2 weeks. Jane asked for a show of hands of people who were supportive of the proposed new policy. The department gave unanimous support to the policy. Policy is attached.

3. Infection control
   Jane conducted the annual review of infection control policies and procedures for the department as per hospital policy. We signed annual review of infection control training confirmation sheets, which Jane will forward to the human resources department for placement in employee files.

4. Parking
   Jane asked for a volunteer to serve on a task force looking at issues around employee parking. The task force will look at existing parking options and consider alternatives for parking in the future. Arica volunteered to serve on the task force. The first meeting is next Friday at 2:30 P.M.

5. Budget request
   Ellie asked if there was any room in the budget for buying the newest revision of the Peabody Motor Scales. Jane said that she would need more information about the cost of the test and ordering information. If we cannot fit it in this year's budget, we should make it a priority for next year's budget.

FIGURE 26.2 Example of Summary Format Meeting Minutes.

You can see that taking minutes like this could lead to writer's cramp. It is a lot of writing, and not all of it is important to note. Perhaps some things would be better left undocumented (e.g., getting cut out of parking spaces by an aggressive lab employee) in departmental meeting minutes. On the other hand, if someone in the department missed the meeting, he or she could have a pretty good idea of what transpired at the meeting simply from reading the minutes.

Another way to take minutes also involves a narrative format, but it uses summaries instead of trying to capture everything that was said. Figure 26.2 is an example of the same meeting, but a different format for the minutes.

You can see that minutes like this take up less space, but they also have less information. The summary format gives minimal information about what was discussed. It is enough to get the essence of what was discussed, but nothing is very substantial.

Minutes can use different numbering systems. Sometimes a typical outline format is used (I., A., 1., a.) but numerical systems are also used (1., 1.1., 1.1.2., 1.2.). While I have seen minutes that were not numbered at all, a numbering system of some kind does make it easier to refer back to specific items.

```
Date: 11-25-13
Present: E. Bay, J. Kay, G. Whiz, and A. Ging

1. Agenda
    1.1. Announcements
    1.2. New patient transportation policy
    1.3. Infection control
    1.4. Parking
    1.5. New budget request

2. Announcements
    2.1. Ellie announced that she would be taking Friday off and a sub would be called in.
    2.2. Jane announced that the United Way fund drive would be starting next week.
    2.3. Gina reminded staff that rounds this week is changed to Thursday at 9:00 A.M.

3. Action Items
    3.1. New patient transportation policy
        3.1.1. The department gave unanimous support to the policy.
        3.1.2. See attached policy
    3.2. Infection control
        3.2.1. We reviewed and signed annual review of infection control confirmation sheets,
               which Jane will forward to the human resources department for placement in em-
               ployee files.
    3.3. Parking
        3.3.1. Arica volunteered to serve on the task force.
    3.4. Budget request
        3.4.1. Ellie will provide Jane with ordering information for the new Peabody Motor Scales.
        3.4.2. It will be ordered if it fits within the department's budget.
```

FIGURE 26.3   Sample Action Format Minutes.

Another format is to list agenda items at the top of the page, and then only document action items. This format definitely saves space. It is sort of a "just the facts ma'am" kind of format. If the minutes from the above meeting were done in an action format, they would look something like Figure 26.3. You can see what a sparse format this is. It is best used for very long meetings.

Another format is a combination of the last two. It summarizes a topic, and then identifies the action item. For example, the parking discussion might look like this:

4. Parking

Jane asked for a volunteer to serve on a task force looking at issues around employee parking. The task force will look at existing parking options and consider alternatives for parking in the future.

Action: Arica volunteered to serve on the task force.

The last format is shown in Figure 26.4. This format requires some preparation before the meeting, but simplifies taking minutes during the meeting (Meetingwizard.org, 2012). Names of the people expected to attend the meeting can be listed on the form and a check-mark placed in front of the ones who attended the meeting (Effectivemeetings.com, 2004). Some places combine the two columns on the right into one action column, but specify the person responsible as part of the action.

There are many other formats. There can be lots of other variations. When taking minutes, the important thing is to listen for the most important information and record it accurately.

OT Department Meeting Minutes

Date/Time: 11-25-08/3:00 P.M.

Members Present ____X____ E. Bay __X__ J. Kay __X__ G. Whiz ____X____ A. Ging

Topic	Discussion	Action	Person Responsible
Announcements	Ellie announced that she would be taking Friday off and a sub would be called in. Jane announced that the United Way fund drive would be starting next week. Gina reminded staff that rounds this week is changed to Thursday at 9:00 A.M.	N/A	N/A
New Policy	The proposed new hospital policy on patient transportation was presented. It was designed to encourage everyone to try to stick to the schedule. The policy is expected to go into effect in 30 days unless there is overwhelming negative feedback. The transportation improvement team is accepting written comments for the next 2 weeks.	The department gave unanimous support to the policy (attached).	Jane
Infection Control	The annual review of infection control policies and procedures for the department as per hospital policy was conducted.	We signed annual review of infection control training confirmation sheets that will be forwarded to HR for placement in employee files.	Jane
Parking	The hospital is looking for a volunteer to serve on a task force looking at issues around employee parking and existing parking options and consider alternatives for parking in the future.	Arica volunteered to serve on the task force.	Arica
New Budget Request	A request was received to buy the newest revision of the Peabody Motor Scales.	Ellie will find information about the cost of the test and ordering options. Jane will see if it fits in this year's budget.	Ellie and Jane

FIGURE 26.4   Sample Meeting Minutes Form.

Exercise 26.1

Summarize the following meeting topics using the combined format (the last one presented):

1. 50th Anniversary Committee Report
   Riva gave an update on the actions of the committee that is planning the 50th anniversary celebration of the hospital. The celebration committee is looking for success stories for a weeklong series (a 4-minute segment each day) on the 11:00 P.M. local news. They would like to highlight a different department each day, but they cannot cover every department in the 5-day series. Rhonda suggested Mr. Sayed who recovered from Guillian-Barré syndrome 2 years ago. He still sends a holiday card each year. Rolanda suggested Mr. Hernandez who had extensive rehab following a head injury, but eventually went home and back to work part time. Robert suggested Mrs. Hellenberger who lost six toes and three fingers to frostbite. The committee is also planning an open house in the cafeteria, and each department can put together a display table promoting programs in the department. After much discussion, the department agreed to talk with the other departments in the rehabilitation area about sharing a segment on Mr. Hernandez. Rhonda volunteered to work with the occupational therapy fieldwork students on a display table for the open house.

Topic	Discussion	Action	Person Responsible

2. Budget
   The head of the department, Barb, said she had noticed a decrease in productivity lately. There has been a downward trend over the last 6 weeks. The company's financial picture is not looking as good as was hoped. Ours is not the only department that is falling below projections. The president of the company is asking each department to develop a plan for cutting expenses for the rest of the year by 10%. Barb would like input from the staff as to what cuts would be the least painful to make. Bob suggested that we could cut out doughnuts and coffee for the morning department meetings. Belinda suggested that we could use coupons and buy generic brands for the occupational therapy kitchen. Becky suggested being more careful about walking off with each other's pens, and try to conserve paper. Bob suggested that they be more conscientious about remembering to bill for adaptive equipment. Barb said those were good suggestions, but they wouldn't come anywhere near 10% of the budget. She asked each person to meet with her privately to discuss other possibilities.

Topic	Discussion	Action	Person Responsible

SUMMARY

Taking accurate meeting minutes is an essential function of any occupational therapy department. There is a delicate balance between recording too much information and too little. The names of the people present at the meeting, the date of the meeting, and the outcomes of the meeting in terms of actions and decisions need to be recorded. There are several formats for recording these meetings. While each has some advantages and disadvantages, choose one that fits your facility's needs.

REFERENCES

Effectivemeetings.com. (2004). *Meeting basics, how to record useful meeting minutes.* Retrieved from http://www.effectivemeetings.com/meetingbasics/minutes.asp

Meetingwizard.org. (2012). *Taking minutes.* Retrieved from http://www.meetingwizard.org/meetings/taking-minutes.cfm

Mosvick, R. K., & Nelson, R. B. (1987). *We've got to start meeting like this! A guide to successful business meeting management.* Glenview, IL: Scott Foresman.

Parlipro.org. (2013). *The minutes.* Retrieved from http://www.rulesonline.com/rror-10.htm#60

RobertsRules.com. (2011). *Changes in the eleventh edition.* Retrieved from http://robertsrules.com/changes11.html

---

Visit **www.pearsonhighered.com/healthprofessionsresources** to access the student resources that accompany this book. Simply select Occupational Therapy from the choice of disciplines. Find this book and you will find the complimentary study tools created for this specific title.

CHAPTER 27

Grant Writing

INTRODUCTION

Occupational therapy services are generally paid for by third-party payers such as Medicare and managed care companies, or provided through school districts. Occupational therapy services provided in emerging practice areas may not have access to third party payment. In any occupational therapy program, there may be clients who cannot afford needed services or equipment. Grants can be written to help underwrite the start-up costs of new programs or to set up fund accounts to help clients pay for services and/or equipment. Rarely will grants be awarded to cover ongoing expenses of existing programs.

▼ WHAT GRANTS ARE ▼

Grants are awards of specific amounts of money for designated purposes. Grants can be awarded by either governmental agencies or private organizations. Regardless of the source of the grant, grants are only awarded to those who apply for them. The organization that awards the grant decides who will be eligible for the grant (Doll, 2010). Grants may be awarded to universities, community agencies, schools, healthcare facilities, or other organizations that meet the requirements for the grant. The organization requesting the grant must demonstrate in writing that there is a purpose and a plan for using the funds that matches the criteria of the grant.

There are different types of grants available, and it is important to match the type of grant to the project for which you are seeking money. A research grant, as you might expect, funds research projects (Doll, 2010). Educational grants fund programs that have as the main goal the education of a group of people. Training grants target the development and implementation of training for designated populations. Planning grants support the planning process for new programs or projects. Demonstration grants provide direct funding for program implementation, especially programs that are known to be successful based on documented evidence (Doll, 2010).

▼ WHERE TO FIND GRANT OPPORTUNITIES ▼

There are several places to look for grant funding opportunities. The Internet has literally millions of sites related to grant writing. Some sites focus more on tips for writing grants, but many others contain specific instructions for applying for particular grants. Table 27.1 lists selected Websites and the type of information found on those sites.

If you work at a facility that has a development office, the people working in that office can be of great assistance. Hospitals and nonprofit corporations often have development offices. The staff of these offices can help you locate funding sources, help you write the grant, and in some cases, actually solicit funds for you. These people have lots of experience working with funding agencies. They know the tricks of the trade. It helps to have a friendly working relationship with development staff if you are going to be seeking grant money from any source. Few things make development staff angrier than staff from other

TABLE 27.1 Grant-Related Websites

WebSite Address	Agency or Organization	Type of Content
www.grants.gov	Federal Government	Searchable listing of federal grant opportunities
www.foundationcenter.org	Foundation Center	Directory of foundations Offers online and classroom training programs on seeking foundation money Has subscription service Has a foundation finder Free tutorials on grant seeking Online library has a glossary of terms used in grant-writing process
www.fundsnetservices.com	Grant Writing Resources	Fundraising and grant-writing resources Grant applications and proposal-writing guides
www.tgci.com	The Grantsmanship Center	Grant information and grantsmanship training Includes grant sources by state search engine
http://grants.nih.gov/grants/oer.htm	National Institutes of Health (federal govt.)	Lots of information on applying for NIH grants
http://www.middlebury.edu/offices/support/grants/grants_index	Middlebury College	Provides advice on grant preparation Links to sites with information on grant writing

departments going out and seeking funds without their knowledge. It is critical that development staff be aware of every time an outside source is asked to make a donation or fund a grant so they can know which funding agency has been asked for what contribution this year. In this sense, they act as gatekeepers for soliciting funds.

▼ GENERAL GRANT-WRITING TIPS ▼

The awarding of grants is a competitive process. Granting organizations usually have less money to award than the total amount requested by grant applicants. This means there will be criteria established to help guide the decision making. It is critical that anyone applying for a grant know exactly what criteria will be used to determine who will receive the grant, and then to use that information in writing the grant (Fazio, 2007). Criteria for awarding grants vary significantly, so it is critical to match the reason you want funding to the criteria used by the funder to make award decisions. For example, if you want funding to help start a program for teenage children of immigrant families to learn work skills, it would be a waste of your time, and the funder's, to apply for a grant for such a program from a funder whose main purpose is to fund programs for adults with chemical dependency. Although some of the teens you propose to serve might have chemical dependency issues, it would be more likely that a funding agency that supported programs focused on self-sufficiency would take an interest in your proposed program.

Agencies and organizations that award grants are called grantors (Doll, 2010). Grantors make it known to the world that they have money to award through a process called a *request for proposals* (commonly referred to as an RFP). The RFP usually spells out the requirements for that grant including the purpose of the grant, types of programs or projects it funds, deadlines for applying for funds, amount of money that may be requested, and the process for applying for the grant (Doll, 2010).

The two most important things to remember when applying for a grant are to follow the instructions and to proofread, proofread, and then proofread some more. While these seem like simple and obvious tips, they are absolutely critical to the grant application process. Granting agencies provide instructions to those interested in applying for grants. There is usually a good reason why they instruct applicants to organize the grant application in a certain way, so even if the applicant thinks it would look better if organized differently; the instructions, including deadlines, have to be followed. You want the reader of your grant proposal to look favorably at your proposal. A grant agency may discard an application without reviewing it if the instructions for submitting the grant were not followed (Doll, 2010).

To the extent possible, reflect the terminology used in the RFP in your grant application (Doll, 2010). Understand what it is the grantor wants to fund and be clear about how your program fits their funding priorities. Be careful to choose words that the funding agency will understand (Doll, 2010). The person reading your grant request will probably not be an occupational therapist, so avoid using a lot of occupational therapy jargon.

Proofreading will ensure there are no typos, no grammatical or spelling errors, and no sloppy formatting or bad copies (i.e., printer running low on ink). As mentioned several times in this book, people form impressions of you and your program based on your written work. To be seen as competent and able to implement the proposed program, you have to write like a competent and polished professional. Not only does the proposal writer need to proofread the proposal, but it is a good idea to get a couple of other people to proofread it as well (Doll, 2010). You want the application to look good.

While specific instructions for the organization of the grant application will vary, a cover letter will usually be the first thing the granting agency representative will read. A cover letter needs to provide enough information to interest the reader and make the reader want to read the rest of the proposal. Be sure your cover letter is addressed to the right person or committee. Be sure the cover letter is on appropriate letterhead and is signed by the person in the highest authority as possible for your program/employer. Try to keep the cover letter to one page. The layout and visual qualities of this page can set the tone of the reader's disposition toward your proposal.

Begin your grant application with an abstract (Doll, 2010). The abstract describes your proposal as briefly as possible. The abstract summarizes the need your proposal intends to address, what the project involves, who will benefit from this project, why this project is important, and the total cost of the project in greatly condensed form. The RFP will specify what content needs to be in the abstract and the word limit for it (Doll, 2010). This is a lot of information to squeeze into one or two pages, but it can be done if you are clear, direct, and do not elaborate on anything. You have the rest of the proposal to do that.

▼ WRITING A GRANT TO FUND A NEW PROGRAM ▼

According to Doll, 2010, in general there are eight key elements that are addressed in the narrative portion of the grant application, as shown in Figure 27.1. In addition to the narrative, most grants also require a budget and supplemental materials. Since every grant is different, additional elements may be included in the narrative, such as budget justification or a description of the program or project team, although for some grantors these may be in separate sections of the grant application. Careful reading of the RFP will tell you what the grantor wants discussed, where to discuss it, and what the word or page limits are (Doll, 2010).

- Background information
- Problem statement (need statement)
- Theoretical foundation (evidence)
- Goals, objectives, activities, and outcomes
- Implementation plan
- Timeline
- Evaluation plan
- Dissemination plan

FIGURE 27.1 Grant Proposal Narrative.
Source: Doll, 2010.

Background

This is where you describe the need for your program, the population it will serve, and the support for your program (Doll, 2010). In this section, you will provide information about the demographics of the population your program will serve. Sometimes, a literature review is part of this section. Be sure to include any references used in the literature review and elsewhere in the grant proposal, using the citation format specified in the RFP (Doll, 2010). Explain the mission of the program. By reading the mission and a description of the proposed program, the reader should have a good idea of what you are hoping to accomplish.

In your grant proposal, you need to explain why your organization is positioned to do what you say you will do (Davis, 2005). Here is where you clearly state your commitment to the proposal. Do not assume the readers will know much about your agency or organization, so tell them why your organization can be trusted to use the grant money efficiently (Davis, 2005). If you have developed other similar projects in the past, explain the success you have had with them.

Most funding agencies need to know that their money is going to support an activity that will benefit some portion of society in some way. It is up to you to clearly demonstrate that your proposed program will do that. It is helpful to know what the mission and goals of the funding agency are, and link your proposal to them (Doll, 2010). You can explain what would happen if the proposal is not funded.

Problem or Needs Statement

The problem or needs statement builds the case for why your program is necessary. According to Doll, 2010 "The problem statement must directly relate to the program" (p. 209). This section has to be very focused on the problem the proposed program addresses. You want to be sure that the people reviewing your application can very clearly see that your program will address this specific need (Doll, 2010). Be sure that the need you hope to address is not so huge that your proposed program could not make a reasonable dent in it. In other words, as a quality improvement coordinator used to tell me, "You can't boil the ocean one teaspoon at a time."

Theoretical Foundation

While not a requirement of all grant application, the theoretical foundation tells the grant reviewers that the approach this program takes is supported by evidence (Doll, 2010). You provide a justification for the strategies your program will employ by naming a theoretical approach and providing evidence to support that approach. This tells the reviewers that you are familiar with the evidence (Doll, 2010). It shows that you are informed and competent.

Goals, Objectives, Activities, and Outcomes

Grantors want to know what your program will do and how you will do it (Doll, 2010). The goals, objectives, activities, and outcomes must clearly relate to each other. The overarching purposes of the program are identified in the goals. There should be a clear link from the goals to the problem or needs statement. A typical grant application will include up to three goals. Objectives are more specific than goals, and describe the steps that will be taken to meet the goals (Doll, 2010). Objectives must be measurable, and can be written in any of the formats described in Chapter 15 of this book. Activities are the specific actions that will occur that will lead to the accomplishment of the program goals and objectives (Doll, 2010). Outcomes are what the implementation of the program will accomplish. The outcomes will be evaluated in the evaluation plan (Doll, 2010).

For example, if you are developing a program for musicians with hand injuries, your goal might be to provide musicians with a program to help their recovery that is sensitive to their unique needs for very precise finger movements. The objectives of the program might be:

- 90% of the musicians participating in the program will rate their satisfaction with the program as very helpful or outstanding.
- 85% will report a decrease of pain while playing of at least two points on a 1–10 scale.
- The reinjury rate will be 20% or less 6 months after intervention ends.

Implementation Plan

This section tells the grant reviewers who the project will serve, what services will be provided, how and where the services will be provided, and when they will be completed (Doll, 2010). This includes how the participants in the program will be recruited, and who the program staff will be. In this section, anticipate possible challenges to implementation and describe how these will be addressed (Doll, 2010).

Include information on space, supplies and equipment, staff, and methods of service delivery. Specify any space, equipment, and supplies that you will need. You can be general and lump similar items into a category. For example, for the musician's rehabilitation program, you could say you need assorted splinting materials and various intervention modalities. This is usually sufficient for small items. For higher-priced items, such as test materials or specialized equipment, list them separately. Describe your space needs in terms of square feet required and the purpose for each required space. If you are so inclined, you can describe your vision of how the space will look. Describe the staff who will implement the grant and how they will do it (Doll, 2010). In other words, describe what you are going to do and who will do it (Davis, 2005). If you are going to use the grant to fund the salaries for the start of the program, explain how salaries will be paid in future years when the grant money is gone. Staff resumés, detailed policies and procedures, and equipment and supply lists can be included in the supplemental materials in appendices to the grant proposal (Doll, 2010).

Timeline

The timeline shows the grant reviewers what will happen and when (Doll, 2010). It shows the chronological order in which actions will occur. It is a helpful and concise way to visualize the program (Doll, 2010).

Evaluation Plan

The evaluation plan tells grant reviewers how you will know if your program is doing what it was designed to do; the effectiveness of the program (Davis, 2005; Doll, 2010). It is a way to hold the program planners accountable. In the evaluation plan, describe the data you will collect to help determine whether or not the program has met its goals, objectives, and outcomes (Doll, 2010). Make sure the evaluation plan relates to the goals and objectives stated earlier in your proposal. Be specific about who will do what as part of the evaluation process.

Dissemination Plan

This section of the grant narrative explains to whom and how program results will be communicated (Doll, 2010). These results may be communicated to program participants, program staff, or the larger community. They may be communicated through a newsletter, a presentation, a scholarly publication, or annual report (Doll, 2010).

Exercise 27.1

Write a goal and two measurable objectives for the following programs.

1. Your clinic is developing a summer program for school-age children who will not be receiving school-based services during the summer break. It will focus on handwriting, movement, and socialization skills.

2. You want to start a not-for-profit agency to help adults with developmental disabilities develop work skills.

3. The hospital would like you to develop a program for women who have had mastectomies and breast reconstruction surgeries.

Budget

The budget section of the grant proposal is equally important as the narrative section. The funding agency may require budget forms to be submitted with the proposal. Every budget item for which you request funding needs to be justified in the narrative portion; there should be no surprises on the budget forms. Your budget is an estimate of costs to deliver the program to consumers. As an estimate, you do not need to record costs down to the last penny; you can round to the nearest dollar, or if you are dealing with large amounts of money, the nearest $100 or $1,000. If some items of the budget for the proposed program will be paid for in some other way (not from the grant), explain the source of that funding. When calculating salaries, remember to include benefits such as health insurance, paid time off, and so on. Do not include any unexplained budget items such as "miscellaneous" or "other" expenses. Never ask for more money than you realistically need.

There are generally two types of expenses to consider in the budget: direct costs and indirect costs (Doll, 2010). Direct costs are those that will be funded by the grant. Indirect costs are not part of the implementation of the grant, but are necessary for daily operations of the organization receiving the grant, such as rent, heating and other utilities, and administrator salaries. Indirect costs are sometimes called overhead or administrative expenses (Davis, 2005).

Some grantors want to see all the sources of income as well as expenses (Davis, 2005). The granting agencies want to know who else is financing this project. Earned income is what you plan to receive in exchange for the services you deliver. For example, if you will ask people to pay for services, the granting agency will want to know how much revenue that will generate. Contributed income can be either cash or in-kind contributions from other sources (other than the granting agency). In-kind contributions are things other than cash, such as donated goods, volunteer time, or discounts. For example, if Target or Walmart agree to sell you cleaning supplies at a 25% discount, you would list the value of that 25% as an in-kind donation (Davis, 2005).

Supplemental Materials

In addition to whatever forms are required by the funding agency and the narrative proposal, you may want to supplement your proposal with supporting materials. These materials belong in appendices at the back of the proposal package. Some of the kinds of items that might be helpful to include in appendices are included in Figure 27.2.

Obviously, it takes careful planning and lots of time to put together a solid grant proposal. The more work you can do before you start writing, the better off you will be in the long run. Understand what the funding agency is looking for in a proposal. If possible, read the proposals of programs the agency has funded in the past. Do not hesitate to ask the funding agency questions throughout the process (Doll, 2010). Always keep copies of everything you send out (Doll, 2010). A paper copy is usually preferred to an e-mailed or faxed one; however, a paper copy can take longer than you think to reach the funding agency. Always allow twice as much time as you think you will need for a paper proposal to be delivered to the funding agency.

- Documents showing the type of business (for-profit, not-for-profit, charitable, etc.) the proposed program will be operated as. This could be in the form of an IRS determination letter to verify tax-exempt status, certificate of incorporation, and by-laws of the organization
- Résumés or biographies of key personnel
- Financial statements from your last complete fiscal year (e.g. income statement, profit and loss statement)
- Letters of support from people outside the organization (only a couple)
- Floor plan for space that will be used for the program
- Equipment and supply lists in detail (summarized in body of proposal)
- Sample forms
- Job descriptions
- Logic model (a diagram showing the relationships among resources, activities, and results)

FIGURE 27.2   Suggested Contents for Appendices.
Sources: Davis (2005); Doll, (2010).

▼ WRITING OTHER TYPES OF GRANTS ▼

Other types of programs for which you might write a grant include setting up a fund for clients who have no insurance to pay for services, a fund to help families buy needed equipment that third-party payers will not pay for, or to help fund research you are planning to do for your thesis or dissertation. You might write a grant to enable your clinic to purchase a particularly expensive piece of equipment. A grant request for these purposes would be less cumbersome to write than a grant to fund a new program.

As with a new program grant, you would begin by following the funding agency's grant application process. You would want to choose your words carefully so that any reader will understand the purpose of your grant proposal. A cover letter and executive summary would accompany the narrative part of your proposal.

The narrative should explain the need for creating the fund or buying the piece of equipment. Provide whatever data you can collect that demonstrate a demand for the services or equipment. You may make both arguments of fact (based on data) and emotions (based on feelings, appealing to the heartstrings) in demonstrating the demand. For example, if you are trying to create a fund for uninsured clients, you could argue on the basis of the percentage of people without insurance in your community, the number of clients who were unable to pay for services. You could also argue that without access to your services, these clients will live in pain, may be more likely to reinjure themselves, and may become a burden to their families.

Since organizations donating money for grants want to know what benefit to the community will result from granting their money to your program, you will need to be very explicit in stating the benefits expected. Perhaps the new equipment will enable you to be more precise in your measurements of dysfunction. Perhaps the fund will enable families to purchase custom-made seating devices for children with multiple disabilities. Perhaps the fund will allow a client to be fully rehabilitated before going back to work, decreasing the likelihood of reinjury.

If you are seeking funding for your research, then your grant application might look a little different. Research is usually for a specific period of time, and there is no need to demonstrate how the program will continue after the funding is discontinued. You will need to explain the purpose of the research, the potential benefits and risks of the research, the cost of the research, where the results will be presented or published, and why you are qualified to do the research. Depending on whether you are applying for a research grant from your college or university, the American Occupational Therapy Foundation (AOTF), or the National Institutes of Health, the amount of information and level of detail required will vary.

Exercise 27.2

1. Visit the AOTF website (www.aotf.org) and locate the grant application for dissertation research.

2. Next, find the research priorities for AOTF.

3. Visit the Minnesota Council of Foundations common grant application form (www.mcf. http://org/mcf/grant/applicat.htm) and locate both the form and the types of information needed for each section of the form.

4. Compare and contrast the two grant applications for both the application process and the types of information each requires.

Exercise 27.3

Which of the following statements are true and which are false, relative to the grant-writing process?

1. _____ In the abstract, take the time to thoroughly explain the purpose of your proposal.
2. _____ Address all the review criteria established by the funding agency in your proposal.
3. _____ It is a good idea to ask lots of questions throughout the process.
4. _____ It is better to present a good-looking proposal than one that is well written.
5. _____ The timeline can be general rather than specific.
6. _____ Goals can be broad and not measurable.
7. _____ Objectives need to meet RHUMBA criteria.
8. _____ You must demonstrate that your project will have an impact on the target population.
9. _____ Program evaluation criteria need to be as detailed as the rest of the proposal.

SUMMARY

When seeking grant money to fund a new program, it is important to present a well-written, thorough, and specific proposal. The proposal needs to contain the information that the funding agency is requesting. While there are some general similarities in the information and format that most funding agencies want, each has some unique requirements, and the proposal needs to be tailored to fit the funding agency. It is vital that someone applying for a grant follow the instructions of the grant funding agency. A cover letter can help create interest on the part of the funding agency in your proposed program. Somewhere in your proposal, you have to be explicit in what you propose to do, why you propose to do it, how you will do it, why you are the one(s) to do it, and how much it will cost to do it. A grant proposal has to be tailored to the funding agency and to the type of grant being requested.

REFERENCES

Davis, B. (2005). *Writing a successful grant proposal.* Retrieved from http://www.mcf.org/system/article_resources/0000/0325/writingagrantproposal.pdf

Doll, J. (2010). *Program development and grant writing: Occupational therapy making the connection.* Sudbury, MA: Jones Bartlett.

Fazio, L. S. (2007). *Developing occupation-centered programs for the community: A workbook for students and professionals* (2nd ed.). Upper Saddle River, NJ: Prentice Hall.

Visit **www.pearsonhighered.com/healthprofessionsresources** to access the student resources that accompany this book. Simply select Occupational Therapy from the choice of disciplines. Find this book and you will find the complimentary study tools created for this specific title.

CHAPTER 28

Policies and Procedures

INTRODUCTION

In any organization there is a need for everyone to understand what is expected of them. People need to know what company policy is and the acceptable ways to do things. This is where policy and procedure manuals come in. They help employees to know what the company wants employees to do without them having to ask a superior before doing anything. Policy and procedure manuals serve to "regulate, direct, inform, and guide" employees (Department of Children's Services [DCS], State of Tennessee, 2013, p. 5). They can be used to train new employees or serve as a reference for more seasoned employees (University of California Davis [UCD], 2011). They can also set or clarify boundaries that also protect employees in the event of an audit or lawsuit (DCS, 2013).

Before facilities, agencies, or programs are credentialed (licensed, certified, or accredited), the surveyors who make the recommendation on credential status will always ask to see policy and procedure manuals. The manuals show what the organization has communicated to employees, in writing, regarding expectations in the workplace. Large organizations may have many policy and procedure manuals. Often, they will have one for human resource policies and procedures, and then one for each department. Smaller organizations may have one manual that has sections for various departments.

Occupational therapy staff usually write their own departmental policies and procedures. There is likely some sort of approval process for the development of new policies and procedures. Organizations in which occupational therapy practitioners are members are also guided by policies and procedures. Medicare, Medicaid, and other payers have policy and procedure manuals that describe what occupational therapy practitioners and the companies that employ them must do in order to submit bills in the right way so the company can get paid.

▼ POLICIES ▼

Policies tell employees what the company's position is on a particular issue. Some policies are required by law or by the credentialing agency. For example, federal law requires that employers have policies on nondiscrimination. A credentialing agency may require a policy on infection control.

In addition to explaining what is expected, policies often state who is responsible for complying with the policy. Individual names are not used, but it might list a job title or state that all employees are responsible for compliance. For example, a policy on infection control would be the responsibility of all employees while a policy on calibration of electronic equipment may be the responsibility of an electrical engineer.

Usually, policies include a statement that explains the purpose of the policy (Page, 2002). The purpose of a policy on safety may be to protect the health of employees. The purposes of a policy on scheduling of clients are to be fair to both clients and staff and to make the most efficient use of resources (staff and space). The purpose is not always explicitly stated. If the policy is the result of a law or a credentialing requirement, the number of the law or standard can be cited in the purpose statement.

Finally, each policy needs an effective date (Page, 2002). Any policy revisions also need to be dated. Sometimes, there is a signature page at the front or back of the manual that the department head or head of the organization signs to indicate that all the policies and procedures have been approved by the organization.

▼ PROCEDURES ▼

Procedures explain, in great detail, what steps need to happen to comply with the policy. A procedure for infection control would include instructions on hand washing, use of protective clothing (e.g., masks, gowns, gloves), disposal of infected waste, cleaning up blood or body fluid spills, and so on. A procedure for scheduling would describe how clients are assigned to a particular staff person, where the schedule is recorded, how appointments are made and canceled, and so on. A policy tells what, a procedure tells how. Because of occupational therapy practitioners' background in task analysis, they are good at breaking down the steps of a task, a necessary skill in writing procedures.

▼ WRITING POLICIES AND PROCEDURES ▼

It is essential that policies and procedures be written clearly, explicitly, and thoroughly to avoid any misinterpretations of policy. Readers should be able to find the important information as quickly and easily as possible. As technology and laws change, it is necessary to revise the policy and procedures. Figure 28.1 shows a sample policy and procedure for timeliness of documentation. Figures 28.2 and 28.3 show sample templates for writing policies and procedures.

Timeliness of Documentation
Occupational Therapy Department

Policy: Documentation will be completed in a timely fashion according to the schedule below.

Applies to: All occupational therapists and occupational therapy assistants.

Responsible party: Occupational Therapy Manager

Purpose: To ensure timely completion of the health record.

Effective date: January 1, 2004; rev January 2, 2009; January 2, 2013

Procedure:
1. Orders will be acknowledged in the client's medical record by an occupational therapist within 24 hours of receipt of the order.
2. Evaluation summaries will be completed by an occupational therapist and filed in the medical record within 48 hours of the first client visit.
3. Contact notes are written at time of the visit by either the occupational therapist or the occupational therapy assistant, whoever conducted the visit.
4. Missed visits will be documented on the same day as the missed visit by the occupational therapist or occupational therapy assistant who was scheduled to work with the client.
5. Reevaluations/revised plans of care will be written by the occupational therapist at least every 90 days.
6. Discharge summaries will be written by the occupational therapist and filed in the medical record within 48 hours of discontinuation.
7. Occupational therapy documentation may be filed by any member of the occupational therapy department or by the unit coordinator on the nursing station.

FIGURE 28.1   Sample Policy and Procedure.

Title of Policy and Procedure		

Title of Policy and Procedure

Effective date (revisions):

Policy:

Applicability:

Responsible party:

Purpose:

Procedure:

FIGURE 28.2   Sample Policy and Procedure Template, Simple.

Title of Policy and Procedure	Number	
	Original date	
	Dates of revisions	
	Approval	
Purpose		
Definitions (*or omit here and put a section for definitions in the back of the manual*)		
Policy		
Positions affected		
Responsibilities		
Procedures		

FIGURE 28.3   Sample Policy and Procedure Template, Formal.
Source: Page, S. (2004).

Notice that the sample policy and procedure is written in straightforward, simple terms. The policy addresses the governing principle, while the procedure describes the tasks required to comply with the policy (UCD, 2011). Make sure you avoid words or names that can become quickly outdated. Any words that may not be understood by a reader (especially a new employee) need to be defined right in the policy. Some people suggest that there be a section on definitions written into each policy, including defining abbreviations and acronyms, as well as technical terms (DCS, 2013; Page, 2004). Others create a section in the policy and procedure manual that provides the definitions of terms and spells out the abbreviations and acronyms used in the manual.

It is useful to begin writing your policy and procedure by gathering up the documents that already exist within the organization, such as the vision, mission, and strategic plan (Page, 2002). An organizational chart will help in determining who reports to whom within the organization. These documents answer questions such as:

- What business are we in?
- Who are our customers?
- What do our customers want?
- What position within the marketplace do we want to be in?

TABLE 28.1 Procedural Word Choices

Degree of Responsibility and Accountability	Verb Used
Requirement	Must
Recommendation	Should
Choice	May
Sequence of events	Does

Source: DCS, 2013.

Best practices suggest that the policy reflects the vision, mission, and strategic plan of the organization (Page, 2002). These documents, along with discussions among leaders and managers within the organization can assist in identifying guiding principles (values and beliefs) for the development of policies and procedures (Page, 2002).

Once you have all the materials that can provide guidance for the development of policies and procedures, you can develop the overall structure of your policy and procedure manual. This is the point at which you need to decide if you want to separate your policies and your procedures in separate manuals or write one combined manual. The rest of this chapter assumes you want a combined policy and procedure manual. It also assumes that you will have a separate section at the end of the manual for definitions, abbreviations, and acronyms.

When writing the procedure it is important to know the degree of responsibility and accountability (DCS, 2013). The degree of responsibility and accountability will be indicated by your choice of words to describe them. A policy can be a requirement, recommendation, choice, or simply a sequence of events. Table 28.1 shows the relationship between procedure word choices and the degree of responsibility and accountability.

Braveman (2006) suggests that policies and procedures, when combined in one document, include the following:

- Statement of the policy
- Purpose of the policy and procedure
- List of types of employees for whom the policy and procedure apply
- Procedures to be followed
- Title of the job of the person who is responsible for overseeing the policy and procedure
- Dates of when the policy and procedure were reviewed

Next, you develop the table of contents. This requires you to name and organize the policies and procedures you need to write. This is done using a drafting process. Only after all the policies and procedures are written and approved will the final table of contents be written, (Page, 2002). Each policy and procedure may also be assigned a number to make locating the policy and procedure easier. Figure 28.4 shows a sample table of contents for a policy and procedure manual for a private practice occupational therapy clinic. Stephen Page (2002), an expert in writing policies and procedures, suggests that you might want to have three tables of contents so that readers have three ways to find the policy and procedure they are looking for:

- Functional categories (e.g., personnel, clinical, documentation)
- Alphabetical by title
- Numerical by policy/procedure number (e.g., I.A. 2, V.12, III-1.5)

Cover page

Approvals

Section I: Supporting Documents
1. Mission statement
2. Vision statement
3. Strategic plan
4. Organizational chart
5. Guiding principles

Section II: Personnel Policies
1. Hiring
2. Background checks
3. Salary and benefits
   a. Pay schedule
   b. Direct deposit
   c. Paid time off (PTO)
   d. Health and dental insurance
   e. Life insurance
   f. Disability insurance
   g. Continuing education
   h. Maternity leave
   i. Jury duty
   j. Leave of absence
4. Drug and alcohol abuse
5. Sexual harassment
6. Overtime
7. Work scheduling
8. Nondiscrimination
9. Conflict of interest
10. Confidentiality
11. Discipline
12. Complaints
13. Workplace civility
14. E-mail and Internet access
15. Performance appraisal
16. Employee safety
17. Keys
18. Dress code
19. Gifts
20. Termination

Section III: Clinical
1. Infection control
   a. Cleaning schedule
   b. Use of cleaning materials
   c. Laundry, gloves, gowns, and masks
   d. Blood or body fluid spills
2. Equipment maintenance
3. Documentation
   a. Referrals/orders
   b. Evaluation
   c. Intervention
   d. Discontinuation

FIGURE 28.4   Sample Table of Contents for a Policy and Procedure Manual for a Private Practice Occupational Therapy Clinic.

4. Communication with physicians, QRCs, and other professionals involved in the client's care
5. Communication with clients
6. Evidence-based practice
7. Charging for services
8. Charging for supplies
9. Program evaluation

Section IV: Administrative
1. Intake
2. Attendance
3. Billing
   a. Services
   b. Supplies
   c. Appeals
   d. Medicare
   e. Medicaid
   f. Managed care
   g. Private insurance
   h. Self-pay
   i. Other payers
4. Services for the uninsured
5. Ordering supplies and equipment
6. Confidentiality of client information
7. Records retention
8. Storage of discontinued charts

FIGURE 28.4 (Continued)

When the draft of at least one format of a table of contents is complete, identify a format for writing each policy and procedure. The format needs to make sense for the type, size, and complexity of the organization for which the policies and procedures are written. The order of the items may be different from one organization to another, but within an organization the order should be uniform and consistent (Page, 2002).

Policies and procedures usually undergo some kind of approval process. Depending on the size and complexity of the organization, the individual policies and procedures may be approved by the owner of the business, a board of directors, or a committee formed for the purpose of approving policies and procedures. The approval may be documented on a cover page for the manual, or on the first page of each policy and procedure.

Exercise 28.1

Write a procedure for the following policy.

Effective date: January 1, 2004; rev. January 1, 2010; January 1, 2013

Policy: Occupational therapy personnel will wash their hands between client visits.

Applies to: All occupational therapists and occupational therapy assistants

Responsible party: Occupational Therapy Manager

Purpose: To try to prevent the spread of infectious diseases.

Procedure:

Exercise 28.2

Write a policy for the following procedure.

> **Effective date:** January 1, 2004; rev. January 1, 2010; January 1, 2013
>
> **Policy:**
>
> **Applicability:** All occupational therapists and occupational therapy assistants.
>
> **Responsible party:** Occupational Therapy Manager
>
> **Purpose:** To ensure that documentation meets with regulatory standards.
>
> **Procedure:**
>
> 1. Document each individual intervention session.
> 2. An occupational therapist or occupational therapy assistant may write and file the visit/contact note.
> 3. The contact note must include a description of the activities or techniques engaged in along with the degree of participation by the client.
> 4. The contact note must include a description of any adaptive equipment, prosthetic or orthotics device that is provided to the client and whether the client or client's caregiver appeared to understand instructions in the use and care of the devices.
> 5. All notes must be signed with first initial, full last name, and credentials of the writer.
> 6. All notes must be dated and the time it was entered into the record noted.
> 7. All notes written by a student must be co-signed by the student's supervisor.

▼ REVIEWING AND REVISING POLICIES AND PROCEDURES ▼

No matter how well written policies and procedures are, they will need to be reviewed and revised on a regular basis, and more often if laws and regulations change that impact the way your work is done or new technologies impact your practice (DCS, 2013). When revising policies and procedures it is helpful to make both the new and the old wording visible to those reviewing the new policy. One way to do that is to use the strikethrough font for the old wording, and red font for the proposed new wording. The track changes feature of most word processing programs will do this for you. (DCS, 2013).

SUMMARY

Policies and procedures tell employees what to do and how to do it. They need to be kept up to date. They are written in simple, direct, and clear wording. Any member of an occupational therapy department may be asked to write a policy and procedure. Some policies and procedures are required by law or by credentialing standards. In addition to complying with laws and standards, policy and procedure manuals can be used as training tools and as resources for questions or problems.

REFERENCES

Braveman, B. (2006). *Leading and managing occupational therapy services: An evidence-based approach.* Philadelphia, PA: F.A. Davis.

Department of Children's Services, State of Tennessee. (2013). *Manual for developing and maintaining DCS policies and procedures.* Retrieved from http://www.state.tn.us/youth/dcsguide/manuals/ManualForDevelopingPoliciesandProcedures.pdf

Page, S. (2002). *Best practices in policies and procedures*. Westerville, OH: Process Improvement Publishing.

Page, S. (2004). *7 Steps to better written policies and procedures*. Westerville, OH: Process Improvement Publishing.

University of California Davis. (2011). *Guide to writing and maintaining campus-wide administrative policy*. Retrieved from http://manuals.ucdavis.edu/resources/GuidetoWritingPolicy.pdf

---

Visit **www.pearsonhighered.com/healthprofessionsresources** to access the student resources that accompany this book. Simply select Occupational Therapy from the choice of disciplines. Find this book and you will find the complimentary study tools created for this specific title.

CHAPTER 29

Job Descriptions

INTRODUCTION

"That's not in my job description."

"I didn't expect to be doing this!"

"She can't really expect me to do all that."

"You want me to do what?"

None of the people who are quoted here seems very happy. They all appear to have a problem related to the reality of their job compared to what they thought their job was. Perhaps they didn't read their job description when they were hired. Perhaps they read a description of their job, but it wasn't a current or accurate one. Maybe no job description exists for their position. Whatever is going on here, it's clear that the supervisor needs to work with the employee to develop or revise the job description. A current and well-written job description can help avoid situations that lead to such comments.

Job descriptions (also called position descriptions) are formal documents that identify the qualifications, duties, and responsibilities of specific positions within a department, organization, or company. They are used in the hiring process to match a candidate for the job to the requirements of the job, and to develop interview questions (Liebler & McConnell, 2012; Mader-Clark, 2007). Workforce Central Florida (2007) says, "For the employee, the job description is a road map and a safeguard" (p. 1). Job descriptions are used in the employee review process to compare employee's performance to the expected performance for that position. Other uses for job descriptions include employee orientation, training, and compensation decisions (Liebler & McConnell, 2012; Mader-Clark, 2007).

Occupational therapists who work in ergonomics, injury prevention and risk management, or functional capacity and worker rehabilitation may be called on to write job descriptions or consult with those writing job descriptions. An essential skill in writing job descriptions is being able to break a task or activity down to its most basic parts. Occupational therapists are excellent at doing this because of our skills in activity (or task) analysis.

▼ LEGAL AND REGULATORY REQUIREMENTS ▼

Job descriptions are legal documents. They can be used in court in lawsuits involving reasonable accommodations (e.g., alleged violations of the Americans with Disabilities Act [ADA]), employment discrimination, termination of employment, and in other employment-related court cases. External accrediting agencies can review a facility's job descriptions as part of the accreditation process. As legal documents, it pays to review existing job descriptions on a regular basis to make sure they are current and consistent with today's practices (Mader-Clark, 2007). Figure 29.1 is a list of dos and don'ts for writing job descriptions that comply with legal and regulatory requirements.

Dos	Don'ts
• Do use action verbs in labeling the job duties • Do be specific, precise, and clear in describing the duties • Do clearly identify which job duties are essential to the position • Do include the physical, mental, and environmental requirements of the job • Do specify the scope of supervisory responsibility of the position (if any) • Do chose your words carefully • Do get feedback on the content of the job description and the wording of it before putting it into use • Do interview people who have similar jobs to help identify the essential functions of the job	• Don't make the list so detailed that it contains every possible task that could be part of it (the kitchen sink approach) • Don't make the job so big it looks impossible for one person to do • Don't include anything that could be contrary to a collective bargaining agreement • Don't use abbreviations that might not be understood by job applicants • Don't include subjective requirements or requirements that only describe one person • Don't make the qualifications so tight they unreasonably restrict who can fill the position

FIGURE 29.1   Dos and Don'ts for Writing Job Descriptions.

Sources: Loy (2007); Workforce Central Florida (2007).

The Fair Labor Standards Act (FLSA) requires employers to document which employees are exempt (professionals) from federal wage and hour regulations and which ones are nonexempt (often paid on an hourly basis) (US Department of Labor [USDL], 2008). To be exempt, professional employees must meet the following criteria:

- The employee must be compensated on a salary or fee basis (as defined in the regulations) at a rate not less than $455 per week;
- The employee's primary duty must be the performance of work requiring advanced knowledge, defined as work which is predominantly intellectual in character and which includes work requiring the consistent exercise of discretion and judgment;
- The advanced knowledge must be in a field of science or learning; and
- The advanced knowledge must be customarily acquired by a prolonged course of specialized intellectual instruction (USDL, 2008 p. 1).

Given this definition, most occupational therapists would be exempt employees, while most occupational therapy assistants and aides would be hourly employees. The best place to document this is in the job description. The more responsibility and independence a position has, the more likely that position is to be exempt.

Federal laws regarding pay equity require that employers prove that jobs requiring similar skill, effort, and responsibility are paid similarly. The skills, effort, and responsibility required for each position within an organization should be clearly spelled out in a job description (Rice University, 2009). Attention also needs to be paid to the qualifications specified for each position description so that laws relating to nondiscrimination (e.g., race, age, gender) are not violated.

Many job descriptions include sections that describe the working conditions, so that employees know what to expect in terms of the work environment. Employees need to know if they will be exposed to any temperature extremes, exposure to toxic chemicals, or loud noises. Not only is this morally correct, but it shows compliance with Occupational Safety and Health Administration (OSHA) regulations. Job descriptions that describe working conditions can serve as a starting point for employee safety training and for the development of safety policies and procedures (Rice University, 2009).

In settings where there are union employees who work under a collective bargaining agreement, job descriptions must not conflict with the collective bargaining agreement (Rice University, 2009). A well-written job description can also help employers properly classify positions into different pay and benefit levels as allowed within the contract.

▼ GATHERING INFORMATION FOR JOB DESCRIPTIONS ▼

If the job description is being written for an existing job, the first step in gathering the needed information is to talk with the people who are currently working in that job/position (Braveman, 2006). Find out how these workers typically spend their day. Ask them what they typically do on an hourly, daily, weekly, or monthly basis. Try to estimate the amount of time spent in each activity, or if exact time varies, estimate the percentage of time spent on each activity on a weekly basis (Braveman, 2006).

One danger in writing a job description for an existing position is that there is a possibility that the job description will be written with a particular person in mind, designing the job to utilize that person's strengths to the maximum extent possible. It is really important, especially to avoid allegations of unfairness, that the position be clearly separated from the person in the position (Drafke, 2002). A job description that is specific to a person will make it very hard to hire a new person when the current person leaves.

If the job description is being written for a new position, start by looking at positions that are similar to the new position and the people who will interact with the new position (Braveman, 2006). Determine what the person in the new position will do on an hourly, daily, weekly, or monthly basis. Make a best guess as to the percentage of time one would spend in each major task. Identify the minimum qualifications for hiring a person to fill this position (education, certification, experience, and special skills). To the ethical and legal extent possible, gather job descriptions from other employers, Web sites, or textbooks that would be similar to the position you are writing about.

The US Department of Labor has a Web site, *Career Onestop* (http://www.careerinfonet.org/jobwriter/default.aspx), which will help you write a job description electronically using a template for hundreds of job titles (USDL, 2007). The site walks you through the process of developing a job description, including the work tasks and activities, contexts, knowledge and skills, and tools and technology. Using a site like this can be a great first step in the process of developing a job description for your work site. While the site offers some options for customization, further refinement of the job description may be necessary. Figure 29.2 shows a sample job description for an occupational therapy assistant and an occupational therapist generated from this Web site.

Title: Occupational Therapist, Pediatric

Reporting Relationships:
1. Reports to Supervisor of Pediatric Rehabilitation
2. Supervises occupational therapy assistant, occupational therapy students, volunteers

Job Specifications:
1. Qualifications
   a. Required:
      1. 1-year experience as a pediatric occupational therapist
      2. Graduate degree in occupational therapy
      3. NBCOT certification
      4. State OT license
   b. Preferred:
      1. 3-year experience as a pediatric occupational therapist
      2. Bilingual (Spanish-English)
      3. SIPT or NDT certification

FIGURE 29.2   Sample Jobs Descriptions.

Sources: Braveman (2006); Liebler and McConnell (2012).

2. Skills
    a. Reading at college level
    b. Writing at professional level
    c. Clinical reasoning
    d. Complex problem solving
    e. Listening comprehension
    f. Public speaking
    g. Time management
    h. Computer (word processing, EHR, spreadsheet, database)
    i. Splinting
    j. Constructing and modifying adaptive equipment
    k. Cooperation, negotiation, persuasion, and social perceptiveness
3. Knowledge
    a. OT theories and frames of reference
    b. Human behavior and performance
    c. Activity analysis
    d. Conditions and diseases
    e. Anatomy and physiology
    f. Teaching and learning theory and techniques
    g. OT intervention strategies appropriate for children

Essential Functions:
1. Evaluates child's level of developmental, physical, behavioral, sensory, and adaptive functions; interprets findings; and generates evaluation/reevaluation reports.
2. Establishes individualized goals to improve child's occupational performance.
3. Develops and implements intervention plans.
4. Develops home programs for children and instructs caregivers on ways to implement the home programs.
5. Documents clinical interventions and the child's response to those interventions.
6. Determines when to terminate services and generates discharge plans and summaries.
7. Provides families with orientation to clinic and clinic policies.
8. Schedules appointments.
9. Directs and supervises occupational therapy assistant in accordance with state law and reimbursement criteria.
10. Orders or fabricates splints, adaptive equipment, assistive technology, and instructs in the use and care of these items.
11. Coordinates service delivery with other team members and outside service providers.
12. Contributes to continuous quality improvement program.
13. Maintains a safe and efficient work space.
14. Informs supervisor of equipment and supply needs.
15. Maintains competency in pediatric occupational therapy.
16. Demonstrates compliance with client health and safety standards.
17. Completes all documentation in a timely manner.
18. Participates in at least 80% of department meetings.

Additional Responsibilities:
1. Attends non-mandatory in-service educational events.
2. Participates in occupational therapy month activities.

Title: Occupational Therapy Assistant, Adult Psychiatry

Reporting Relationships:
1. Reports to Occupational Therapy Supervisor.
2. Supervises occupational therapy assistant students, volunteers.

FIGURE 29.2 (Continued)

Job Specifications:
1. Qualifications
   a. Required:
      1. 1-year experience as an occupational therapy assistant
      2. 2-year degree in occupational therapy assistant
      3. NBCOT certification
      4. State OT license
   b. Preferred:
      1. 2-year experience in mental health setting
2. Skills
   a. Grade 12 reading level
   b. Writing at professional level
   c. Complex problem solving
   d. Listening comprehension
   e. Public speaking
   f. Time management
   g. Computer (word processing, EHR, spreadsheet, database)
   h. Cooperation, negotiation, persuasion, and social perceptiveness
3. Knowledge
   a. Psychiatric OT frames of reference
   b. Human behavior and performance
   c. Activity analysis
   d. Psychiatric conditions and diseases
   e. Teaching and learning theory and techniques
   f. OT intervention strategies appropriate for adults with mental illness

Essential Functions:
1. Contributes to the evaluation of client's level of developmental, physical, behavioral, sensory, and adaptive functions.
2. Contributes to the establishment of individualized goals to improve client's occupational performance.
3. Implements intervention plans.
4. Instructs caregivers on ways to implement the home programs.
5. Documents clinical interventions and the client's response to those interventions.
6. Contributes to the determination of when to terminate services and the generation of discharge plans and summaries.
7. Provides families with orientation to clinic and clinic policies.
8. Schedules appointments.
9. Directs and supervises OTA students in accordance with state laws, reimbursement criteria, and AOTA fieldwork evaluation criteria.
10. Coordinates service delivery with other team members and outside service providers.
11. Contributes to continuous quality improvement program.
12. Maintains a safe and efficient work space.
13. Informs supervisor of equipment and supply needs.
14. Maintains competency in psychiatric occupational therapy.
15. Demonstrates compliance with client health and safety standards.
16. Completes all documentation in a timely manner.
17. Participates in at least 80% of department meetings.

Additional Responsibilities:
1. Attends non-mandatory in-service educational events.
2. Participates in occupational therapy month activities.

FIGURE 29.2 (Continued)

▼ PARTS OF JOB DESCRIPTIONS ▼

Job Title

The job title is the formal name of the position for which the description is being written. The title should be as clear and specific as possible, and indicate the skill level of the job duties (Liebler & McConnell, 2012). If there is only one occupational therapist at the place of work, then the simple job title of occupational therapist may be sufficient. If there are multiple occupational therapy practitioners, and the work duties required of each is different, then the title may need to be more specific. Examples of job titles include:

- Occupational therapy aide
- Occupational therapy assistant I
- Occupational therapy assistant II
- Staff occupational therapist—Med/Surg
- Staff occupational therapist—Rehab
- Lead occupational therapist
- Occupational therapy specialist
- Occupational therapy supervisor
- Occupational therapy manager

The title is usually just a few words long. It is possible for several people to have the same job title, but be differentiated by a specialty practice area or unit name after the title. A hospital might have eight staff occupational therapists, but some might work primarily in rehabilitation, while others work primarily in mental health. In this instance, some of the staff occupational therapists might call themselves "staff occupational therapist—rehabilitation," while others call themselves "staff occupational therapist—mental health." Officially, they could all have the job title of staff occupational therapist.

Job Purpose

The job purpose (sometimes called the job function, job objectives, or job summary) provides an overview of the job and explains why this position exists: the purpose of the job (Mader-Clark, 2007). It should only be a sentence or two long, describing the scope of the position, without a lot of detail. It should contain just enough information to provide an overview of the position and to distinguish it from other positions in the organization (Liebler & McConnell, 2012). The details of the job will be described elsewhere in the job description, so keep this as concise as possible.

Reporting Relationships

In this section, identify which job title/position the person in this position will report to and which job titles/positions will report to this person (Braveman, 2006; Liebler & McConnell, 2012). Do not name names, since people change jobs fairly often, and you do not want to rewrite the job description every time a supervisor or supervisee leaves. Most often, the reporting relationships can be found on the organizational chart for the organization, business, or agency (Liebler & McConnell, 2012).

Job Specifications

This is where you provide detail about the qualifications required for this position, the working conditions, level of responsibility and autonomy, and types of equipment the person in the position will need to be proficient in using (Liebler & McConnell, 2012). In some organizations, the working conditions may be identified on a checklist attached to the job description. Figure 29.3 contains a list of possible working conditions that an occupational therapy practitioner may have to work under.

1. General Physical Requirements

❏ Sedentary work: Mostly (90–100%) sitting; occasional walking or standing; occasional lifting, pushing, pulling, or carrying up to 10 lbs.

❏ Light work: Mostly (75–89%) sitting; occasional walking or standing; occasional lifting, pushing, pulling, or carrying up to 20 lbs.

❏ Medium work: Some sitting (50–74%); some walking or standing; occasional lifting, pushing, pulling, or carrying up to 50 lbs; frequent lifting, pushing, pulling, or carrying up to 20 lbs.

❏ Heavy work: Mostly standing or walking (75–89%); occasional sitting; occasional lifting, pushing, pulling, or carrying up to 100 lbs.; frequent lifting, pushing, pulling, or carrying up to 50 lbs.

❏ Very heavy work: Mostly standing or walking (90–100%); occasional sitting; occasional lifting, pushing, pulling, or carrying in excess of 100 lbs.; frequent lifting, pushing, pulling, or carrying in excess of 50 lbs.

2. Physical Activities

❏ Bending
❏ Climbing
    ❏ Stairs
    ❏ Ladders
    ❏ Ramps
❏ Crouching
❏ Crawling
❏ Fingering
❏ Grasping
❏ Kneeling
❏ Leaning
❏ Lifting
❏ Maintaining balance
❏ Placing
❏ Pulling
❏ Pushing
❏ Reaching
❏ Standing
❏ Stooping
❏ Talking
❏ Touching
❏ Turning or twisting
❏ Walking

3. Mental/Intellectual Activities

❏ Attention to detail
❏ Categorization
❏ Complex mathematics
❏ Cooperating following directions
❏ Generalization
❏ Listening
❏ Memory
    ❏ Short-term
    ❏ Long-term
❏ Prioritizing
❏ Problem solving
❏ Reading at _____ grade level
❏ Sequencing
❏ Simple mathematics

FIGURE 29.3 Sample Working Conditions Checklist.

Sources: Wake Forest University (2000); AOTA (2014).

4. Environmental conditions
- ❏ Atmospheric conditions
  - ❏ Dust
  - ❏ Fumes
  - ❏ Gases
  - ❏ Odors
  - ❏ Poor ventilation
  - ❏ Steam or mist
- ❏ Exposure to infectious diseases
- ❏ Exposure to sharp instruments (e.g., needles, scissors, knives)
- ❏ Exposure to toxic chemicals/agents
- ❏ Extreme cold indoors (below 32 for 1 hr. or more)
- ❏ Extreme heat indoors (above 100 for 1 hr. or more)
- ❏ Exposure to weather extremes outdoors (e.g., wind, humidity)
- ❏ Frequent temperature changes
- ❏ Loud noise
- ❏ Proximity to electrical current
- ❏ Proximity to moving mechanical parts
- ❏ Proximity to moving vehicles
- ❏ Vibration
- ❏ Working in high places (e.g., on scaffolding)
- ❏ Work with volatile people (e.g., people with head injuries, mental illness, or prisoners)
- ❏ Work in small, enclosed places

FIGURE 29.3 (Continued)

There are two types of qualifications that are used to determine whether an applicant is a good fit for a particular job. Required qualifications reflect the minimum education, skills, and experience necessary for anyone to possess in order to do the job. Preferred qualifications are those that the employer would like an employee to possess above and beyond those that are required. For example, a job as a lead occupational therapist may require 2 years of clinical experience, but 5 years of experience would be preferred. An entry-level occupational therapist position might require a master's degree in the field, but a doctoral degree may be preferred.

When writing a job description, it is very important to carefully evaluate the education, skills, and experience necessary to do the job. As each qualification is identified, it is helpful to ask, "Is this really necessary, or is this something it would be nice to have?" Do not set the required qualifications so high that it will limit the number of applicants, particularly if it would eliminate all people of a certain age, gender, or race, but not so low that everyone meets all the qualifications (Western Kentucky University, n.d.). The qualifications need to be commensurate with the level of responsibility the job carries. Types of qualifications can include (Liebler & McConnell, 2012):

- Minimum education level
- Licensure, certification, or registration required
- Amount and type of experience
- Specific knowledge required
- Physical skills required
- Communication skills required

Be as specific as possible in listing qualifications. Avoid vague terms such as *good skills*, *appropriate degree*, and *several years*. Describe the kind of work experience and mention the number of years—for example, 3 years of experience working with children and families, 1 year of hospital experience. When listing the types of skills required or preferred, be sure they are job related. While it might be nice to have only optimists working in your department, optimism is not usually a job-related skill. Be wary of listing skills that are overly broad and open to interpretation, such as being a team player or of good character.

Essential Functions

The ADA defines essential functions as those functions that an employee is required to do, or are fundamental to the job such that the nature of the job would change if it was removed (Equal Employment Opportunity Commission [EEOC], 2005; Workforce Central Florida, 2007). If it is something that a person spends very little time doing or it is done rarely (once a year), then it is not essential. The ADA requires that the essential functions be identified (although the ADA does not specifically require written job descriptions); this information is used in determining if discrimination has occurred. If a candidate is otherwise qualified, and can perform the essential functions of the job with or without accommodations, that person is protected under the law (EEOC, 2005). This does not mean the employer has to hire that person, but only that the person's disability or perceived disability cannot be used as a reason not to hire the person. An employer can hire the most qualified applicant for a job (EEOC, 2005).

The EEOC (2005) does provide some guidance for determining the essential functions of the job. In addition to the criteria already discussed, the EEOC also considers the level of specialization required, the number of other employees among whom a particular task could be divided or reallocated, the work experience of current and previous employees in the same position, and the terms of the collective bargaining agreement if that position is covered under a union contract (EEOC, 2005; Loy, 2007).

In some places, the essential functions, along with marginal functions or additional responsibilities, are listed as job duties (Braveman, 2006; Workforce Central Florida, 2007). Job duties sometimes include specific tasks that may or may not be essential. Depending on the nature of the job being described, this could be a very long list. Some suggestions are to list the job duties in order of importance, by separating the routine duties from the periodic duties (Braveman, 2006), or by separating the essential functions from the marginal functions or additional responsibilities (Loy, 2007; Workforce Central Florida, 2007). Describe the job duties using action verbs (Workforce Central Florida, 2007).

Some people recommend using a "catchall" or "elastic" sentence in order to avoid having employees claim a particular task is not in their job description (Workforce Central Florida, 2007). This seems to run counter to all the advice to be specific and clear. This is an example of a catchall sentence: Performs other duties as assigned by supervisor. While on the one hand this might cover just about anything a supervisor could throw at a supervisee, it might be vague enough that it could be challenged in court.

SUMMARY

Job descriptions are an essential part of any employment situation. They outline what an employee is expected to do. They help guide hiring, performance review, compensation, and disciplinary actions of employers and provide employees with a clear set of performance expectations. A well-written job description should include the job or position title, purpose of the position, reporting relationships, job specifications (qualifications, working conditions, equipment used, and responsibility and autonomy), and essential functions or job duties.

REFERENCES

American Occupational Therapy Association. (2014). Occupational therapy practice framework: Domain and process (3rd ed). *American Journal of Occupational Therapy, 68*(Suppl. 1), S1-S48. http://dx.doi.org/10.5014/ajot.2014.682006

Braveman, B. (2006). *Managing and leading in occupational therapy: An evidence-based approach.* Philadelphia: F. A. Davis.

Drafke, M. W. (2002). *Working in health care: What you need to know to succeed.* Philadelphia: F. A. Davis.

Equal Employment Opportunity Commission. (2005). *The ADA: Your responsibilities as an employer.* Retrieved from http://www.eeoc.gov/facts/ada17.html

Liebler, J. G., & McConnell, C. R. (2012). *Management principles for health professionals* (6th ed.). Sudbury, MA: Jones and Bartlett.

Loy, B. (2007). *Job descriptions.* Retrieved from http://www.jan.wvu.edu/media/JobDescriptions.html

Mader-Clark, M. (2007). *Writing and using job descriptions.* Retrieved from http://www.nolo.com/article.cfm/ObjectID/7D40564D-E366-49E5-8F7C42399A6D071F/

Rice University. (2009). *How to hire handbook: Guidelines for writing job descriptions.* Retrieved from http://people.rice.edu/jobs.cfm?doc_id=7333

US Department of Labor. (2007). *Career onestop.* Retrieved from http://www.careerinfonet.org/acinet/JobWriter/default.aspx

US Department of Labor. (2008). *Fact Sheet #17D: Exemption for professional employees under the fair labor standards act* (*FLSA*). Retrieved from http://www.dol.gov/whd/overtime/fs17d_professional.pdf

Wake Forest University. (2000). Checklist for determining the general physical requirements, physical activities, visual acuity, and working conditions of staff positions. Retrieved from http://hr.wfu.edu/files/2011/10/gen-physical-req-checklist.pdf

Western Kentucky University. (n.d.). *How to hire handbook: Guidelines for writing job descriptions.* Retrieved from http://www.wku.edu/CareerServ/welcome/students/handouts/hiring.pdf

Workforce Central Florida. (2007). The importance of a properly written job description [electronic version]. *Workforce Watch, 1*(47), 1–2.

Index

qualities of good, 70, 70f
school system, 204–235
word list use, 14
Doll, J., 258, 259, 260, 261, 262, 263, 264
Domain, *Occupational Therapy Practice Framework: Domain and Process*, 40–46, 40f
Drafke, M. W., 277
Dunn, W., 121, 127
Duration, 149
change measurement, 142b
intervention, 110, 153
in sample evaluation reports, 128–133
Durfee, M. J., 11

▼ E ▼

Ecology of Human Performance model/ framework, documentation influence, 52t
Education, 40
Education records, 79
Education-related abbreviations, 35b
Edwards, A. M., 104
Edwards, J. N., 106
Electronic documentation, as plagiarism, 88
Electronic health record (EHR), 99–108
communication skills, 103
confidentiality of, 102–103
core functions of, 100b
health information exchange (HIE), 104
history of, 99–100
human positions, 102
informatics and quality improve- ment, 106
locating and entering information in, 104–105
meaningful use, 105
practical considerations of, 101–103
purpose advantages and disadvan- tages of, 100–101
standards, 105
user behavior, 102
Electronic medical record (EMR), 73, 99
E-mail, 7–9
"commandments,", 8
tips, 8b–9b
Environmental statement, IFSP services, 221
Environments, *Occupational Therapy Practice Framework*, 45
Equal Employment Opportunity Commission (EEOC), 283
Essential functions, ADA definition, 283
Established plan of care, Medicare term, 154
Ethical considerations, 89–90
Ethical responsibility, 74
Evaluation
IEP services, 226–227
IFSP services, 216–217
Medicare definition, 113f
new program grant proposal, 263
notice and consent, educational services, 216
occupational therapy definition, 46
process, 122–123, 122f
purposes, 120
Evaluation Report and Initial Intervention Plan, 129f, 133e–134e

Evaluation reports
components, 123–125
data interpretation, 126–127
exercises, 133e–134e
format, 128–133
role delineation, 119–120
writing, 125–126
Evaluative statements, 126, 126e, 126t
"Evidence-based," as buzzword, 14
Evidence-based practice, 121
Evidence of an altered health record, 68f
Exceptions, CARE documentation system, 62, 62b, 63b
Existing position, job description, 277

▼ F ▼

Fair Labor Standards Act (FLSA), job description, 276
Fair use, 89
Family Education Rights and Privacy Act (FERPA, 1974), 79–80
Family information, IFSP, 217
Fancott, C., 9, 10
Fazio, L. S., 259
Federal criminal penalties, 78
Federal False Claims Act, 84
Federal Register, 75, 79
Findings (F)
evaluation report, 128, 129f–133f
intervention plan, 156, 163f–164f
Fischer, H. H., 11
Flow sheets, progress reporting, 190–193, 190f–192f, 191f–192f
Follow-up recommendations, discharge summaries, 198
Formal writing, examples of, 3t
Frames of reference
description, 49
documentation influence, 50t–55t
in evaluation, 120
Fraud
Abuse and, 83–86
AOTA Code of Ethics on, 85
identification exercise, 86e
Fremgen, B. F., 66, 67, 73, 75, 80, 83, 84, 91, 95, 97, 115, 188
Frequency
abbreviations, 17, 19b
intervention, 110
Function
as buzzword, 14
Functioning and disability, ICF structure, 38
Functions, job descriptions, 283

▼ G ▼

Gartee, R., 26, 35, 73, 74, 78, 99, 100, 104
Gately, C.A., 26, 33, 95, 96, 97, 144, 172, 175, 176, 177, 178, 179, 198
Georgetown University Honor Council, 90, 91
Ginosar, D., 11
Glaser, T., 193
Glomstad, S., 248
Goal directions, 138f
Goals
and frame of reference compatibility, 57e
IEP services, 229–231, 230e, 231f

IFSP services, 218f–219f, 220f
intervention planning, 155, 156
long-term, 139, 157
new program grant proposal, 262
short-term, 140, 157
written, 15
Goal, ultimate of occupational therapy, 151
Goal writing
ABCD, 143–145
COAST, 145–146
directions, 137–140
formats, 143–151
long-term, 139
RHUMBA, 146–149
role delineation, 137
short-term, 140
SMART, 149–151
Google.com™, 90
Gordon, J., 144, 172, 175
Government Accountability Office, 243
Grant, P. D., 239
Grant proposal, new program, 260–261
background, 261
budget, 263–264
dissemination plan, 263
evaluation, 263
goals, objectives, activities and outcomes, 262
implementation plan, 262
problem or needs statement, 261
supplemental materials, 264
theoretical foundation, 261–262
timeline, 262
Grants
appendices content, 264f
proposal narrative, 261f
related websites, 259t
sources, 258, 261f
Grant writing, 265e, 266e
new program, 260–264
other types, 265–266
Griffiths, R., 70
Guido, G. W., 67, 68, 96, 97, 239, 240, 241
Guise, J., 9, 10

▼ H ▼

Habilitative goals, 138
"Health care operations," 79
Health informatics of EHR, 106
Health information exchange (HIE), 104
Health Information Technology for Economic and Clinical Health (HITECH) Act (2009), 100
Health Insurance Portability and Ac- countability Act (HIPAA, 2003), 73, 75–79
HealthIT.gov., 99, 104
Health promotion, goals, 140
Hersh, W., 106
Hinijosa, J., 55, 56, 120, 121,
HIPAA Privacy Notice, 78
Home-based services, IFSP, 221, 222
Home health care, evaluation, 135
Honor code exercise, 90e
How long, RHUMBA goal format, 146, 148e
Human position, EHR and, 102